Well Beings

Well Beings

A Guide to Health in Child Care

Third Edition

Editors:
Danielle Grenier, MD, FRCPC
Denis Leduc, MD, FRCPC

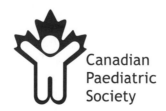

Canadian
Paediatric
Society

ISBN 978-0-9781458-9-7 (English)
ISBN 978-1-926562-00-1 (French)

Printed and bound in Canada

This book is printed on a recycled, acid-free stock.

Library and Archives Canada Cataloguing in Publication

Well beings : a guide to health in child care / editors, Danielle
Grenier, Denis Leduc. — 3rd ed.

Issued also in French under title: Le bien-être des enfants.
Includes bibliographical references and index.
ISBN 978-0-9781458-9-7

1. Children—Health and hygiene—Handbooks, manuals, etc. 2. Day care
centers—Health aspects—Handbooks, manuals, etc. 3. Family day
care—Health aspects—Handbooks, manuals, etc.
I. Grenier, Danielle, 1951- II. Leduc, Denis, 1947- III. Canadian
Paediatric Society

RJ101.W44 2008   362.198'92   C2008-904530-0

This book is available in both English and French, and may be ordered from the publisher:

Canadian Paediatric Society
2305 St. Laurent Blvd.
Ottawa, Ontario K1G 4J8
Tel.: 613-526-9397
Fax.: 613-526-3332
www.cps.ca, www.caringforkids.cps.ca

Acknowledgement: This project is funded in part by the Government of Canada's Social
Development Partnerships Program. The opinions and interpretations in this publication
are those of the author and do not necessarily reflect those of the Government of Canada.

Please note: The information found in this book should be used to support, not to replace,
the advice given by a physician, other health professional, or any provincial/territorial child
care licensing body. Information is not intended, and should not be used, to contradict
specific laws or policies in any jurisdiction. All medical content has been developed by the
Canadian Paediatric Society and reviewed by experts.

Phone numbers and website addresses are current as of August 2008.

Contents

Chapter 1: Early Learning and Child Care in Canada   **1**

Chapter 2: Healthy Activities   **9**

Chapter 3: Nutrition   **25**

Chapter 4: Dental Health   53

Chapter 5: Keeping Children Safe   59

Chapter 6: Transportation Safety   **111**

Chapter 7: Common Conditions   **127**

Chapter 8: Preventing Infections   **141**

Chapter 9: Managing Infections   **167**

Chapter 10: Chronic Medical Conditions   235

Chapter 12: Children's Emotional Well-Being   293

Chapter 13: Including Children with Special Needs   315

Chapter 14: Protecting Children from Maltreatment   353

Chapter 15: Caregivers' Physical Health   **365**

Chapter 16: Caregivers' Emotional Health   **389**

Tables

Figures

Text boxes

Preface

Choosing child care is one of the most important decisions that parents will make for their children in the early years. It's also one that more Canadians than ever are faced with: More than 70 per cent of mothers with young children are in the paid labour force, requiring the availability of some form of care. Above all, when parents look for child care, they want to ensure that their children are safe and protected. And more than ever, they seek an environment where children will be nurtured, stimulated, valued and part of a caring community. Increasingly, quality child care is seen as a critical element of preparing children for school entry and for success later in life. The expectations of people who plan and deliver child care have never been greater.

With so many preschool children spending their day outside the home, ensuring a broad base of health and safety knowledge in child care settings is critical. Child care practitioners—whether they work in a large centre or family home—must have appropriate training and access to resources to help them design their programs, manage their daily activities, and handle unexpected situations. That's where *Well Beings* comes in.

When *Well Beings* was first published in 1992, it was ground-breaking. Dr. Lee Ford-Jones, the book's editor, and an extensive team of contributors and reviewers were visionary in their belief that promoting health and safety in child care settings requires distinct knowledge, skills and behaviours—and that this information should be delivered in a way that practitioners could integrate into their daily practices.

Thanks to their vision and commitment, *Well Beings* became Canada's definitive resource on health and safety in child care. A fixture in centre- and home-based settings alike, it is also an essential text for early childhood education students and instructors as well as local/regional public health professionals who license and set policy on child care. Many physicians and other health care providers keep a copy in their office as a valuable reference when working with parents. This provides community-based physicians involved in the medical care of these children with an additional resource when making recommendations regarding the impact of certain medical problems on the child care setting. In these situations, it is comforting to know that the same guidelines are shared by both the medical community and child care providers.

When the Canadian Paediatric Society set out to produce a third edition of *Well Beings*, we knew several things from the start. First, we had to preserve what people in the field told us were the most important features of the original book—its authoritative evidence base, its comprehensiveness and its practicality. Second, we had to reflect the current reality of child care in Canada—incorporating new information about the early years, up-to-date medical knowledge, and an understanding of the changing face of child care, both among the children and the providers themselves. Finally, it was critical that this updated edition be relevant to people in the field, which is why we strengthened our collaboration with the child care and public health communities.

Two fundamental principles are integral to *Well Beings*. The first is that the well-being of children is paramount. Their health and safety are the starting points for everything in this book. All children have the potential to thrive in and benefit from quality early childhood care. And all children in care settings have the right to the advantages of a nurturing and stimulating environment. It is not enough to simply "look after" children while parents are away. Child care now goes hand-in-hand with opportunities for early learning, which helps children maximize their developmental potential. By integrating health promotion and safety practices into their daily care, providers can focus on the core aspects of their work—ensuring that the children in their care are learning, growing, and having fun.

The second principle that guided us in developing this book is that high quality child care is a partnership between families and practitioners. Many children spend more time in a care setting

Notes on style and nomenclature

Child care practitioner: There are many terms to describe the person who works with children every day, from the professional "early childhood educator" to the informal "caregiver." We've chosen "child care practitioner" as the most inclusive, with "caregiver," "practitioner," and "staff" as variants.

Gender: Where we couldn't keep our child care practitioner gender-neutral, she is always female. This is simply because women are a majority of the child care sector, though we acknowledge that male colleagues play an increasingly important role. When discussing individual children, we generally alternate between "she" and "he," or refer to children in the plural.

Parents and families: Finally, when we refer to a child's parents, in the plural, we mean *any* primary caregiver and every configuration of family. The term "family" is a second choice for referring to that child's own household.

than at home. Ongoing communication with families, which promotes their involvement, is a cornerstone of quality care. Practitioners who take the time to understand children in the context of their family as well as in a care setting are able to provide a level of care that enhances each child's growth and development. We encourage you to share this book with families, as you build a unique relationship with each child in your care.

Well Beings is intended to complement—not replace—local, regional and provincial/territorial regulations and policies. Our goal is to present the gold standard of care and practice. The policies and regulations in your jurisdiction may differ somewhat, and we encourage you to consult them as appropriate.

Because health information is not static, we know that material in *Well Beings* will evolve over the coming years. To ensure that users of the book stay up-to-date, we've created a special section on the Canadian Paediatric Society's website, Caring for Kids, to provide new information and allow users to share their feedback. You'll find links to valuable documents for parents on Caring for Kids that you can download, print, and share with the families you work with. These documents—which cover virtually every aspect of care in the preschool years—are especially important when there is an illness in your program, or when you want to share information about developmental milestones or behavioural issues. We've also posted print-friendly versions of many of the forms and resources from *Well Beings*, as well as links to additional resources from other organizations. Be sure to visit www.caringforkids.cps.ca and let us know what you think.

The development of *Well Beings* over a three-year period involved a network of experts in paediatrics, child care, public health, and many other disciplines—leading authorities in their respective fields. Our gratitude to the many people who reviewed and contributed to this book cannot be overstated. They are acknowledged by name in the following pages, which somehow seems inadequate given the time and energy they devoted to this initiative. We were truly fortunate to work with each and every one of them.

To the thousands of child care practitioners across Canada, we commend you for the work that you do and for incorporating this resource into your daily practice. We hope that it not only enhances your professional lives, but ultimately the lives of the children and families that you serve.

Danielle Grenier, MD, FRCPC
Medical Affairs Officer
Canadian Paediatric Society
Gatineau, Que.

Denis Leduc, MD, FRCPC
Past President
Canadian Paediatric Society
Montreal, Que.

About the Canadian Paediatric Society

Our mission

The Canadian Paediatric Society is the national association of paediatricians, committed to working together to advance the health of children and youth by nurturing excellence in health care, advocacy, education, research and support of its membership.

Who we are

As a voluntary professional association, the CPS represents more than 2,500 paediatricians, paediatric subspecialists, paediatric residents, and other people who work with and care for children and youth.

What we do

To fulfill its mission, the CPS is active in several major areas:

- **Professional education:** The CPS supports the continuing professional development needs of paediatricians and others involved in providing health care to children and youth through position statements, a peer-reviewed journal, and educational opportunities such as an annual conference and regional courses.
- **Advocacy:** The CPS works to identify gaps in and promote improvements to public policy that affects the health of children and youth.
- **Public education:** The CPS works to increase public awareness and education about the health needs and health care of children and youth. Our goal is to help parents make informed decisions about their children's health by producing reliable and accessible health information.
- **Surveillance and research:** The CPS monitors rare diseases and conditions through the Canadian Paediatric Surveillance Program, and ensures continued research into vaccine-associated adverse reactions and vaccine-preventable diseases through IMPACT (Immunization Monitoring Program, ACTive).

Because the needs are so great, the CPS also collaborates with other many other organizations to promote the health of children and youth.

On the Internet

www.cps.ca: This is the primary online home of the Canadian Paediatric Society. Visit this site to access position statements on a range of topics affecting the health of children and youth, as well as information about professional development and joining the CPS.

www.caringforkids.cps.ca: Caring for Kids is the CPS website for parents and caregivers. On Caring for Kids, you'll find a special section devoted to *Well Beings*, including content updates, links to information for sharing, print-friendly versions of many of the forms and resources in this book, and much more.

Acknowledgments

The Canadian Paediatric Society extends its thanks to everyone involved in the development of this book. First and foremost, we are grateful to the *Well Beings* Editorial Board, who reviewed and contributed to multiple drafts of the manuscript. Their expertise was always a given, but their dedication to this project—from 2005 to 2008—has been inspirational.

In addition to the contributions of the Editorial Board, each chapter in *Well Beings* was rigorously reviewed by people from many disciplines, with particular involvement of the public health and child care communities. These committed reviewers provided their insight and expertise every step of the way. Similarly, volunteer experts within and outside the Canadian Paediatric Society generously gave of their time, experience and knowledge, often contributing text of such quality that it now appears in these pages.

Editorial Board

CO-EDITORS

Danielle Grenier, MD, FRCPC
Community Paediatrician
Medical Affairs Officer, Canadian Paediatric Society
Gatineau, Que.

Denis G. Leduc, MD, FAAP, FRCPC
Associate Professor, Paediatrics
McGill University Hospital Centre
Montreal, Que.

Members

Cecilia Irene Baxter, MD, FRCPC
Professor, Paediatrics
University of Alberta
Paediatrician, Royal Alexandra Hospital
Edmonton, Alta.

Margaret P. Boland, MD, FRCPC
Associate Professor, Paediatrics
University of Ottawa
Paediatric Gastroenterologist
Children's Hospital of Eastern Ontario
Ottawa, Ont.

Linda M. Casey, MD, FRCPC, MSc
Assistant Professor, Paediatrics
University of Alberta
Paediatric Physician Nutrition Specialist
Stollery Children's Hospital
Edmonton, Alta.

Anne Fenwick, RN, BScN
Director, Family Health
Region of Peel – Public Health
Brampton, Ont.

T. Emmett Francoeur, MD, FRCPC
Associate Professor, Paediatrics
McGill University
Director, Child Development Program
Montreal Children's Hospital
Montreal, Que.

Joanne M. Langley, MD, MSc, FRCPC
Professor, Paediatrics
Dalhousie University
Halifax, N.S.

Anne Maxwell, BA
Senior Director, Projects,
Programs and Services
Canadian Child Care Federation
Ottawa, Ont.

Dorothy L. Moore, MD, PhD, FRCPC
Associate Professor, Paediatrics
McGill University
Division of Infectious Diseases
Montreal Children's Hospital
Montreal, Que.

Elizabeth Moreau, BA, MM
Director, Communications and Public Education
Canadian Paediatric Society
Ottawa, Ont.

Michelle G. Ponti, MD, FRCPC
Community Paediatrician
Medical Director, London-Middlesex
Children's Aid Society
London, Ont.

Sarah Emerson Shea, MD, FRCPC
Associate Professor, Paediatrics
Dalhousie University
Halifax, N.S.

Richard S. Stanwick, MD, MSc, FRCPC, FAAP
Chief Medical Health Officer
Vancouver Island Health Authority
Victoria, B.C.

Jennifer Strickland, BA
Publications Coordinator
Canadian Paediatric Society
Ottawa, Ont.

Lynne J. Warda, MD, FRCPC, PhD
Assistant Professor, Pediatrics and
Child Health
University of Manitoba
Medical Director, IMPACT – Injury Prevention
Centre
Children's Hospital
Winnipeg, Man.

Reviewers and contributors

Shazhan Amed, MD, FRCPC
B.C. Children's Hospital
Diabetes and Endocrinology
Vancouver, B.C.

Yvonne Andrade, RN, BScN, IBCLC
Public Health Nurse, Family Health
Region of Peel – Public Health
Brampton, Ont.

David Aoki, PHN, RN, BNSc, BSc
Public Health Nurse, Communicable Disease
Control Team 1
Region of Peel – Public Health
Brampton, Ont.

Debbie Birkenbergs, RN, BScN
Public Health Nurse, Family Health,
Child Health
Region of Peel – Public Health
Brampton, Ont.

Irena S. Buka, MB, ChB, FRCPC
Associate Clinical Professor, Paediatric
Environmental Health Specialty Unit
University of Alberta
Edmonton, Alta.

Julie Butler, BA ECE
President, Association of Early Childhood
Educators of Quebec
Member Council, Canadian Child Care
Federation
Pointe Claire, Que.

Risa Cashmore, RN, BSc, CIC, CCHN(c)
Infection Control Specialist
Region of Peel – Public Health
Brampton, Ont.

Zave H. Chad, MD, FRCPC
Past Chair, Canadian Allergy, Asthma
and Immunology Foundation
Associate Professor, Paediatrics
University of Ottawa
Ottawa, Ont.

Karen Chandler, BA ECE, MA
Professor, School of Early Childhood
George Brown College representative
Member Council, Child Care Human
Resources Sector Council
Canadian Child Care Federation
Toronto, Ont.

Laurel Chauvin-Kimoff, MDCM, FRCPC,
FAAP
Medical Director, Child Protection, and Chair,
Child Protection Committee
Montreal Children's Hospital
Associate Professor of Paediatrics
McGill University
Montreal, Que.

Ruth Collins RN, CIC
Infection Control Specialist
Communicable Disease
Region of Peel – Public Health
Brampton, Ont.

Kim Cornish, PhD
Professor and Canada Research Chair in
Developmental Neuroscience and Education
Director, Child Laboratory for Research and
Education in Developmental Disorders
McGill University
Montreal, Que.

Lana Crossman, Communications Manager
Canadian Child Care Federation
Ottawa, Ont.

Michael T. Dickinson, MD, FRCPC
Head of Pediatrics
Miramichi Regional Hospital
Miramichi, N.B.

Andrée Durieux-Smith, PhD, FCAHS
Vice-Dean, Professorial Affairs and Professor
of Audiology, School of Rehabilitation Sciences
Faculty of Health Sciences, University of Ottawa
Ottawa, Ont.

April Duxbury, RN, BScN
Public Health Nurse, Chronic Disease and
Injury Prevention
Region of Peel – Public Health
Brampton, Ont.

Samantha Earl, RN, BScN
Nurse Consultant
Hepatitis C Secretariat
Ministry of Health and Long Term Care
Toronto, Ont.

Mark E. Feldman, MD, FRCPC
Assistant Professor, Paediatrics
University of Toronto
Toronto, Ont.

Sue Fernane, RN, BScN
Research and Policy Analyst, Communicable
Disease Division, Healthy Sexuality Program
Region of Peel – Public Health
Brampton, Ont.

Marcia Frank, RN, MHSc, CDE
Clinical Nurse Specialist, Diabetes Service
Hospital for Sick Children
Toronto, Ont.

Nancy Geronazzo, RD
Public Health Dietitian, Family Health
Region of Peel – Public Health
Brampton, Ont.

Andrea Gingras, RN (retired)
Home Child Care Provider
President, Child Care Provider's
Resource Network
Ottawa, Ont.

Joanna Hastings, RN
Family Health Supervisor
Healthy Babies Healthy Children Program
Region of Peel – Public Health
Mississauga, Ont.

Beata Hilliard, BAA, CPHI(C), COHS
Public Health Inspector, Environmental
Health, Support Programs
Region of Peel – Public Health
Brampton, Ont.

Harold E. Hoffman, MD, CCFP, FRCPC,
FACOEM
Adjunct Associate Professor
University of Alberta
Edmonton, Alta.

Pat Hogan
Director, Dartmouth Pre-school
Dartmouth, N.S.

Sharon Hope Irwin, EdD, LLD (Hon.)
Senior Researcher
SpeciaLink: The National Centre for
Child Care Inclusion
Sydney, N.S.

Les Johnson
National Director Training and Client
Services
St. John Ambulance
Ottawa, Ont.

Carla Kane, BScN
Practice Consultant, Community Care
Facilities Licensing Program
Vancouver Island Health Authority
Victoria, B.C.

Jennifer Kay, RN, BScN
Public Health Nurse, Chronic Disease
and Injury Prevention
Region of Peel – Public Health
Brampton, Ont.

Kathy Kitka, RN, BScN
Public Health Nurse
Chronic Disease and Injury Prevention
Region of Peel – Public Health
Brampton, Ont.

Caryn LaFlèche, ECE III
Director, Les enfants précieux inc.
Board Member, Manitoba Child Care
Association
Member Council, Canadian Child Care
Federation
Winnipeg, Man.

Lisa Lamarr-O'Gorman
Manager, Algonquin College Early
Learning/ECE Faculty
Ottawa, Ont.

Monique Laprise
Psychoeducator, Teacher
Department of Early childhood education
diploma, Cégep de Saint-Jérome,
Manager, Growing together project
Fondation Lucie et André Chagnon
Montreal, Que.

Claire M.A. LeBlanc MD, FRCPC, Dip.
Sport Medicine
Department of Pediatrics
Division of Rheumatology
Stollery Children's Hospital
Edmonton, Alta.

Emily Lecker, MSc, OT
Occupational Therapist
MAB-Mackay Rehabilitation Centre
Montreal, Que.

Alison Leduc, MSc, OT (OT Reg NS)
Occupational Therapist
Halifax, N.S.

J. Victor Legault, DDS
Executive Director
Canadian Academy of Pediatric Dentistry
Montreal, Que.

Cynthia Lindsay, RN, BScN
Public Health Nurse, Family Health
Region of Peel – Public Health
Brampton, Ont.

Hélène Lowell, RD
Office of Nutrition Policy and Promotion
Health Canada
Ottawa, Ont.

Nicola Lyons, RN, BScN
Public Health Nurse
Homelessness Initiative, Reproductive
and Homelessness Team
Region of Peel – Public Health
Brampton, Ont.

Karen Macklon
Society of Yukon Family Day Homes
Whitehorse, Yukon

Christine K. MacLeod
Licensed Family Child Care Provider
Instructor/Coordinator Family Child Care Training
Kwantlen University College
Delta, B.C.

Jason Marquez, BASc, CPHI(C)
Public Health Inspector, Environmental Health
Support Programs
Region of Peel – Public Health
Brampton, Ont.

Tammy Martin
Canadian Child Care Federation
Ottawa, Ont.

Kelly Massaro-Joblin, ECE, C.
Executive Director, Schoolhouse Playcare Centre
President, AECEO
Thunder Bay, Ont.

David L. McGillivray, MD, FAAP, FRCPC
Montreal Children's Hospital
Montreal, Que.

Robin McMillan, BA ECE
Canadian Child Care Federation
Ottawa, Ont.

Andrea Meeker, RN, BScN
Public Health Nurse, Family Health
Division/Child Health Program
Region of Peel – Public Health
Brampton, Ont.

Angelo Mikrogianakis, MD, FRCPC
Department of Paediatrics, Division of
Emergency Medicine
Hospital for Sick Children
Assistant Professor of Paediatrics
University of Toronto
Toronto, Ont.

Golda Milo-Manson, MD, MHSc, FRCPC
VP Medicine Academic Affairs
Bloorview Kids Rehab
Associate Professor of Pediatrics
University of Toronto
Toronto, Ont.

Eunice Misskey, RD, MCEd
Health Promotion, Population and Public
Health Services
Regina Qu'Appelle Health Region
Regina, Sask.

Deb Mytruk
Manager of Provider Services, Calgary
Family Day Home Agency
Alberta Family Child Care Association
Canadian Child Care Federation
Calgary, Alta.

Trudy Norton
Researcher/writer (Retired)
Special Health Care Project
Vancouver, B.C.

Nicole O'Donnell, RN, BScN
Public Health Nurse, Family Health
Region of Peel – Public Health
Brampton, Ont.

Dan F. Otchere, BDS, DDPH, MSc
Dental Consultant, Chronic Disease
and Injury Prevention
Region of Peel – Public Health
Brampton, Ont.

Jeanine Plamondon, BA
Project/Program Coordinator
Certified Early Childhood Educator
Canadian Child Care Federation
Ottawa, Ont.

Carolyn Pullen, RN, BScN, MEd
Director, Knowledge Translation
Canadian Cardiovascular Society
Ottawa, Ont.

Lucille Repetski, RN, BScN
Public Health Nurse, Chronic Disease
and Injury Prevention
Region of Peel – Public Health
Brampton, Ont.

Michael J. Rieder, MD, FRCPC, PhD
Department of Paediatrics, Division of
Clinical Pharmacology
Children's Hospital of Western Ontario
London, Ont.

Leslie Rourke, MD, CCFP, MClinSc, FCFP
Associate Professor, Discipline of Family
Medicine
Memorial University of Newfoundland
St. John's, Nfld.

Robert Schroth, DMD, MSc
Assistant Professor
Faculty of Dentistry, University of Manitoba
Winnipeg, Man.

Lisa Semple, RN, MN
Canadian Cystic Fibrosis Nurses'
Interest Group
Cystic Fibrosis Clinic, Alberta Children's
Hospital
Calgary, Alta.

Audrey Shaw, RN, MScN
Manager, Communicable Disease Program
Vancouver Island Health Authority
Victoria, B.C.

Trent J. Smith, MD, FRCPC
Community Paediatrician
Kamloops, B.C.

Dale M. Stack, PhD
Professor, Department of Psychology and
Centre for Research in Human Development
Concordia University
Staff Psychologist, Montreal Children's
Hospital
Montreal, Que.

Nancy Stevens, RN, BScN
Public Health Nurse, Communicable Disease
Control
Region of Peel – Public Health
Brampton, Ont.

Sara Tarle, BComm
Canadian Child Care Federation
Ottawa, Ont.

Lee Tidmarsh, MD, FRCPC
Psychiatrist, Developmental Disabilities
and Mental Health Services
Fraser Health Authority
Vancouver, B.C.

Debbie Valickis, RN, BScN, CIC
Infection Control Specialist, Communicable
Diseases
Region of Peel – Public Health
Brampton, Ont.

Charmaine S. van Schaik, BSc, MSc, MD, FRCPC
Southlake Regional Health Centre
Newmarket, Ont.

Michelle Ward, MD, FRCPC
Consultant Pediatrician, Division of Pediatric Medicine
Child and Youth Protection Service
Children's Hospital of Eastern Ontario
Ottawa, Ont.

Susan Zivkovic, BA (Hons)
Health Promotion Officer
Communicable Disease Division
Region of Peel – Public Health
Brampton, Ont.

Contributors to the French edition

Well Beings is available in French under the title *Le bien-être des enfants : Un guide sur la santé en milieu de garde.* Our thanks to translator Dominique Paré and reviewer Martine Leroux for their superb rendering, and to these French-language medical experts who contributed with both sense and style.

Anne-Claude Bernard-Bonnin, MD, FRCPC
Paediatrics, CHU Sainte-Justine
Department of Paediatrics
Université de Montréal
Montreal, Que.

Marie Gauthier, MD, FRCPC
Paediatrics, CHU Sainte-Justine
Department of Paediatrics
Université de Montréal
Montreal, Que.

Pascale Gervais, MD, FRCPC
Paediatrics, Centre Mère-Enfant du CHUQ
Department of Paediatrics, Université Laval
Quebec, Que.

Élisabeth Rousseau-Harsany, MD, FRCPC
Paediatrics, CHU Sainte-Justine
Department of Paediatrics
Université de Montréal
Montreal, Que.

Participants in the 2001 review of *Well Beings*

In 2001, this book underwent a thorough content review by a committee of experts, chaired by Dr. Lee Ford-Jones. They lay the groundwork for the present edition, and we thank them for pointing the way.

Dr. Anne-Claude Bernard-Bonnin
Dr. Maurice Bouchard
Dr. Margaret Cox
Dr. Simon Dobson
Dr. Joanne E. Embree
Dr. Victor C. Goldbloom
Dr. Danielle Grenier
Dr. Robert M. Issenman
Dr. Barbara J. Law
Dr. Denis Leduc
Dr. Noni MacDonald
Dr. Stuart M. MacLeod
Trudy Norton
Dr. W. Donald Reid
Dr. Reginald S. Sauvé
Dr. David Fraser Smith
Dr. Richard Stanwick
Dr. Joseph Telch
Dr. Lynne J. Warda
Dr. David W. Warren

Development and production

Project Coordinator: Jennie Strickland

Project Manager: Elizabeth Moreau

Writing and editing: Christine Langlois, Judith Whitehead, Jenny Wilson

Cover and book design: Fairmont House Design

Translation and review: Dominique Paré (Le bout de la langue), Martine Leroux (SMART Communications)

Index: Heather Ebbs

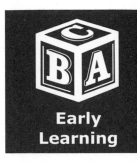

c h a p t e r

1

Early Learning and Child Care in Canada

If you're reading this edition of *Well Beings*, you are obviously interested in providing a healthy, safe environment for the children in your care. Whether you work in a child care centre, a family child care home, a preschool or other community program, you play an important role in healthy child development. Yet while you likely seek information on a regular basis, you may find a lack of up-to-date sources that you can trust and apply in everyday practice. That's why the Canadian Child Care Federation is pleased to collaborate with the Canadian Paediatric Society on this practical guide to health and safety in child care, which will support you in providing high quality early learning and care.

This latest edition of *Well Beings* reflects significant changes in knowledge and practice since the original version was published in 1992. Recent research on brain development, for example, has shed light on the impact that children's experiences in the early years have on their success in school and throughout their lives. Much more is known about what constitutes quality child care and the role that it plays in supporting healthy child development.

Our thanks to the Canadian Child Care Federation for contributing this chapter.

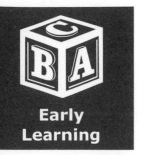

Families rely on child care services more than ever—in 2005, fully 70 per cent of children aged 6 months to 5 years were in some form of non-parental care, with about half in regulated services. And the face of the early learning and child care "classroom" has evolved, better reflecting the diversity of Canada. Children are more likely to be from different cultural backgrounds or to have varying physical and mental capabilities. Child care practitioners look for ways to best meet the needs of these children and their families and to offer them the quality care that all children deserve.

How child care is delivered in Canada

Early learning and child care services are offered in a variety of settings to suit family and child preferences, work demands or schedules, or cultural needs. These settings include:

- Child care centres (regulated): Located in purpose-built spaces or facilities that have been adapted for child care. Care can be offered on a profit or non-profit basis.
- Family child care (regulated and unregulated): Located in the child care provider's home. This can be offered through individuals or through a profit or non-profit agency.
- Nanny care (unregulated): Located in the child's home, this type of care can be offered by individuals or through a for-profit agency.
- Care by a relative (unregulated): Located in the child's home or that of a relative by private arrangement.
- Preschools and nursery schools (the latter are unregulated in some jurisdictions).

The range, quality, and accessibility of services can vary widely, even within jurisdictions. Provincial/territorial ministries or agencies are responsible for regulating areas such as health and safety, staff qualifications, staff-to-child ratios, group size, programming and parental involvement in licensed settings. However, legislated standards are also uneven across the country. With the exception of some cities in Ontario and Vancouver, B.C., municipalities have almost no role in regulated child care.

Almost all provinces and territories require at least some of the staff working in child care centres to have training in early childhood education. Regulated services also include site visits to ensure programs comply with minimum health and safety standards. However, due to factors such as a lack of regulated spaces, most child care in Canada continues to be unregulated, provided by a relative, family child care provider or in-home caregiver (nanny). Care for children under the age of 5 years (or 4 years in Ontario, which provides junior kindergarten for 4-year-olds in most regions) is considered a responsibility of the family, not the government.

Although the federal government is generally not involved in providing early learning and child care services, it does assume responsibility for programs serving populations for whom it has a fiscal responsibility. Examples include programs for First Nations and Inuit children (Aboriginal Head Start) and for military families, as well as financial assistance for child care while immigrant and refugee parents take language training.

Quality child care and child development

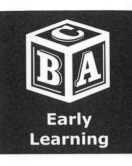

Studies show that quality care can further a child's physical, social, intellectual and emotional development. Research also shows that quality child care can improve school readiness (especially memory and language skills), provide early intervention for children at risk and—by enabling parents to work—can help reduce child poverty. Further, it is clear that quality child care can benefit all children, both advantaged and disadvantaged. Studies show that children who receive quality care during the preschool years have better cognitive and social skills, even after taking family situation into account.

Although provincial/territorial government regulations set minimum requirements for ratios of children per adult, group size, physical space and practitioner training, these vary across Canada. This is especially true for ratios. For example, provincial/territorial regulations for the ratio of child care staff to children aged 12 months to 24 months range from 1:3 in Newfoundland, to 1:6 in Nova Scotia, to 1:8 in Quebec for children 18 months to 4 years (1:5 for children 18 months or younger). The Canadian Child Care Federation's *National Statement on Quality Child Care* goes beyond minimum requirements to suggest that quality child care requires the following nine elements, working together:

- the child at the centre,
- collaborative partnerships with families,
- quality indoor and outdoor physical and learning environments,
- a purposeful learning program,
- a supported workforce,
- leadership at the program level,
- effective administrative practices at the program level,
- an effective infrastructure that includes a vision of an early learning and child care system, government policies and processes based on evidence, system-wide planning and resources, public funding for operating and capital costs, adequate wages and parent fees, research and evaluation, and communication of the research, and
- skilled and knowledgeable child care practitioners.

The CCCF statement provides in-depth information on each of these components of quality.

The child care practitioner plays a vital role

Of all the elements of quality, the role of skilled and knowledgeable practitioners is paramount. Research has consistently shown that it is the practitioner's level of knowledge and skill that affect children's experience the most.

The early learning and child care sector has continued to improve itself. Led by the Canadian Child Care Federation, the sector has developed occupational standards, outlining the minimum requirements of those working with children. The *Occupational Standards for Child Care Practitioners* has been widely distributed and is used in training institutions and individual centres to guide practitioner development. These occupational

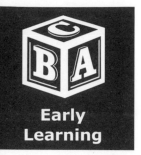

standards form the basis of the following sections that elaborate on the vital role of child care practitioners.

Health and safety responsibilities

The primary concern for all child care practitioners is to keep the children in their care healthy and safe. Practitioners need to be aware of and apply current, relevant provincial/territorial health regulations. In general, these regulations should ensure that the child care environment minimizes the risk of infection or food contamination. In daily practice, practitioners identify potential or immediate health hazards in the child care setting and take appropriate action to address them. Good safety and hygiene practices are explained to the children in a way they can understand and modelled so the children will adopt them.

Practitioners must also maintain up-to-date knowledge of first aid procedures, CPR, fire safety, and illness and injury prevention strategies. They maintain safe indoor and outdoor spaces, and are able to identify situations or materials and items that are unsafe and take appropriate action. They know the signs and symptoms of possible neglect or abuse and can report it.

Practitioners protect and promote children's physical health and well-being by understanding their nutritional needs and providing healthy, balanced snacks and meals, and monitoring and recording children's food intake when necessary—particularly for children with feeding issues.

Increasingly, practitioners evaluate child care environments from the perspective of environmental health. Because young children are still developing and because they often explore the world through their mouths, they are particularly vulnerable to environmental toxins. Practitioners make themselves aware of toxins in building supplies, detergents and play materials that could affect children's health.

To best protect the health of children in their care, practitioners need to maintain detailed and up-to-date records for each child.

The basics: Staff-to-child ratios, group size and age mix

The relationship between the number of adults caring for children in a child care centre and the number of children in their care—specifically, the number of children each practitioner is responsible for—is called the **staff-to-child ratio**. Along with staff education and training, this ratio is a leading determinant of quality child care. That is because it affects every aspect of service in centre-based programs: how well staff are able to supervise children, how effectively they maintain healthy routines, and how much personal attention they can give to each child.

A second, related indicator of quality care in centres is **group size**. This refers to the number of children—usually of about the same age—who are being cared for together in a defined space. In Canada, provincial/territorial regulations govern both staff-to-child ratios and group size in child care centres. They also specify the maximum number of children allowed in

---

home-based programs, which differs from group size since the children in care can vary widely in age. Thus, the **age mix** of children, which is also regulated for home settings, is another determinant of quality child care. In both centre and home settings, staff can provide better care to smaller groups, whether children are of the same or of different ages.

Research shows that when child care practitioners are responsible for fewer children, in smaller groups, programs can:

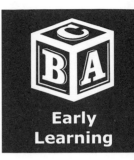

Early Learning

- increase the frequency and language level of interactions between staff and children,
- promote the quality of interactions (e.g., by giving personal attention),
- help children talk and play among themselves,
- allow children greater autonomy as they move through their programming day,
- provide a more appropriate level of stimulation for children of different ages and stages,
- support learning, and social and emotional development for each child, and
- strengthen attachments between children and child care practitioners.

These positive dynamics benefit the whole group.

While staff-to-child ratios and group size vary with the setting, the program, and the ages of the children, a general rule applies: The wider the age spread among children, and the younger they are, the smaller the group needs to be for child care practitioners to provide quality care for all. Evidence-based recommendations for staff-to-child ratios by age and group size for child care centres have been developed by the U.S. National Association for the Education of Young Children. The American Academy of Pediatrics has also developed standards for home-based child care in *Caring for Our Children*. According to the Canadian Council on Learning, an optimal adult-to-child ratio in any setting is about 1:3 for children under 2 years, 1:6 for children 2 to 3 years, and 1:8 for preschoolers. These ratios change with circumstances, such as when children needing special medical or developmental support are included, or when special services are being offered (e.g., overnight care).

In home settings, the staff-to-child ratio and the maximum allowable group size are combined. Usually, one or perhaps two child care practitioners make up the entire staff, caring for a maximum number of children of stipulated ages. The more children there are in a home setting, the more physical contact among them there is likely to be—a dynamic that can result in the spread of infection. The presence of children in diapers increases that risk.

There are advantages to mixed-age groups, which are overwhelmingly the norm in home settings. A mixed-age program can:

- accommodate the care of siblings within the same group,
- when small, have a more natural, "family-like" character,
- allow older children to be role models for younger ones, which may foster self-confidence in older children.

However, the needs of children of different ages conflict at times. Common challenges for mixed-age groups include:

- toy requirements. Toddlers need a safe play environment with no play materials that present a choking hazard. Preschoolers benefit from playing with toys that often have small parts.
- activity levels. Preschoolers need the freedom to be physically active in ways that younger children may find intimidating.
- play patterns. Toddlers might enjoy sweeping objects off a tabletop or dumping them out of containers. This can be frustrating for preschoolers trying to build, assemble or put toys away.

Children have a right to quality care in any setting, whether at home, in a child care centre or in a home-based program. While the right ratio, group size and age mix do not in and of themselves guarantee quality care, they are definitive, especially when combined with staff education, in-service training, and strong leadership.

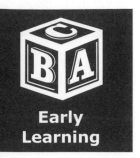

Finally, practitioners must provide a psychologically nurturing environment for all children. They understand the stages and milestones for social and emotional development and create appropriate environments to support children. Sometimes, children who demonstrate demanding behaviour can expose themselves or other children to risk of injury. Child care practitioners are skilled at recognizing potential hazards and acting appropriately to protect children. They also understand that culture, religious values and socio-economic status may influence the way children communicate and behave.

Relationships with children and families

For most child care practitioners, the most rewarding aspect of their work is the relationships with children in their care. Caring involves both love and labour. It is at the core of the practitioner's work and is reflected in all interactions with children. Practitioners respond to each child's expression of need, provide children with experiences that build trust, and express verbal and non-verbal warmth, affection, consideration and acceptance. They show a genuine interest in children's activities, ideas, opinions and concerns. They respect each child and encourage them to find safe ways to express their feelings. The bond between children and practitioners can be very strong, lasting well beyond their time together in care.

In quality programs, practitioners and parents work in partnership—sharing expertise and experiences—to ensure children's optimal development. Practitioners make sincere efforts to understand each family's needs, cultural and/or religious practices and preferences related to child-rearing. Before a child enters the program, practitioners discuss the program's philosophy, policies and procedures and the child's daily routines.

Once a child is in the program, practitioners and families work together to help the child settle in and establish initial developmental goals. In the beginning, adjustments to routines, food and activities may be made, where possible, to reflect family practices and respect family preferences.

Children in full-time care spend most of their day outside the family home and away from parents. The practitioner's ability to observe children's skills, abilities, interests and needs and communicate these developments to parents is an important way for families to stay informed. Trained practitioners can recognize the signs and symptoms of physical, emotional or developmental delays or challenges, and can take appropriate action.

Relationships with colleagues

Child care practitioners often work as part of a team and share responsibility with others for program planning, implementation and assessment. Everyone benefits from supportive, collaborative working relationships, and from discussing issues and opinions in an open, frank and respectful manner. Child care practitioners share relevant information about children and families with colleagues in a way that respects each family's dignity and privacy.

Home-based child care providers don't often work with other staff on a daily basis. However, they can also benefit from networking, sharing ideas and discussing challenges with other family child care providers.

Collaboration with other child-serving organizations

Practitioners often work with members of community organizations as part of a service-provision team to help further the health and development goals of the children in their care. They maintain a balance between sharing information to help children and families and respecting principles of privacy and informed consent.

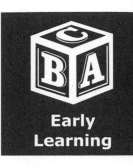

Early Learning

Networking with other professionals can lead to rewarding partnerships that further caregivers' knowledge and understanding of their own practice. Community or provincial/territorial organizations can offer additional opportunities for collaboration and learning.

Training and professional development

Training ensures that practitioners have the knowledge and experience to provide a high level of care, based on developmentally appropriate and inclusive practices.

Early childhood learning and child care education is offered at Canadian colleges and universities through certificate, diploma and undergraduate programs as well as post-graduate degrees. The depth, level and quality of training vary widely among different schools and across the country. There are no national standards for basic, entry-level training in early childhood education.

Professional development is an ongoing process. Even trained practitioners can identify areas of strength and areas where more knowledge or skills are needed. They regularly reflect on their knowledge, skills and attitudes and how they might enhance their relationships with children, families and colleagues. Training institutions and child care organizations offer a wide variety of workshops, seminars and other programs for practitioners to enhance their work and improve knowledge or skills.

The many lenses of child care

As Canadian society becomes more and more diverse, so does the early learning and child care setting. In any one child care or early learning program, practitioners may encounter many languages, ethnicities and cultures. Meeting the needs of families from different backgrounds is part of providing quality child care. This can pose a variety of challenges and opportunities to practitioners.

Caring for children who have not yet fully mastered English or French can be a challenge but encouraging children to speak their first language can be beneficial. Children who master their first language will learn a second language more easily. In the child care environment, children who share the same first language benefit from using it when they interact. Practitioners can compile a bilingual list of basic words or phrases, such as "toilet" and "mommy will be back soon," to facilitate communication.

Culture, like language, has a significant influence on a child's development. Practitioners need to encourage and integrate cultural elements into their program. They also need to be aware of different values and beliefs about how to care for children. For instance, certain cultures value the well-being of the group over the needs of the individual. This can affect

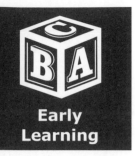

Early Learning

the level of independence granted to children. Some parents form a close bond with their child by feeding, carrying or taking him along everywhere they go—often past the age at which this attachment would be considered appropriate in North America.

Cultural values can also affect communication (direct versus indirect) and learning styles (through questioning, talking and analyzing versus observing and imitating). It is helpful for the practitioner to explain the program's philosophy to parents to see if it is a good match for their beliefs and goals. However, it's not always possible for immigrants or minority parents to find a program that reflects their values, culture, or language to the extent that they would prefer. In this case, practitioners can be respectful by being open and understanding, offering books and toys that reflect diversity, and planning inclusive activities.

Quality early learning and child care programs are also successful at integrating children with special needs. Practitioners work with parents and health professionals or other resource personnel to create a more inclusive environment by developing a plan that addresses the needs of all children in the program. Sometimes this requires extra training for practitioners, adapting program content and structure, or rearranging the physical environment to make it accessible to all children.

Selected resources

American Academy of Pediatrics, American Public Health Association, and National Resource Center for Health and Safety in Child Care. 2nd Ed., 2002. *Caring for Our Children: National Health and Safety Performance Standards; Guidelines for Out-of-Home Child Care*. Elk Grove Village, IL: AAP.

Doherty, Gillian. 2003. *Occupational Standards for Child Care Practitioners*. Ottawa, Ont.: Canadian Child Care Federation.

Friendly, Martha, Jane Beach, Carolyn Ferns and Michelle Turiano. 7th ed., 2006. *Early Childhood Education and Care in Canada*. Toronto, Ont.: University of Toronto, Childcare Resource and Research Unit.

Government of Newfoundland and Labrador, Department of Health and Community Services. 2004. *Standards for early childhood programs in centre-based child care*. www.health.gov.nl.ca/health/childcare

Kaiser, Barbara and Judy Sklar Rasminsky. 1999. *Partners in Quality 2: Relationships*. Ottawa, Ont.: Canadian Child Care Federation.

Kaiser, Barbara and Judy Sklar Rasminsky. 1999. *Partners in Quality 4: Communities*. Ottawa, Ont.: Canadian Child Care Federation.

Miller, Robin. 2006. *Why is high-quality child care essential? The link between quality child care and early learning*. Montreal, Que.: Centre of Excellence for Early Childhood Development. www.ccl-cca.ca/CCL/Reports/LessonsInLearning/20060530LinL.htm.

National Association for the Education of Young Children (U.S.). 2005. Teacher-child ratios within group size. www.naeyc.org/academy/criteria/teacher_child_ratios.html.

chapter

2

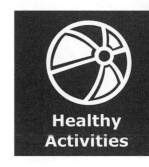

Healthy Activities

P hysical activity is a key determinant of children's healthy development. Children need movement and active play—each and every day—to develop physically, emotionally and cognitively. Providing children with opportunities to move and offering a safe and encouraging play environment are core elements of quality child care.

While most children are naturally active from an early age, societal changes and technological advances have resulted in less physical activity. Babies are confined to car seats for long commutes, toddlers and preschoolers spend hours a day watching TV, and family lifestyles limit the amount of time children have to play outdoors. As a result, many Canadian children—some as young as 2 years old—are not physically active enough to build strong bones and muscles or to maintain a healthy body weight. This lack of activity also affects children's cognitive and social development as well as their future health. Child care practitioners need to ensure that children engage in regular physical activity each day through play, games and other fun activities.

Daily physical activity

Babies and young children learn through movement—by doing. Activity, which is essentially playing, is how they develop cognitively as well as physically. Daily physical activity may also improve the way children eat and sleep.

Healthy Activities

10 ways to encourage young children to be active

1. **Create and ensure safe access to play environments, both indoors and out.** Children need to develop their physical abilities in safe and comfortable settings.

2. **Be an active facilitator.** Adult participation in any physical activity increases the interest and enjoyment of children.

3. **Encourage appropriate dress.** Let families know that informal clothing that allows free movement and is appropriate to the season is preferable to outfits that need to be kept neat and clean.

4. **Offer opportunities for physical activity every day,** not just on special days. Active play that is as regular as lunch and nap time will help ensure that physical activity remains a natural part of children's daily lives.

5. **Plan activities that match children's abilities,** so they experience a sense of achievement. Recognize and praise improvement.

6. **Post images** of children moving and playing actively.

7. **Walk** to points of interest rather than going by vehicle. Model and share in the fun of walking to a park or playground for a spell of vigorous play.

8. **Emphasize fun, not competition,** and build basic skills with varied activities. Offer praise and encouragement.

9. **Practice fairness.** Avoid comparing individual children's abilities or relating gender with particular activities.

10. **Offer children a choice** of activity whenever possible, and lots of opportunities for unstructured play. Invite children to tell you what they'd like to do.

Regular physical activity:

- enhances healthy growth and development,
- builds strong muscles and bones,
- strengthens the heart,
- maintains flexibility,
- helps achieve and maintain a healthy weight,
- promotes good posture, coordination and balance,
- improves overall fitness,
- builds confidence, and
- helps children relax.

Active children learn to run, jump and kick while playing. As they develop, basic skills help to support a positive body image and facilitate recreational and sports activities later in life. Inactive children who don't develop these skills may lack confidence or feel awkward during physical activities as they get older. These feelings can contribute to a sedentary lifestyle as children mature and increase the risk of early obesity.

Children with more opportunities to be physically active tend to make positive, healthy choices in other areas of life as they mature. Studies show they eat more nutritious foods and are less likely to smoke, use drugs or abuse alcohol. Physical activity is also associated with better mental health because it helps children express intense emotions in a constructive way. Exercise and having fun alleviate stress.

Another important reason for children to be physically active is because they enjoy play. For some children, enjoyment is enhanced by competition; for others, active play is a pleasure in and of itself. Child care practitioners are ideally situated to instill the pure fun of different physical activities long before competition becomes an issue. Physical activity is also a way of socializing with peers and bonding among family members.

Steps to physical development

Infants

Young children's physical development happens gradually, in stages, and progresses from the centre of the body outward. When one new skill or movement is mastered, it sets the stage for the next. For example:

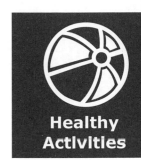

Healthy Activities

- Infants first learn to lift and control their head, strengthening neck muscles.
- Next, they gain control of muscles in their torso, used for sitting.
- Then they begin to use arms and legs for crawling and, eventually, walking.
- Finally, they develop fine motor control by learning to use smaller muscles in their fingers, wrists, toes and ankles.

As babies move through each stage of physical development, they can be gently encouraged to begin the next. However, don't rush them to the next step before they have mastered the previous stage. Children know best when they are ready to try something new.

REMEMBER

Although there are patterns of development, children vary widely in terms of what new task they'll perform and when. You can help families recognize, respect and celebrate individual differences.

Sitting up

Starting at about 6 months, a baby begins to sit up, at first with support and only for a few seconds. Give her lots of floor time to practice. Help her learn to balance by placing her in a sitting position surrounded by pillows to ensure a soft landing when she topples. However, be sure to remain with her, supervise her closely around any soft surface to prevent suffocation, and provide a steadying hand while she reaches for a toy. Even if she can't achieve a sitting position on her own, she'll reach up to ask for help. Once a baby can sit by herself, she can play independently for brief periods. She will then begin to lunge forward to grab a toy in front of her. Lunging is a new movement that strengthens her muscles in preparation for the next step: crawling. You can encourage lunging by placing a toy almost out of reach.

Crawling

Once a baby can roll over, at about 6 months, he begins to rock back and forth on his tummy. This rocking is usually a prelude to crawling. How babies crawl varies widely. Some pull themselves along the floor, others go backward before they go forward or scoot around on their behinds. Some babies don't crawl at all but go straight to pulling themselves up on the furniture and "cruising" to get around. Form is less important than the effort it takes to move and explore. Encourage a baby to move by giving lots of supervised floor time, placing interesting objects just beyond reach and creating gentle "obstacle courses" to navigate, such as a pile of pillows to crawl over or a cardboard box to explore. **Actively supervise an exploring baby at all times.**

Soon he will want to climb. Provide close and constant back-up for a baby climbing stairs—a favourite activity. He will need extra help backing down but will practice for hours, given the opportunity.

Standing and walking

Well before a baby can stand by himself, he enjoys being supported in a standing position for bouncing or "stepping." At about 7 months, he has the strength to stand for a second or two with support. Then, usually between 9 and 12 months, he learns to pull himself up to a standing position by grabbing onto furniture or your leg. At first he is tentative, hanging on tight and needing help to sit back down. Then he learns to steady himself, stepping around furniture while holding on. Once he has enough strength in his legs to stand freely, he will take that exciting first step.

Toddlers and preschoolers

Once a child is toddling, physical strength increases quickly as she moves from walking to running, then jumping. As both gross and fine motor skills improve, she is keen to try new ways of moving. Provide a safe, nurturing and minimally structured play environment for this age group. Supervised walks in the neighbourhood, unorganized free play outdoors, and visits to a park or playground all develop children's enjoyment of outdoor physical activity and unstructured exploration under close and constant supervision.

There is not enough evidence to recommend exercise programs or classes for babies and toddlers as a way of promoting increased physical activity or preventing obesity in later years. But you can encourage parents to limit their child's screen time (e.g., watching TV, playing computer or video games) to less than 1 hour a day. Setting limits early encourages more activity and less passive snacking.

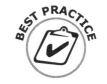

Sedentary "screen time" should not be part of the regular child care routine. Minimize or eliminate TV viewing and discourage access to computer games.

Once the basics—walking, running, jumping—are mastered, a child is ready to learn new skills: kicking a ball, throwing, catching, riding a tricycle, balancing and climbing. Encourage free play with an emphasis on fun, spontaneity, exploration and experimentation, always providing a safe environment and equipment, and proper supervision. Preschoolers thrive on active play that is unorganized and largely child-led, with adult instruction limited to a show-and-tell format, on play surfaces that are level and relatively free of clutter. Appropriate activities might include running, water play (e.g., under a sprinkler), tumbling, throwing and catching. Walking tolerable distances to an interesting destination like a playground or park should be a regular program and family activity. (For information on safe play, see Chapter 5, *Keeping Children Safe*.)

You can help children reach their physical potential and enjoy vigorous activity by scheduling time for movement, planning engaging activities, and making sure they have challenging and age-appropriate equipment on hand.

How much activity?

Exactly how much activity young children need every day isn't known, and probably varies from child to child. *Canada's Physical Activity Guide for Children*, developed by Health Canada, includes recommendations for children and youth 6 years and older, but not for younger children. What is known is that active play comes naturally to children and has many benefits, even if these are difficult to measure scientifically.

Movement and activity are important virtually from birth:

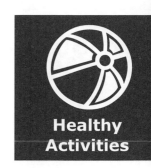

Healthy Activities

- Babies need to explore by touching and tasting. They develop motor skills and large muscle movement through daily interaction with caregivers, objects and environments.
- It's important not to restrict babies' potential for movement, though active supervision is critical.
- Limiting the time babies spend in strollers, playpens and car seats means more time for play.

Some experts say that toddlers and preschoolers need to spend at least 60 minutes and preferably up to several hours a day taking part in supervised **unstructured play**, both indoors and out. Here's what is known:

- Unstructured or uninterrupted free play, at children's leisure and at their own pace (play for the sake of play), is important to children's development.
- Toddlers and preschoolers shouldn't have to stay still for more than 60 minutes at a time, except when sleeping.
- Toddlers need some structured physical play in short intervals throughout the day. **Structured play** includes more organized activity, such as circle games (e.g., Ring Around the Rosie), interactive songs (e.g., the Hokey Pokey), throwing sponge balls and simple games like Simon Says. Short, structured physical activities should be part of programming throughout the day, with lots of unstructured playtime between games.

How to engage children in physical activity

Build more physical activity into your program by following the natural activity patterns of the young children in your care. These tend to be spontaneous and intermittent, so encouraging physical activity and facilitating children's movement skills will mean playing in short spurts, on demand, staying "in the moment" and allowing children to stop or change play as their interests and abilities develop. What's most important when taking part in children's games or free play is sharing their enjoyment. Children participate more fully in any play activity when an adult joins in, even indirectly. By taking part in play, adults validate children's

REMEMBER

Facilitate play, be an active role model, provide lots of feedback and introduce an occasional surprise or challenge. You don't need to control children's activity.

(and their own) sense of fun. Try activities that you think children will enjoy and be prepared to change quickly if they resist or lose interest.

As with other interactions between children and caregivers, it's important to observe the stage of development each child has reached before introducing a new activity. Children develop at different rates—for example, one child may walk at 9 months and another at 16 months—but they will respond enthusiastically to activities that are suitable for their developmental stage.

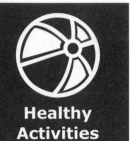

Healthy Activities

Assessing children's motor skills

As you engage children in physical activity, pay attention to the motor skills they are developing and plan activities that enhance them.

- **Body awareness** is a child's understanding of how his body moves. It promotes a general sense of physical well-being.
- **Spatial awareness** is the child's awareness of his body in space, which helps orient and guide him as he moves through his environment.
- **Locomotor skills**, such as crawling, walking, running and jumping, enable a child to move.
- **Non-locomotor skills** enable a child to move while staying in place: bending and stretching, pushing and pulling, twisting and turning, falling and rising, swinging and swaying.
- **Manipulative skills** are the abilities that children develop to control objects—by catching, kicking, striking, rolling, tossing and bouncing.
- **Directional skills** enable a child to move in all directions—forward and backward, side to side and upside down.

> **How to engage children in physical activity**
>
> 1. Make it fun.
> 2. Keep it interesting.
> 3. Set small, achievable goals.
> 4. Incorporate activities that emphasize basic motor skill development, such as running, rolling, climbing, throwing, catching and kicking.
> 5. Plan activities in short bursts with frequent breaks.

Physical development through active play

Babies need to squirm and wiggle, movements that gradually develop into touching, grabbing, rolling and crawling. **Supervised tummy time** helps babies strengthen muscles in their neck, back, arms and legs.

- Encourage a baby's impulse to roll, which helps develop balance, strength and vision.
- Roll a ball to her or blow bubbles nearby while she watches.

Once a baby is crawling, give her lots of floor time to explore her surroundings. A baby is developing her brain, muscles and visual skills as she uses opposing arm and leg movements to crawl.

Children respond to music from birth. As they gain control over their limbs, they will follow an adult's lead and respond to it through movement. Moving to music helps develop coordination as children try to follow a beat.

- Introduce babies to singing play with songs and rhymes with actions, such as finger games.
- Encourage bobbing up and down to music, which is the first step to learning to jump.
- Teach toddlers and preschoolers songs that involve actions and movement, like Ring Around the Rosie, and Head and Shoulders, Knees and Toes.
- Have a regular music time. Play favourite music and encourage toddlers and preschoolers to dance. Teach 4- and 5-year-olds simple dances like the Hokey Pokey.

Toddlers love to walk, run and jump. Make sure your program keeps toddlers and preschoolers active for a portion of every day.

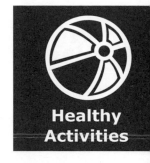

- Provide toddlers with lots of opportunities to walk on different surfaces, both indoors (carpet, tile, wood flooring) and out (grass, gravel, concrete, sand), and to go barefoot where it is safe.
- Make time for toddlers to stop and pick up pebbles and twigs while they walk. Examining things en route is fun and instructive.
- Initially, hold a child's hand while he practices walking up and down stairs or goes up and down hills.
- Play chasing games. Take turns chasing children, then letting them chase you. Chase around objects indoors and around trees outside. Change direction often.
- Hold hands while children walk along a low wall or raised curb, or as they jump off a bottom stair or step.
- Practice walking backward and sideways. Think up walking games, like walking from one maple tree to the next in the park.
- Go on "exploring" walks.
- Give children lots of room to walk and run. Take 4- and 5-year-olds on short walks with a purpose—to do shopping or mail a letter.

ALERT

Be careful not to pull or swing too hard on a toddler's extended arm. This can cause an arm-pull injury (sometimes called nursemaid's elbow).

- Encourage jumping. Put something soft on the floor and invite children to jump over it. Make an obstacle course using simple objects: unrolled socks can be presented as something to jump over in different ways. Encourage jumping backward and sideways, or in a pattern: front, side, back.
- Take "jumping" walks, where children can jump over (or into!) every puddle or across every crack in the sidewalk.
- Dance and jump to music, each child separately, then joined in a circle. **Try introducing music and dances from different cultures, so every child gets a chance to show how his family might dance at home.**

Swinging, spinning and rocking

These movements develop balance, which is the basis for many kinds of activity as children grow. **When playing spinning games, go slowly and spin in both directions. Avoid pulling too hard on a child's extended arm.**

- Lift a child and swing her gently back and forth in the air. You can also do this to music. Lift her up and down, side to side. Slowly spin round and round, then spin the other way.

- Rock a child on your lap, backward and forward, and side to side.
- Let a child sit on your ankles or knees while you're in a chair. Bounce her up and down.
- Play the airplane game. Lie on your back on the floor with your feet in the air. Have a toddler lie on her tummy on the soles of your feet and hold her hands while she "flies."
- Have a child sit on a blanket on a slippery floor. Spin her around slowly one way, then the other, while she hangs on.

Take children to the playground to use the swings on age-appropriate play structures. Constant supervision and holding a child steady until she has the strength to hold on herself are important for younger children. Make sure there is nothing in a child's way while she is swinging, including other children.

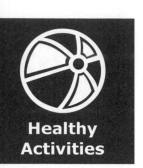

Healthy Activities

Climbing and hanging

Children develop upper-body strength by using their hands and arms to hold their own weight. Give them lots of opportunities to use age-appropriate climbing structures, at your local playground or on an indoor play structure. Be sure to supervise and support them until they are able to hold themselves up safely.

- Let a child hang or swing from monkey bars. Supervise, offer support and, once he's got a good grip, encourage him to swing from bar to bar, alternating hands.
- Teach a child the wheelbarrow walk. Hold on to his legs while he walks on his hands, keeping his back straight.
- Teach him the "bear walk": walking on his hands and feet with his behind in the air.

Catching, throwing and kicking

Children love to catch, throw and kick balls, actions that develop hand-eye and foot-eye coordination. Ball activities can be an enjoyable part of spontaneous play and develop a child's sense of timing, which is important for all kinds of activities.

- Start with slow-moving bubbles and scarves. During tummy time, blow bubbles away from a baby's face so she can watch them float by. Throw a light scarf in the air so it lands close to her. As a baby gains mobility and control, she'll try to catch bubbles and grab a scarf.
- Roll a large soft ball toward a baby or from side to side, so she can observe these motions.
- Sit on the floor with a baby (or toddler) sitting between your knees and facing another caregiver (who may also have a baby sitting with her). Roll a ball between you. Lift the child's leg or draw her legs together to stop the ball when it comes her way.
- Give toddlers and preschoolers lots of opportunities to throw, kick and chase soft balls, inside and out of doors. Offer balls in a variety of sizes, textures and degrees of bounciness. Show 4- and 5-year-olds how to kick a soccer ball.
- Encourage toddlers and preschoolers to blow and chase bubbles. Blow bubbles for them to jump over, kick, catch and chase. Have them try to catch a bubble on their shoe, with a finger, on a knee.

- Play games involving building up and knocking down stacks of light objects (e.g., empty cardboard boxes, plastic blocks). Toddlers and preschoolers can knock over the stack by throwing a ball or kicking it over.
- Play "toss the laundry." Have children throw rolled-up pairs of socks into the laundry basket.
- Help children create an obstacle course of everyday household objects and then roll a ball through it.

Building strength and dexterity through play

Having strong hands and fingers is important in nearly every aspect of a child's life. Play that builds strength and dexterity can start early, to the accompaniment of song, nursery rhymes or simple conversation.

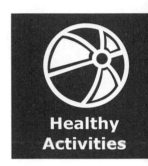

Healthy Activities

- Gently open and close a baby's fists. Play hand games like Round and Round the Garden, Pat-a-Cake and Itsy Bitsy Spider.
- Introduce various kinds of play with sand, play dough, finger paints and water to help develop hands and fingers. Pouring or scooping, playing with a water wheel or cylinder all support the development of fine motor skills.
- Introduce age-appropriate crafts that involve gluing, using safety scissors and plasticine. Give 4- and 5-year-olds smaller craft items to manipulate.
- Play games and activities that involve cross-patterning, where one side of the body does something different from the other side. This kind of movement improves coordination. Marching is a simple activity that involves cross-patterning.

Getting active outside

Children benefit tremendously from daily physical activity outdoors, in different kinds of weather throughout the year, including winter cold. Running, jumping, climbing and playing happen naturally in large outdoor settings. Children need time for both unstructured and structured play outside. Yet despite the importance of outdoor play, children spend little time outside. Recent research suggests that the lack of outdoor play contributes to rising childhood obesity rates and poor concentration, and dampens curiosity and creativity.

Whenever possible, children should be given time to play freely outdoors where they can run in the grass and on uneven ground, climb hills, and examine and collect natural objects. Children tend to prefer playing actively outdoors, and child care practitioners need to create daily opportunities for children to take part in active play outside. Active play might entail a walk to the park or along a nearby nature trail, but could also simply mean supervised time spent in a backyard or in a centre's outdoor play area.

Child care practitioners who work in urban and suburban locations may not have easy access to wilderness areas. However, small children can still explore nature by searching for caterpillars in the garden or building a play-fort under the backyard hedge.

Having outdoor toys, such as balls, pails and shovels, encourages children to play and stay active outside for longer periods. Structured games that toddlers and preschoolers enjoy indoors, such as marching games, scavenger hunts and circle games, can be played outside.

Consider ways to create natural spaces and opportunities for children to play outside.

- Create a garden suitable for small children. They can help to plant and water the garden, and learn the names of the plants they grow.
- Leave part of the outdoor play area or yard in a natural state for children to explore.
- Make sure there is a shady area where children can find shelter from full sunlight in summer.
- Give children time and opportunities to "play in the dirt" or "play in the snow" and investigate whatever interests them in the natural world.

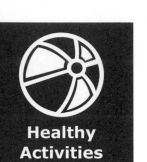

Healthy Activities

Choosing outdoor equipment and toys

Children also benefit from play on safe, age-appropriate playground equipment. When buying outdoor equipment for your home setting, choose a structure that complies with the latest Canadian Standards Association guidelines and is specifically designed for the age range of children in your care. (See *Selected resources* at the end of this chapter.) Low one- or two-step climbers, low balance beams, and open-ended objects like tires or fabric-covered tunnels encourage safe active play.

Tricycles and other ride-on toys help develop large motor skills and are appropriate for children 3 years of age and older. Having a range of ride-on toys available in different sizes helps ensure a safer fit and minimizes competition for them, which is important for both safety and enjoyment. Children should use ride-on toys only on level surfaces inside a fenced area. Closely supervise those who are riding, and make sure they wear a helmet. (For more about ride-on toys and tricycles, see Chapter 5, *Keeping Children Safe*.)

Planning indoor activities

Children also need space and time for both unstructured and structured physical activity indoors. Structured activities, such as marching together to music or playing circle games, require little or no equipment, while other types of activity may require specialized play equipment or facilitation. Good indoor activities include:

- dancing to music—let children choose their favourite music,
- following along with a movement video,
- having a scavenger hunt,
- rolling and jumping on soft mats or pillows on the floor,
- climbing on indoor play structures,
- throwing soft balls or bean bags,
- waving rhythmic scarves,
- doing group activities with a large sheet or parachute (children lift it together, hide under it, etc.), and
- having ride-on toys inside.

Children are always imagining new ways of seeing and using their everyday surroundings. A couch is not just for sitting; it's also for hiding behind, perching, turning into a fort and bouncing on. A hallway is more than a way to get to the next room; it's an open invitation to run. When children interact with their environment in creative ways, they are learning. Child care practitioners can nurture the imaginative use of everyday things. However, not all spaces are appropriate for every behaviour. Designing a play space for physical activity should take into account children's needs for:

- **Movement**: The space should invite children to move in safe ways with a minimum of restriction or frustrating obstacles.
- **Comfort**: The space should offer varying levels of stimulation, with some areas for loud, exuberant, active play and other areas for quiet breaks from the action.
- **Competence**: Within the space meant for their use, children should feel free to manage and manipulate whatever materials and equipment are provided there.
- **Control**: Children need to feel mastery over their space and be given opportunities to experiment.

Children tend to move more and stay engaged longer in spaces designed with child-sized furniture and equipment. Always consider how to make activities safer—constant supervision is key, but removing obstacles or objects in the environment that might harm a child on the go is important too.

From 3 to 5 years of age, children are learning basic skills such as throwing, running and jumping, which form the basis for many sports activities. Their balance improves and their vision matures. However, children of this age have difficulty judging or following the direction and speed of moving objects. As well, their attention span tends to be short.

Although preschoolers might enjoy watching other children play organized sports, they are still too young to participate. Introducing sports can begin in middle childhood, from 6 to 9 years of age, once their attention span lengthens and their ability to combine actions (e.g., running and throwing) is more developed.

When planning active indoor play, consider that children continually interact with their environment in imaginative, creative ways.

Young children enjoy mastering skills in fun ways without any emphasis on competition. You can instill the pure fun of physical activity long before competition is an issue.

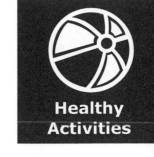

Healthy Activities

Engaging children with special needs

Children with special needs have the same enthusiasm and the same right to be physically active as other children, and benefit equally from opportunities to take part in daily activities. In fact, being physically active is especially important for children with a disability because movement counters some effects of their disability.

Benefits include:

- improving physical stamina and self-confidence, which can bring greater independence.
- maintaining or achieving a healthy body weight and building strength. Both help a child using a wheelchair or other mobility device to get around with less effort, increasing mobility.
- improving circulation, which reduces blood pooling and swelling in the lower limbs.
- increasing strength and flexibility, making daily tasks easier.
- improving posture, which reduces discomfort that can accompany long periods of sitting.

Creating an inclusive environment where all children can take an active part involves modifying certain activities and providing assistance where necessary. Many children's games and activities can be adapted to include children with a disability. If you have questions about the safety of a particular game or activity for a child with special needs, seek information and approval beforehand from that child's treating physician. (See Chapter 13, *Including Children with Special Needs* and *Selected resources* at the end of this chapter.)

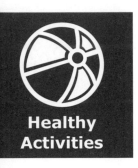

Healthy Activities

All children, including those with a disability, need opportunities to take risks, make choices and mistakes, and work toward increasing independence (as well as interaction) through physical activity and play.

The right clothes and shoes for activity

Clothing should not be a barrier to full participation in active play. Advise parents to choose children's clothing, shoes and boots for ease of movement, including putting on and taking off. Encourage children to be comfortable about getting their clothes dirty. Shoes and jackets with Velcro closures, simple pull-on toques and slip-on boots all allow children and their caregivers to get active quickly. Footwear should be non-slip. In cold weather, children need clothing that keeps them warm and dry while allowing for ease of movement. If a child's hands and feet are warm in cold weather, his clothing is probably adequate. Be sure to come prepared for active play by dressing comfortably yourself.

In warm weather, babies and young children move most easily when they are wearing light clothing. Where it is safe, going barefoot or wearing non-slip socks helps to exercise feet and develop children's sense of touch.

Encouraging healthy physical activity within families

Child care practitioners can play a vital role in encouraging families to be physically active together. You can do this by "setting the pace."

- Share information about the physical activity component of your program with parents at the time of enrolment. Include this information in the package given to new parents, and display posters and photographs of children at play. Encourage parents to introduce new activities at home.

- Let parents know what physical activities their child enjoys.
- Build physical activity into events. On family night or whenever families are invited to visit your facility, include a demonstration of activities that the children enjoy. Get the adults up and moving too. Teach them the words and moves to activity songs. Offer handouts that describe games or words to activity songs for parents to try at home.
- Encourage parents to organize an active play group. It can be as simple as meeting in the park on Sunday afternoons so that their children play outdoors together.
- Share information about the importance of daily physical activity and the need to limit a child's screen time at home to no more than 1 hour a day.
- Encourage parents to contact their local public health unit to learn about programs in the community that promote free or low-cost physical activity ideas (e.g., community or early learning centres, parent–child groups).

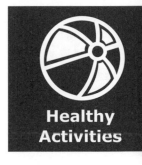

Healthy Activities

Active games to play with toddlers and preschoolers

Have lots of activities ready to keep young children moving. This selection of fun and adaptable games can be used as a starting point and changed to suit children's abilities. Once children are old enough, let them take turns leading the group.

Keep games interesting by asking children to suggest adaptations or new ways to play. Seeking out and incorporating their tastes and interests will enhance the duration and popularity of any game.

For toddlers

Jack-in-the-Box: Children curl up in a ball, each in an imaginary box. When you pretend to lift the lid, up they pop! You can play this game to music. When you stop the music, all "jacks" pop up.

Follow the Leader: Children follow you and your actions as you lead them around the facility. This can be done with or without musical accompaniment.

Up and Down: Children follow your actions—squat down, stand up, lie down, sit up, kneel down, stand up, lie down, legs in the air, stand up, arms in the air, "shake it all about." Have them practice falling safely and loosely, dropping down slowly to the front and rolling, then to the back.

Big and Small: Children follow your instructions to make themselves big, make themselves small, make big circles with their arms, make small circles with their arms, make big jumps, make small jumps, etc.

Log Roll: On a gentle incline, children roll down like logs with their bodies stretched out, legs together and hands together above their heads.

For preschoolers

Games involving creative movement, with or without music, are favourite pastimes for children this age.

Laughing Statues: Designate boundaries to play within, then choose one child to be the leader. When the leader calls "go," players race around the yard, dancing, spinning and leaping. When the leader shouts "freeze," they pretend to be statues, standing as still as they can. The leader then walks to each player, stares and says "Ha!" If a "statue" moves or laughs, he joins the leader and together they attempt to make the other statues laugh, visiting each remaining player. The last one to stay successfully frozen is leader for the next round.

Animal Chase: Children form a circle. One stuffed animal is handed around the circle. While this stuffed animal goes around, a second one is introduced. The object of the game is for the second animal to catch up with the first. More stuffed animals can be added.

Visiting the Zoo: Children walk around a space and transform themselves into animals as you name them. They can slither on the floor as snakes, make themselves small and scamper on all fours like mice, stretch their necks and walk tall like giraffes.

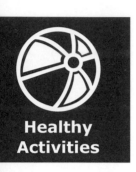

Healthy Activities

Active programming

Active child care programs ensure that children play energetically for a portion of every day. They encourage and support physical learning and the impulse to play. Both are essential to child development, and healthy activities bring pleasure and benefit to all who participate.

Selected resources

Activities

Active Living Alliance for Canadians with a Disability. Activity fact sheets. www.ala.ca

Barbarash, Lorrain. 1997. *Multicultural Games: 75 Games from 43 Cultures.* Champaign, IL: Human Kinetics.

Best Start Resource Centre, Physical Health Resource Centre and the Nutrition Resource Centre. 2005. *Have a ball! A toolkit for physical activity and the early years.* www.beststart.org

Dietitians of Canada. 2007. *Healthy Start for Life. Keeping active together planner: Activity planning for preschoolers.* www.dietitians.ca

Lansky, V. 2001. *Games Babies Play from Birth to Twelve Months.* Minnetonka, MN: Book Peddlars.

Ontario Public Health Association (Nutrition Resource Centre). 2007. *Busy bodies: Creative food and play ideas for your preschooler (ages 3 to 5).* www.nutritionrc.ca

Rappaport-Morris, Lisa and Linda Schultz. 2nd ed., 1991. *Creative Play Activities for Children with Disabilities: A Resource for Teachers and Parents.* Champaign, IL: Human Kinetics.

Sanders, S.W. 2002. *Active for Life: Developmentally Appropriate Movement Programs for Young Children.* Champaign, IL: Human Kinetics.

Silberg, Jackie. 1998. *500 Five Minute Games: Quick and Easy Activities for 3–6 Year Olds.* Castle Hill, Australia: Pademelon Press.

Toronto Public Health. 2000. *Fun and physical activity: For families and caregivers with children 0–4 years.* www.toronto.ca

———. 1999. *Moving on the spot, Family fun in 5 minutes, Daily physical activity.* Booklet and posters, with some movement sessions for families in Tamil, Chinese and Spanish, and for classroom use. www.toronto.ca

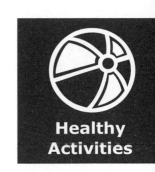

Healthy Activities

Resources for child care practitioners

Calgary Health Region, Alberta Cancer Board, Three Cheers for the Early Years. 2006. *Snacktivity box: Activities for promoting healthy eating and active living habits for young children.* www.calgaryhealthregion.ca

Canadian Child Care Federation. www.cccf-fcsge.ca

———. 2006. Bringing back physical activity play in childhood. Resource sheet #79.

———. 2006. Quality environments and best practices for physical activity in early childhood settings. CD.

———. 2004. *Moving and growing 1: Physical activities for the first two years.*

———. 2004. *Moving and growing 2: Physical activities for twos, threes and fours.*

———. 2003. *Outdoor play in early childhood education and care programs.*

———. 2001. Musical playtime. Resource sheet #8.

———. 2001. Healthy habits include fitness. Resource sheet #11.

———. 2001. Exploring nature with children. Resource sheet #43.

———. 2001. Supporting your child's physical activities. Resource sheet #52.

Canadian Standards Association. 4th ed., 2007. *Children's Playspaces and Equipment.* Mississauga, Ont.: CSA.

Government of Nova Scotia, Health Promotion and Protection, Active Kids Healthy Kids. 2005. Active living for early childhood. www.gov.ns.ca

National Association for Sport and Physical Education (U.S.). 2002. Active start: A statement of physical activity guidelines for children; Birth to five years. www.aahperd.org

———. 2000. Appropriate practices in movement programs for young children ages 3–5. www.aahperd.org

Resources for families

Active Healthy Kids Canada. www.activehealthykids.ca

Canadian Paediatric Society. www.caringforkids.cps.ca

———. 2005. When is my child ready for sports?

———. 2002. Healthy active living for children and youth.

Public Health Agency of Canada. 2002. Canada's physical activity guide for children. www.phac-aspc.gc.ca

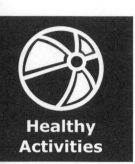

Healthy Activities

Websites

Alberta Government, Healthy U. www.healthyalberta.com

Canadian Association for Health, Physical Education, Recreation and Dance. www.cahperd.ca

Canadian Fitness and Lifestyle Research Institute. www.cflri.ca

Canadian Society for Exercise Physiology. www.csep.ca

Canadian Standards Association. www.csa.ca

Evergreen Learning Grounds Program. www.evergreen.ca

Heart and Stroke Foundation of Canada. www.heartandstroke.ca

chapter

3

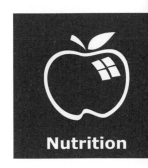

Nutrition

Nutrition

Feeding children healthy food in ways that nourish both body and mind is at the heart of caregiving. Food provides nutrients crucial to physical growth and good health, and eating is an important developmental process, changing as babies and children move from one stage to the next. Enjoying mealtimes with other children and caregivers is a vital way for a child to feel loved and secure within a caring community.

A comprehensive picture of the physical and social developmental milestones connected with feeding that children reach during infancy and early childhood appears in Table 3.1. Understanding these physical and social steps helps child care practitioners and families recognize normal eating patterns and behaviours. Through nurturing and responding appropriately, child care practitioners can reinforce healthy attitudes toward food.

TABLE 3.1

Developmental milestones related to feeding from birth to age 5

Age	Physical	Social
Birth to 4 months	• opens mouth wide when nipple touches lips • sucks and swallows	• recognizes source of milk by about 10 weeks
4 to 6 months	• has increased sucking strength • brings fingers to mouth	• socializes during feeding
6 to 9 months	• drinks from a cup held by an adult • eats soft food from a spoon with a "munching" chew (an up-and-down motion) • enjoys holding food and finger feeding	• loves to be included at the table for meals • begins to show likes and dislikes for certain foods
9 to 12 months	• tries to use a spoon • starts to finger feed with a more advanced grasp • feeds at regular times	• is conscious of what others do • imitates others
12 to 18 months	• grasps and releases food with fingers • holds spoon but use is awkward • turns spoon in mouth • uses a cup but may dribble	• wants food that others are eating • loves performing • understands simple questions and requests
18 to 24 months	• begins rotary chewing (in a circular motion) • has decreased appetite • likes eating with hands • likes trying different textures	• is easily distracted • prefers certain foods • considers ritual important
2 to 3 years	• holds a glass • places a spoon straight into mouth • spills a lot • chews a variety of foods but choking is still a hazard	• likes to help in the kitchen • has definite likes, dislikes and rituals (such as shape of foods) • insists on doing it "myself" • dawdles • has food jags, eating only one or two foods for extended periods
3 to 4 years	• holds a cup by the handle • pours from small pitcher • uses a fork • chews most foods	• has improved appetite and interest in food • requests favourite foods • relishes (or not) the shape and colour of foods • makes choices between foods • is influenced by TV commercials • imitates food preparation
4 to 5 years	• uses knife and fork • drinks from a cup easily • self-feeds easily	• prefers talking to eating • continues with food jags • likes to help around the house • is interested in types of food and where they come from • is increasingly influenced by peers

Nutrition

General principles

Three important principles apply to feeding children of all ages. Every child in any care setting should be offered food in a quantity and quality that:

- meet individual metabolic and nutrient needs, as well as promoting normal growth,
- are age-appropriate, safe and consistent, and
- are culturally appropriate, promoting feelings of love and security.

Feeding and mealtimes should be relaxed and pleasurable for both children and their caregivers. Food is to be enjoyed. Feeding babies and children well means learning to read their hunger cues, offering food when they are ready to eat and letting them decide when they are satisfied. From birth, letting a child take the lead about how much she needs to eat is the basis for appropriate feeding as she grows. Good eating habits learned in childhood can last a lifetime, and child care practitioners are in an ideal position to help families instill those good habits.

Understanding food security

Food security means having access to enough healthy food without experiencing difficulty in meeting other basic family needs. Not all families you encounter will have enough safe, nutritious food to feed their children throughout the month. Along with nutritional and health consequences, food insecurity has both psychological and social consequences for children.

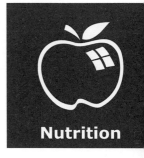

Nutrition

Policies that encourage mothers who breastfeed and support them in out-of-home settings are especially positive, because breastfeeding is an important aspect of food security for babies and their families. By providing nourishing food in a comfortable setting, child care practitioners can reduce the negative impact of food insecurity on particularly vulnerable children. If you suspect that some children are arriving in the morning without having had a nourishing breakfast, you'll want to plan a healthy snack for early in the day. As well, child care services can be a hub for information about community resources and local food security initiatives, such as community kitchens and gardens.

Creating a nutrition policy

A nutrition policy outlines how you will provide a well-balanced diet for all children in your program. Your policy needs to conform to any provincial/territorial regulations that address nutrition in child care settings. Where applicable, these regulations may specify:

- how often meals and snacks are served,
- how food is prepared and stored,
- how food brought from home is labelled,
- how often menus are prepared, recorded and presented to parents,
- that written feeding instructions must be provided by parents for all children under the age of 1 or with special dietary needs,

- that the names and pictures of children with food allergies, what they are allergic to, and how to manage a reaction are to be posted in both the cooking and serving areas. (See Chapter 10, *Chronic Medical Conditions*, and *Selected resources* at the end of this chapter.)

Some child care facilities do not provide food for children and require parents to supply their child's food each day. These facilities still require a nutrition policy outlining which foods and beverages are acceptable and how they are to be labelled, stored and served.

As part of your nutrition policy, keep a contingency or back-up supply of basics at the centre in case a child arrives without food or must stay longer than expected because of bad weather or other circumstances.

Collaborating with families

When a child care practitioner takes on the responsibility of feeding children, she needs to work closely with families to ensure that what is offered in the program complements what the child is eating at home. The food she serves should meet each child's individual nutritional and developmental needs and be compatible with the family's religious and cultural views. In any given facility, there may be children who are vegetarians, have food restrictions based on religion, or are allergic to certain foods. It takes careful planning to provide for such a wide range of needs. Having children from many cultures in a program presents a rich opportunity to explore—in collaboration with parents—a range of cuisines when planning menus. While offering specific suggestions is beyond the scope of this chapter, there are great resources to help you learn more about different food patterns and traditions. (See *Selected resources* at the end of this chapter.)

Sharing your nutrition policy with parents before enrolment is important for ensuring a good fit, and there are occasions when a parent may legitimately request a menu change for health reasons. Share nutrition updates with all parents and refer to your policy if you and a parent disagree about a food issue. You may want to organize an information night for families or distribute brochures and posters from your local public health agency to parents. In some communities, you can refer to a registered dietitian for additional information and support. **Remember: all parents want to feed their children well.**

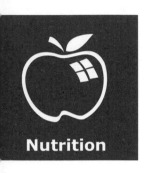

Nutrition

Feeding babies from birth to 12 months

As a child care practitioner, you need to know how to feed children through all the developmental stages of their first year. Infants usually start with breast milk and move on to their first "complementary" foods (so-called because—ideally—they complement continued breastfeeding) at about 6 months. The shift to solids while infants continue to breastfeed happens slowly, over many months. Gradually, infants learn to eat foods that are varied in texture, flavour, temperature and shape.

Together, you and an infant's parents will work out a plan for feeding. This schedule may involve giving the child one or more bottles of expressed breast milk when the mother is unavailable to breastfeed or offering formula when the mother is away. Regardless of the type of milk feeding, as you get to know the child you'll learn to recognize hunger cues and respond accordingly. Hunger cues include rapid eye movement, waking, stretching, stirring, hand-to-mouth activity, and oral activities such as sucking, licking and rooting (seeking the nipple when held). Try to feed an infant "on cue," before she reaches the crying stage. However, not all crying is a demand to eat. Try to follow the infant's home routine as much as possible, staying alert to changes as the child reaches a new stage of development. Where possible, it's helpful for one child care practitioner to consistently feed a given child. This feeding relationship allows the caregiver to learn and respond to the child's hunger cues while building the child's sense of security.

Make feeding time unhurried and a chance for closeness. Cradle the infant in your arms, changing his position occasionally. Talk to him quietly. Hold the bottle so the nipple is always full to prevent him from swallowing too much air. Remember that feeding is a time for social contact.

ALERT

Never prop a bottle in an infant's mouth. Not only does bottle propping deprive a child of the physical contact that should accompany every feeding, but it increases the risk of choking, aspirating milk into the lungs, ear infections and early childhood tooth decay.

Let infants self-regulate their milk intake. Watch for the cues and respond appropriately. How often an infant feeds and how much she takes at one feeding can vary a lot from day to day. The amount also depends on her activity level and growth rate. Infants have appetite spurts at about 2, 3 and 6 weeks and at 3 and 6 months. They may want extra feedings at these times. Follow the infant's lead, and don't coax her to finish a bottle. Discuss their child's feeding schedule daily with parents and record the times and amounts of each feeding while the infant is in your care.

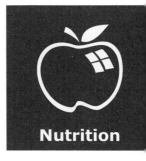

Nutrition

Offering breastfeeding support

Breast milk is the optimal food for infants because it has the right composition of nutrients for growth and brain development, is easy on the digestive system, and contains antibodies and other immune factors that help babies fight off illness. Exclusive breastfeeding with vitamin D supplementation for the first 6 months of life has been shown to reduce the occurrence of gastrointestinal and respiratory infections. Since breast milk is tailor-made by each mother for her own baby, the infant has less exposure to foreign proteins. Breastfed babies also have a lower incidence of sudden infant death syndrome (SIDS). Breastfeeding may continue into the second year and beyond, providing benefits for both baby and mother. Complementary iron-rich foods should gradually be introduced at about 6 months, while breastfeeding continues.

Child care settings play an increasingly vital role in supporting and facilitating parents in their decision to breastfeed successfully. The Baby Friendly Initiative is a WHO/UNICEF program that helps promote, protect and support breastfeeding. Child care practitioners can participate by:

- having a written policy on how breastfeeding is supported in their facility and including it in the information package,
- providing a comfortable place on site for mothers to breastfeed and express milk,
- promoting breastfeeding on site with wall posters and free brochures,
- encouraging staff members to discuss breastfeeding with current and prospective parents and to refer them to breastfeeding community supports and resources,
- including fathers in breastfeeding discussions.

Develop an individual breastfeeding support plan for each breastfed baby in your care. This plan should include how breast milk will be stored and offered, and what staff should do if the baby is hungry and a designated supply of expressed breast milk is gone or a mother is running late. Your policy should be flexible enough that mothers can meet their babies' needs in a variety of ways. One mother may prefer to nurse just before leaving the facility and will want the child eager to feed again when she arrives at pick-up time. Another might wish to nurse once she arrives home and will ask staff to feed her infant before she arrives for pick-up. Some mothers want their child to receive only breast milk and express enough milk for the day. Others may breastfeed only at home and have you give the infant formula when he's in your care. Your role is to support each parent's choice in a non-judgmental way.

Storing and handling breast milk

Breast milk doesn't look or smell like formula or cow's milk. It can have a blue, yellow or even brown tinge and normally separates into layers of cream and milk. It may turn more yellow when frozen. Breast milk is perishable and needs careful handling and storage.

Ask parents to bring fresh bottles of expressed milk for their child each day. They should also supply extra milk that can be kept frozen at the child care facility for contingency use. Screw-cap glass bottles, hard plastic cups or bottles with tight caps, or sterile freezer bags designed for storing breast milk are considered safe containers. Don't store expressed breast milk in regular plastic freezer bags or bottle liners designed for holding formula, as these can easily leak, spill or split when frozen. Ask parents to label the supply with their child's name, the amount of milk and the date of expression. Store expressed breast milk in the refrigerator or freezer as soon as it is prepared or received.

The label on expressed breast milk should be carefully checked (preferably by two people) before every feeding. It is important to avoid giving breast milk to the wrong baby as there is a very small risk of a blood-borne virus being present. If it is, the child to whom the milk belongs may have antibodies acquired from her mother and be somewhat protected, but another child may not be. Your facility should have a protocol for managing breast milk errors. Both the mother who produced the breast milk and the parents of the baby who was given the wrong milk must be advised if an error occurs, and public health authorities contacted without delay. Blood tests may be required and the baby who received the milk may require immunization against hepatitis B.

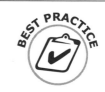

To prevent microbial growth:

- Discard any leftover breast milk in a bottle that has had contact with a child's mouth.
- Don't add warm expressed milk to milk that has been chilled or frozen.

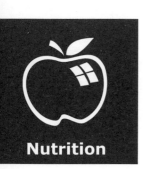

Nutrition

Parents may want any fresh, unused breast milk returned to them at the end of the day. Breast milk can be used for up to 2 days if it is kept refrigerated. Freshly expressed then frozen breast milk can be kept for different lengths of time depending on the type of freezer:

- 2 weeks in your refrigerator's freezer compartment
- 2 to 3 months in a stand-alone fridge-type (upright) freezer
- 6 months in a separate chest-type freezer (at a temperature below -20°C [-4°F])

Do not use the stove-top or a microwave to thaw or warm frozen expressed milk. To thaw frozen breast milk, loosen the lid and place the container in the refrigerator several hours before the milk is needed or under cool running water to thaw more quickly. Keep thawed breast milk refrigerated and use it within 24 hours. Do not refreeze thawed breast milk.

To warm breast milk, place the container or bottle in a pan or bowl of warm water. Milk warmed in a microwave may contain "hot spots" that can scald a baby's mouth, and overheating milk on the stove will destroy its nutrients. Before feeding, shake the bottle gently to mix separated layers and test the milk on the inside of your wrist to make sure it isn't too warm.

Commercial formula

Where breast milk is not an option, a store-bought, cow's milk-based formula with sufficient iron (at least 4 mg/L) is recommended for healthy full-term infants. If a child care practitioner needs to prepare a supply of formula each day, Table 3.2 may be useful for gauging amounts. There is no comparable chart for breast milk, expressed or otherwise, because watching for a baby's hunger cues and feeding on demand is the best feeding plan in any setting. A child's growth and weight gain, and daily indicators like the number of wet diapers are the best measures of a feeding plan's success. The following suggested amounts of formula are only guidelines. **Remember: every baby is different.**

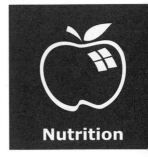

Nutrition

TABLE 3.2

Average amounts of formula per feeding (30 mL = 1 oz.)

Age	Number of bottles each day	Amount in each bottle
Birth to 2 weeks	6–10	60–90 mL (2–3 oz.)
2 to 8 weeks	6–8	90–120 mL (3–4 oz.)
2 to 3 months	5–6	120–180 mL (4–6 oz.)
3 to 5 months	5–6	150–180 mL (5–6 oz.)
5 to 7 months	5–6	150–180 mL (5–6 oz.)
7 to 9 months	4	180–240 mL (6–8 oz.)
9 to 12 months	3–4	180–240 mL (6–8 oz.)

Source: HealthLine and Health Link protocols (Saskatchewan, Alberta).

Most commercial formulas are made from cow's milk protein, but specialized formulas are available for infants diagnosed with a gastrointestinal or metabolic disease. Evaporated milk, whole cow's milk and goat's milk are not recommended for infants under 12 months of age. **Any alternative formula should be used only with a doctor's approval and direction.**

Formula is available as a ready-to-serve liquid, a concentrated liquid or a powder. All forms of formula, when they are prepared according to package directions, are identical in their nutritional content. Ready-to-serve formula is the most convenient but also the most expensive. You can require parents to provide fresh bottles of formula each day or prepare it yourself. If preparing **liquid formula** on site, make only what you'll need for the next 24 hours at one time. Label bottles of formula with the child's name and time of preparation, and store them in the refrigerator. Be aware that **powdered formula is not sterile**: prepare only enough formula for one feeding at a time, immediately before each feeding.

To prepare formula: Wash your hands with soap and water. Thoroughly wash bottles and nipples, removing all milk residue with a brush. Until an infant is 4 months old, sterilize bottles, nipples and utensils by boiling them for 2 minutes. After 4 months, cleaning them in the complete wash/rinse/dry cycle of a dishwasher is sufficient. If you're using disposable bottle liners, wash and rinse the holder before each use and sterilize the nipples. **Disposable bottle liners should never be reused.**

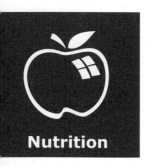

Nutrition

Measure and mix formula according to the directions on the label. Concentrated liquid or powdered formula should be prepared **exactly** according to the manufacturer's directions. Too much or too little water can be harmful, and the water must be clean and free from contamination. Types of water generally appropriate for mixing formula include municipal (city) tap water (only from the cold water tap), well water that meets standards of safety, and suitable commercially bottled water (except for carbonated, mineral or distilled water). **For infants under 4 months old, all types of water must be boiled for at least 2 minutes and cooled before mixing, to ensure they are pathogen free.** Boiled water will keep 2 to 3 days in the refrigerator, or for 24 hours at room temperature, as long as it's stored in a sterile, closed container.

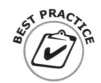

To prevent microbial growth:

- Prepare powdered formula just before a feeding and don't store it in the fridge.

- Don't leave any formula unrefrigerated for more than 1 hour.

- Never reuse a bottle of formula or milk once an infant has drunk from it: always discard leftover milk.

Store concentrated liquid formula in the refrigerator once it's been opened. Store unmixed powdered formula on a shelf in a sealed container in a cool place and use it up within the period specified on the label, or 30 days, whichever is sooner.

Until an infant is 4 to 6 months old, it's common practice to warm a bottle to remove the chill. Although this step isn't necessary, infants tend to prefer warm milk. Place the bottle in a pan or bowl of warm water or use a bottle warmer, and test the formula temperature on the inside of your wrist before feeding. **Don't use a microwave to warm a bottle.** Record the amount of formula that an infant consumes so that parents can track daily intake.

Water and juice

Infants who are breastfeeding exclusively from birth to age 6 months do not require supplemental water. Nor do healthy formula-fed infants. However, an infant who has fever or diarrhea may need extra fluids such as additional breast milk and/or an oral rehydration solution (ORS). (For more about diarrhea, see Chapter 7, *Common Conditions*, and Chapter 9, *Managing Infections*.) When a baby begins to eat complementary foods at about 6 months, water may be offered occasionally. Water used in the feeding of children, either for drinking or for preparing food and other beverages, must be clean and free from contamination. Water run from the cold water tap is less likely to contain lead, copper and other non-biological contaminants, so avoid using water from the hot water tap for food preparation.

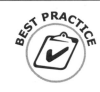

Beverages such as fruit drinks, sweet powdered drinks reconstituted with water, soda pop, teas and energy drinks are not suitable for infants or young children and should not be offered in the child care setting.

Fruit juice is not necessary or recommended until children are older than 6 months and eating a variety of foods. Then, offer only 100% fruit juice in a cup (never a bottle), and only as part of a meal or snack. Limit the quantity to 60 to 120 mL (2 to 4 oz.) per day. Too much juice causes diarrhea and early childhood tooth decay (ECTD) and can decrease a child's appetite for more nutrient-rich foods, including breast milk.

Complementary foods

Readiness

Exclusive breastfeeding is recommended for healthy full-term infants for the first 6 months of life. At about 6 months, most babies are ready to try other foods while continuing to breastfeed. Formula-fed babies are also ready for complementary foods at about 6 months.

Babies are ready for complementary foods when they seem hungrier than usual, are interested in food when others are eating, vocalize, and generally let you know they'd like some too. They are able to sit without support and have good control of their neck muscles. They pick up food and try to mouth it, open wide when food is offered on a spoon, and hold a bit of food in their mouth without pushing it out with their tongue (the extrusion reflex). An equally important social cue is that they can show lack of interest in food by leaning back, closing their mouth, or turning their head away.

By sharing information and working together, child care practitioners and families can ensure children get enough nutrient-rich food every day. For babies whose mothers wish to sustain breastfeeding for as long as possible, the transition to complementary foods happens slowly over many months, so that solids do not replace breast milk too quickly.

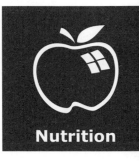

Nutrition

Amounts and textures

Continue to follow a child's cues for how much food to offer. Start by offering a teaspoon or two, and don't rush. Some babies will need to try a food many times before accepting it. Try to pick a time of day when the child seems alert and interested. Don't coax a baby to eat more or try to trick him by playing a game or by offering a sweetened food. A child who is allowed to follow his own hunger cues is much less likely to overeat later in life.

Slowly, add a variety of more textured foods (and more food) as the baby develops and learns to handle different foods in the mouth. Encourage self-feeding. The transition to a family diet should be made at about 12 months of age. Breastfeeding can be sustained, topping up solid foods until a child is 2 years of age and beyond. If you are formula feeding, gradually add solid foods while continuing with formula until the baby is about 12 months old.

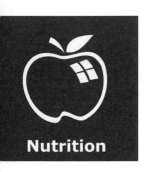

Nutrition

TABLE 3.3

Textures: which, when and how often

Child's developmental stage	Complementary food (how often)	Food consistency and texture
Sitting with support	2 to 3 times a day*	• puréed, mashed and semi-solid foods
Sitting unassisted	2 to 3 times a day*	• healthy family foods • small amounts of soft-mashed foods without lumps
Crawling	3 to 4 times a day*	• healthy family foods • ground or soft-mashed foods with tiny, soft lumps • crunchy foods that soften, such as whole grain crackers
Walking	3 meals and 2 to 3 snacks a day*	• coarsely chopped foods • foods with more texture • bite-sized pieces of food • finger foods

* Plus breast milk, formula or whole cow's milk, depending on the child's age.

Nutrient-rich complementary foods

Follow the family's lead when offering foods to children for the first time and develop your menus with nutrient needs and diversity in mind.

Foods containing iron are recommended as the first to be introduced. Iron is essential not only for brain development but to form hemoglobin, the substance that carries oxygen in the bloodstream. A lack of iron can result in anemia, impaired learning ability, poor growth and irritability.

Here are some key points to remember:

• Single-grain, iron-fortified infant cereals have traditionally been the first complementary foods offered to babies in Canada, but meat and alternatives can also be introduced at about 6 months depending on the family's preference and cultural tradition. Meats, cooked and mashed egg yolk (but not the egg white), poultry and de-boned fish, as well as tofu and well-cooked dried peas, beans and lentils, are sources of iron. Iron from meat is better absorbed than iron from other foods.

- De-boned fish is an important protein choice. Refer to Health Canada's most recent advisory on types and amounts of fish appropriate for young children at www.healthcanada.gc.ca.
- You can offer dark green, orange and yellow vegetables soft-cooked or baked (these are high in vitamins A and C) and puréed or mashed fruit. Limit fruit juice to no more than 120 mL (4 oz.) per day and offer only in a cup.
- After a child reaches 9 months, you can offer calcium- and protein-rich milk products such as yogurt (3.25% fat content [MF] or higher), cottage cheese and other cheeses. Some milk products contain vitamin D, which is listed on the label.
- To help prevent iron-deficiency anemia, you should wait until a child is a year old before offering pasteurized whole cow's milk. Drinking too much milk (more than 720 mL [24 oz.] per day) may lead to a reduced intake of other nutrient-rich foods, although there is no hard evidence that offering milk before or after solids makes a difference to intake. Offer milk in a cup. While cow's milk is a poor source of vitamin C and iron, it's a very good source of calcium, protein and concentrated calories needed for energy and growth; 500 mL (16 oz.) of fluid milk also provides 5 μg (200 IU [International Units]) of vitamin D.
- Potatoes, rice, plain oatmeal or smooth porridges and pasta are good sources of energy. These can be cooked, mashed and served to infants as part of a healthy diet.
- You can share plain healthy family foods with babies. "Plain" means no added salt, sugar, spices or coatings. Canned or frozen plain vegetables, like legumes, may need to be well rinsed to remove salt.

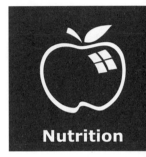

Nutrition

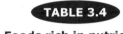

TABLE 3.4

Foods rich in nutrients

Protein/Iron/Zinc (Helps build and heal tissue)	Vitamin A (Aids cell growth and immune system development)	Vitamin C (Strengthens tissue, bones and teeth)	Folate (Helps brain and nervous system development and builds healthy blood cells)
• lamb, turkey • beef, bison • liver (chicken, beef) • venison, wild meat • chicken, pork • de-boned fish* • egg yolk • infant cereal • tofu, lentils, legumes	• egg yolk • liver • avocado • sweet potato, carrot • squash, pumpkin • spinach, chard • broccoli • mango, apricot • cantaloupe	• cantaloupe • broccoli • kiwi • orange • 100% fruit juice • tomato • squash, spinach, mango • strawberry • watermelon	• liver (chicken, beef, pork) • green pea, spinach • lentils, legumes, tofu • avocado • egg yolk • orange, cantaloupe • beet greens, broccoli, chard • pasta, bread

Note that foods don't need to be introduced in this order.

*Refer to Health Canada's most recent advisory on types and amounts of fish appropriate for young children at www.healthcanada.gc.ca.

Vegetarian diets
Babies on vegetarian diets should follow the same timing for the introduction of solid foods. Discuss with parents what protein sources are appropriate, depending on the form of

vegetarianism the family follows. Types of vegetarian diets include lacto-ovo (eating eggs and dairy products, no meat), ovo-vegetarian (eating eggs, no dairy products or meat), lacto-vegetarian (eating dairy products, no eggs or meat) and vegan (eating food from plant sources only). When working with a vegan family, encourage parents to consult with a registered dietitian for advice about the best way to meet a child's nutritional needs, which include protein, iron, zinc and vitamin B12.

Tips for introducing complementary foods

- **Follow the child's lead** on how much food to offer. The best guide is the child's appetite. Children vary enormously in their size and growth rate. It's rare for a child to eat too little, although he may not be eating as much as his parents or caregiver think he should.
- **Encourage self-feeding.** Learning to self-feed is an important developmental milestone that a baby reaches through much practice and considerable mess-making. A baby who finger feeds is responding to his own hunger cues, in effect taking responsibility for how much he wants to eat. Let a child hold the spoon as you guide food to his mouth. Offer small amounts of finger food for him to explore with his fingers and work to put into his mouth. Supervise mealtimes closely, sitting within arm's reach at all times.
- **Introduce new foods one at a time**, preferably after they've been tried at home, and allow 3 to 5 days before trying another new food. That way, if there's an allergic reaction or sign of intolerance, it's easier to pinpoint which food might have caused the problem.
    - ➤ If a problem with a particular food is known or detected, **defer to parents' instructions** and/or encourage them to consult with their doctor or a registered dietitian for guidance.
    - ➤ **Start with single foods and avoid mixtures** until all component foods have been tried on their own.
    - ➤ **Wait until a baby is 1 year old** before introducing egg whites, because of the risk of allergies, and honey, because of the risk of infant botulism.
- **Keep to the recommended limits for milk and milk alternatives.** The recommended daily intake of milk and alternatives is up to 720 mL or 24 oz. per day for children 24 months and older. After 2 years of age, two servings of whole milk or alternatives (e.g., cheese, yogurt) is all a child usually needs per day. Lower fat milk (1% or 2% MF) can be offered between the ages of 2 and 5 and skim milk after children are 5 years of age.
- **Prevent choking hazards** by making foods safe or avoiding them if they are unsuitable for a child's age or stage of development.
- **Know your role.** The child care practitioner decides which food to offer and when. Each child's role is to decide whether and how much to eat.

Commercial or homemade food?

Offering homemade baby food has the advantage of allowing a more gradual transition from purée to solid textures according to each baby's need. Commercial food is convenient for parents and child care practitioners but is more costly than homemade food.

If parents are preparing homemade food, ask them to provide you with a daily supply. Keep this food covered in the refrigerator and be sure to serve it within a day or two.

Nutrition

Alternatively, you can ask parents to prepare and freeze food that you can transfer to the freezer at your facility for future use. Ask parents to freeze homemade food in ice-cube trays and supply you with the food cubes in freezer bags, labelled with their child's name, the date of preparation and what the food is. Care should be taken in transporting frozen food from home so that no thawing occurs. Frozen puréed fruit and vegetables can be kept in the freezer for 3 months, and frozen puréed meat for 1 month.

To serve frozen food, take one cube or more from the freezer just before mealtime. Thaw and heat it in a double boiler or small bowl of hot water. Stir the food and check its temperature carefully before offering it to children. **Never refreeze food once it's been thawed.**

Feeding children 1 to 5 years of age

A baby who is 1 year old is ready to take part in regular meal and snack times with you and other children in your care. Meals are important social times in a child's day, times when learning about food combines with observing and interacting with other children and caregivers. The child care practitioner's role is to make those mealtimes relaxed and enjoyable. Eating in a positive atmosphere helps children to develop healthy attitudes to food, themselves and other children.

At 1 year of age, a child can eat most of the foods that older children eat as long as they aren't a choking hazard.

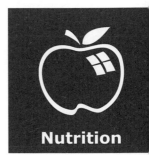

Nutrition

To prevent choking:

- observe children's chewing and swallowing abilities and serve foods appropriate for their age and stage of development,
- sit down for snacks and meals, and supervise while eating by sitting at the same table as the children,
- do not allow children to feed other children,
- ensure children sit upright while eating, and
- discourage talking while children have food in their mouths.

Foods that may cause choking, especially for children under 4 years old, are:

- hard and/or round foods (e.g., hard candies or cough drops, nuts, pieces of raw vegetable, whole grapes, raisins, wiener slices, rice, peas and corn),
- foods with pits, seeds, bones (e.g., fish), popcorn husks that can be aspirated,
- sticky foods (e.g., peanut or other nut butters served alone or on a spoon, marshmallows),
- chewy foods (e.g., meat not cut into small enough pieces, wiener slices, gum or gummy bears), and
- any food served with toothpicks or skewers.

Make food safer by:

- grating raw vegetables to aid chewing,
- slicing grapes into quarters or halves,

- removing pits or seeds,
- gently cooking or steaming hard vegetables to soften them,
- spreading sticky foods, like nut butters, thinly on pieces of cracker or toast, rather than on sliced bread,
- chopping or scraping stringy meat and adding broth to moisten it,
- de-boning fish, and
- cutting wieners lengthwise, in small pieces.

Timing meals and snacks

Toddlers and preschoolers need to eat often—they need three meals a day and two or three snacks (morning, afternoon and possibly before bed). Together with parents, plan the timing of meals and snacks so that children are offered the right amount of food at about 2-hour intervals. Take each family's schedule into account. For example, if there is a long commute home at the end of the day, serving a snack in late afternoon may be more appropriate than in mid-afternoon. Try to offer a snack at least 1½ to 2 hours before the next meal.

REMEMBER

Anticipating a child's hunger and having a meal or snack ready is crucial at this age—and an important strategy for preventing temper tantrums.

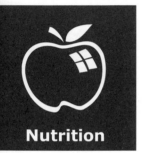

Nutrition

Provincial regulations and occupational guidelines specify what food must be offered and how often, depending on a child's age and the number of hours spent in care. Here's a basic routine to follow regardless of the age of children in your care:

- For 2- to 4-hour sessions (either morning or afternoon), provide a snack 1½ to 2 hours before the next planned meal.
- For 4- to 6-hour sessions, provide one meal and one snack.
- For 7- to 8-hour sessions, provide one meal and two snacks.
- For 9- to 10-hour sessions, provide two meals and two snacks.

Following *Canada's Food Guide*

Every child needs a daily balanced diet that consists of foods from all four food groups— vegetables and fruit, grain products, milk and alternatives, and meat and alternatives. Young children have small appetites and need energy for growth and development. This means that what you offer at snack times is just as important as the food you serve at meals.

Canada's Food Guide recommends daily:

4 servings of vegetables and fruit for children 2 to 3 years old and 5 for children age 4 to 8. Choose at least one dark green and one orange vegetable or fruit. Vegetables and fruit are a source of vitamins, minerals and fibre.

3 servings of grain products for children 2 to 3 years old and 4 for children age 4 to 8. Make at least half of the grain products whole grain. Grains are an important source of energy from carbohydrates.

2 servings of milk and alternatives for all children 2 through 8 years old. After children turn 2 years of age, lower fat milk (1% or 2% MF) or milk alternatives may be offered, and skim milk may be served after children turn 5. Milk is a nutritious source of calories, as well as calcium and vitamin D, for growing children. Some milk alternatives (e.g., fortified soy beverage) have vitamin D added. Check labels for calcium and vitamin D content.

1 serving of meat and alternatives for all children 2 through 8 years old. Choose a variety of lean meat, poultry, and de-boned fish, eggs, tofu, dried peas, beans and lentils. Meat and alternatives are an important source of iron and protein.

As anyone who feeds toddlers and preschoolers knows, some children eat much more than others and actual amounts can also vary widely from day to day. Serving sizes for this age group can be very small—as little as 60 mL (2 oz.) of juice or ¼ of a bagel, for example, though portion sizes generally increase with age. A 1-year-old may eat 30 g (1 oz.) of chicken and a 3-year-old might eat twice that amount. Children's appetites fluctuate in relation to growth patterns. You can't encourage a child's growth by encouraging eating. Growth fuels appetite, so when a child is having a growth spurt she will be hungrier and let you know.

Your job is to offer a proper balance of appropriate foods: from at least three of the four food groups at mealtimes, and from at least two of the four food groups for each snack during the day. When introducing a child to a new food, try to offer it alongside a familiar one. So if you want a child to try scrambled eggs, serve them with his favourite toast. Introduce melon pieces along with his tried-and-true banana.

Don't stigmatize food by suggesting that chocolate bars are "bad" and apples are "good." Rather, talk about "everyday foods" like vegetables and fruit, whole grain cereals and breads and "sometimes foods." "Sometimes foods" are the high-sugar cereals, sweets, heavily salted and high-fat processed meats and snack foods that can be an occasional addition to a meal but are not everyday fare.

Sugar and sugar substitutes

Encourage children to eat more wholesome foods without added sugar or sugar substitutes by choosing to eat them yourself. Limit honey, molasses, syrups, and brown and refined white sugars, which all have similar caloric content

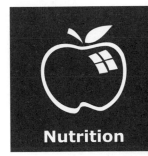

Nutrition

The golden rules of feeding children

- Offer meals and snacks at regular intervals.

- Provide a variety of food, in accordance with *Canada's Food Guide*.

- Have a comfortable place to sit and eat.

- Supervise and share in mealtimes by eating with the children.

- Offer food in forms children can manage easily (i.e., cut into pieces or mashed) to prevent a choking hazard.

- Provide devices or utensils—a booster seat, a cup or a small spoon—that help children to feel included and eat more independently.

- Teach age-appropriate table manners.

- Make mealtimes pleasant.

Allow children to:

- Choose to eat or not to eat the meal.

- Eat as much or as little as they want.

and contribute to tooth decay. Sugar substitutes such as aspartame and sucralose have been used instead of natural sweeteners in most processed foods for many years. They are a safe, calorie-saving alternative to sugar and do not contribute to early childhood tooth decay. However, artificial sweeteners also have no intrinsic nutritional value and do not contribute to a well-balanced diet.

Juice and water

Serve vegetables and fruit more often than fruit juice. Drinking fruit juice and fruit drinks can lead to children consuming less milk than they need. Offer water, especially between planned meals and snacks, when children are thirsty. Limit juice to one serving (120 mL [4 oz.]) of 100% unsweetened juice per day. Serving fruit instead of fruit juice has the added benefit of supplying necessary fibre to a child's diet.

Dietary fibre

Dietary fibre, which is the undigested parts of food plants, is an important element in a child's diet. There are two types of fibre: insoluble and soluble. **Insoluble fibre**, found mainly in wheat bran, vegetables, and the peels of fruit and vegetables, promotes healthy bowels and helps prevent constipation. **Soluble fibre**, found mainly in fruit, oat products and legumes like beans, helps to regulate blood sugar and cholesterol levels. Children who are eating according to *Canada's Food Guide* will receive the fibre they need.

Here are some tips for ensuring your menu includes adequate fibre:

- Serve a variety of whole grain bread and pasta products.
- Choose cereals with at least 4 to 6 grams of fibre per serving.
- Serve fruit and vegetables with their skins on. Wash them thoroughly.
- Serve brown rice.
- Substitute up to half the white flour with whole wheat flour when making homemade pancakes or muffins.

What about fat?

Children 1 to 5 years old continue to need enough calories for growth and development. Offer a variety of nutritious foods, including some choices that contain concentrated sources of energy from fat, such as pasteurized whole milk and peanut butter.

Healthy fats are also found in most vegetable oils, salad dressings, soft margarines and

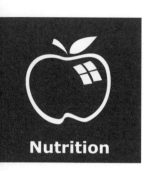

Nutrition

Encourage children to eat well

- Serve a variety of foods and include at least one nutritious choice on the table that you know children will eat.

- Encourage children to help in the kitchen. They are more likely to eat salad if they have helped to tear up the lettuce.

- Offer food in interesting shapes. Use a cookie cutter to turn ordinary sandwiches into stars.

- Let children dip softer vegetables and fruit in yogurt.

- Talk positively about food and avoid discussing your own dislikes or dieting efforts at the table or within earshot of children.

- Eliminate distractions by turning off the TV and make a rule about no toys at the table.

- Banish junk food from the pantry so that no one (yourself included) is tempted to eat something that will spoil their appetite for the next meal. Be a good role model.

- Avoid conflicts about food.

- Avoid offering food as a reward or incentive for eating.

mayonnaise, though these are best served in small amounts. Healthy fats contain essential fatty acids like omega-3 and omega-6 that cannot be made in the body and must come from the diet. Cook with vegetable oils such as canola, olive and soybean. Choose soft margarines.

Fats that are solid at room temperature contain more trans and saturated fats associated with increased risk of heart disease. Therefore, limit butter, hard margarines, lard and shortening. Read labels and avoid serving trans or saturated fats found in some commercial products, such as cookies, donuts and crackers.

Limit processed meats, such as wieners and luncheon meats, which are also high in fat.

Getting through the picky stage

Many children go through stages of refusing to eat certain foods, being easily distracted at mealtimes and seeming to "eat like a bird." As a child care practitioner, you may see less of this behaviour than their families. Parents often comment that their children will eat food in the child care facility that they won't touch at home. Positive peer example may have something to do with this phenomenon.

Recognize that children, when offered a variety of nutritious foods, will probably eat what they need, even if their appetites vary widely. An infant who is growing rapidly in the first year may have a stronger appetite than a toddler in his second or third year, whose growth normally slows down while mobility and autonomy increase.

Your strategy, when a toddler or preschooler is refusing certain foods or whole meals, is to let him make that choice. At the same time, stick to the rule that the kitchen won't reopen until the next planned snack or meal.

Don't serve a snack 15 minutes after a child refuses lunch. You may have to deal with some crankiness, but don't give in and stay positive. The child will be ready to eat when the regular snack time comes around, and other children will learn by example.

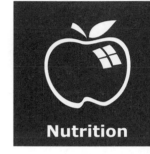

Nutrition

Special feeding issues

You're sure to encounter a range of special feeding issues while caring for children. Because every child is different, your approach to these issues needs to be personal, flexible and collaborative. However, some basic guidelines apply.

Food allergies

A food allergy involves an immune reaction triggered when a certain food or food additive (the allergen) is eaten and, in serious cases, is merely present in minute amounts. An allergic reaction can be very sudden and severe, even life threatening. If a child in your care has a food allergy, your role is to take every reasonable precaution against exposure to the trigger food and to be ready to respond to an allergic reaction. (For more on food allergies, see Chapter 10, *Chronic Medical Conditions*, and Chapter 11, *Emergencies*.)

Food intolerances

A food intolerance is different from an allergy in that it doesn't involve an immune reaction. A child who has an intolerance to a food may experience bloating, loose stools, gas or other symptoms after eating a certain food. In some cases of food intolerance, that food can be avoided. For example, if a child has loose stools after drinking apple juice, it can be easily decreased or eliminated from her diet.

Lactose intolerance occurs when the body doesn't produce enough of the enzyme lactase to fully break down the sugar (lactose) found in most dairy products. It is extremely rare in children this young but may be a short-term problem following a gastrointestinal infection. While children from certain cultures, including First Nations and Asian children, are known to have higher rates of lactose intolerance, the condition usually develops later, after at least 3 years of age. For these children, calcium can be obtained from broccoli, fortified soy milk, canned salmon and sardines with edible bones, oranges or fortified orange juice, almonds, lactose-free or lactose-reduced milk, and pinto beans. Pay special attention to foods that need to be modified to prevent choking.

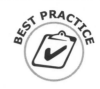

Any recommendations about substitutions for milk in a child's diet, including offering lactose-reduced milks, should be made by the child's family doctor or paediatrician.

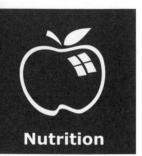

Nutrition

Feeding a child with a developmental delay

Although many children with a developmental delay have no difficulty eating, some do. They may, for example, have more difficulty chewing and swallowing, and might aspirate food into their lungs more easily if the amount taken is too large or given too rapidly. While each child's needs are unique, here are some general guidelines:

- **Learn from parents**. They will have figured out the best way to help their child eat. If possible, have a parent feed the child in your facility at least once with an assigned caregiver present, to observe feeding strategies.
- **Be very patient**. Allow the child to chew her food completely before offering more, and never rush her.
- **Encourage self-feeding** as much as possible, even though it may be messier or take longer.
- **Designate one caregiver** to help feed the child. She will get to know and trust this caregiver, who will also learn the child's special feeding techniques. Other staff will also need to be familiar with the child's needs, for times when the primary caregiver isn't available.
- **Ensure that the child feels part of the group at mealtimes**.
- **Do not allow other children to feed the child**.

Feeding an overweight or obese child

With almost one quarter of children age 2 to 5 in Canada either overweight or obese, the issue of feeding children to maintain a healthy weight is important. First of all, don't confuse temporary chubbiness with a weight problem. Chubby toddlers often transform into thin preschoolers.

If you suspect that a child is overweight, discuss your concerns with the parents. They may wish to consult their doctor or a registered dietitian about next steps. Together, you, the family and a health care professional can make a plan for achieving the child's healthy weight. Here's how to help:

- Evaluate your menus to be sure you're offering all children in your care a balanced diet that contains appropriate amounts of healthy fat.
- For children over 2 years old, consider serving lower fat milk (1% or 2% MF) or skim milk and alternatives like lower fat yogurt and cheese some of the time. In particular, assess the menu to ensure that you aren't serving too many processed foods that are high in fat, such as cookies, chips, luncheon meats, or packaged cracker and processed cheese combinations.
- Don't focus attention on the child's weight in any way (e.g., by encouraging him to eat less or offering him different foods from his peers).
- Don't compare children by weight or make comments about how much or how little they eat. Encourage all children in your care to follow their own hunger cues and to eat as much or as little as they want.
- Create lots of opportunities every day for children in your care to take part in physical activity that burns energy.
- Encourage parents to set short time limits on passive activities such as watching TV or playing computer games and avoid these pastimes in your program.
- Be a good role model. If children in your care see you choosing an apple as a snack and chasing a ball with them in the park, they will be more likely to make their own healthy choices. If children hear you speak negatively about food or body shapes and sizes, they will learn from that too.
- Promote a positive body image by choosing games, stories and activities that encourage self-esteem.

Nutrition

Meal planning

The time spent planning nourishing and enjoyable meals is an important part of the child care routine. Planning ahead in a home setting is especially important because, between preparing, serving and cleaning up, a lot of time is already spent in the kitchen. A well-thought-out meal plan saves time and stress and helps avoid last-minute shopping trips.

Getting started

Choose a weekly menu planning form. If required, use the form stipulated by your provincial/ territorial child care regulations. You can also use the checklist below or one provided by Dietitians of Canada or other health organizations.

Here's some advice about successful menu planning from the Healthy Start for Life program, a collaboration between Dietitians of Canada and nine other organizations:

For each meal:

Include a serving from at least three of the four food groups. For example:

- Choose a serving from the grain products group (e.g., pasta),
- Add a serving from the vegetables and fruit group (e.g., tomato sauce),

- Select a serving from the milk and alternatives group (e.g., pasteurized milk), or
- Offer a serving of meat, poultry, de-boned fish, eggs or meat alternatives such as beans, lentils or tofu.

For snacks:

- Include a serving from at least two different food groups.
- Choose nutritious snack foods such as vegetables, fruit, breads, cereals, milk, cheese or yogurt.
- Limit juice to one serving (120 mL [4 oz.]) per day. Serve water when children are thirsty.
- Avoid sticky, sweet foods such as dried fruit, which can stick to the teeth and cause cavities (unless children can brush their teeth right after).

To help preschoolers enjoy your meals:

- Involve them in menu planning.
- Choose foods that are easy to eat and suited to their personal and cultural preferences.
- Choose foods that can be served separately on a plate more often than mixed dishes.
- Include some finger foods.
- Offer child-sized servings.
- Present food in attractive, fun and interesting ways. Use foods of different colours, shapes and flavours.

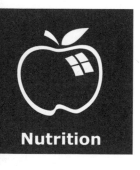

Nutrition

What else should you keep in mind?

- Encourage variety by including some "new" foods, in small amounts at first.
- Limit low-nutrient foods that are high in salt, fat, sugar or caffeine (e.g., chips, chocolate, candies, soft drinks).
- Balance higher fat foods with lower fat foods. For example, avoid having higher fat choices such as pizza, hot dogs and chicken nuggets all in the same week.
- When higher fat choices are served, balance them with more vegetables and fruit.

Meal plan checklist

Use this checklist to plan daily menus. If your menu is complete, it includes:

- ❑ food choices that children will eat and enjoy and that are safe to eat,
- ❑ meals and snacks with foods of different colours, flavours and textures,
- ❑ 4 servings per day of vegetables and fruit for children 2 to 3 years of age and 5 servings for children age 4 to 8. Provide one dark green and one orange vegetable and (at most) one serving of juice,
- ❑ 3 servings per day of grain products for children 2 to 3 years of age and 4 servings for children age 4 to 8. Provide at least half of these as whole grains, such as whole wheat bread or cereals, buns, bagels, tortillas, pita bread or brown rice,
- ❑ 2 servings of milk and alternatives each day,
- ❑ 1 serving of meat, poultry, de-boned fish, eggs, cooked dried peas, beans or lentils, tofu or peanut butter (if nuts and nut butters are permitted in your facility), and
- ❑ nutritious snacks that don't cause dental cavities.

TABLE 3.5

Sample one-day menu for a child 3 years of age

	Recommended daily *Food Guide* servings			
	Vegetables and fruit	**Grain products**	**Milk and alternatives**	**Meat and alternatives**
Child 2 to 3 years of age	4	3	2	1

Foods	Number of *Food Guide* servings				
	Vegetables and fruit	**Grain products**	**Milk and alternatives**	**Meat and alternatives**	**Added oils and fats**
Breakfast					
½ bowl of whole grain cereal (15 g)		½			
125 mL (½ cup) of 2% milk			½		
Snack					
60 mL (¼ cup) carrot sticks and broccoli florets with salad dressing	½				✔
water					
Lunch					
½ salmon sandwich on whole wheat bread (made with 30 g [1 oz.] of canned salmon and mayonnaise)		1		½	✔
60 mL (¼ cup) red pepper strips and cucumber slices	½				
125 mL (½ cup) milk			½		
1 peach	1				
Snack					
½ bowl of oat rings cereal (15 g)		½			
125 mL (½ cup) milk			½		
Dinner					
125 mL (½ cup) spaghetti with tomato and meat sauce (about 40 g [1½ oz.] of meat)	½	1		½	✔
125 mL (½ cup) milk			½		
125 mL (½ cup) applesauce	1				
Snack					
½ banana	½				
Total *Food Guide* servings for the day	**4**	**3**	**2**	**1**	

Source: Health Canada, *Eating Well with Canada's Food Guide: A Resource for Educators and Communicators*, Appendix A (Sample one-day menus), p. 44.

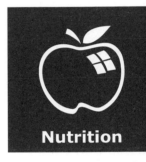

Nutrition

Build up your weekly menus until you have 3 or 4 weeks worth of menus that you can then rotate and share with parents. Post and/or circulate your menus to help parents plan family meals and minimize repetition. Rotating the menu ensures variety and helps you to avoid repeating a food too often. By planning 3 or 4 weeks ahead at a time, you'll reduce the time it takes to order, purchase and prepare food and have accurate information about food costs. You may want to use the menus to create a master shopping list of regularly purchased items.

Mark up a copy of your menu with children's responses to it and any preparation issues that crop up, so you can revise it as needed. When you alter a menu, review it against the checklist to ensure you've covered everything.

Preventing food-borne infections

Food-handling practices are one of the most closely regulated areas in the child care profession, and with good reason. Food-borne illnesses are common, potentially very serious and can occur within half an hour of or up to 2 weeks after eating food contaminated by harmful bacteria (e.g., salmonella, shigella, *Escherichia coli*), viruses (e.g., norovirus), or germs carried by insects and rodents. Safe food-handling and storage protocols are essential for preventing both the spread of infection through food contamination and food poisoning, which results from eating food contaminated by bacteria that thrive in moist, warm substances like food. These bacteria can double in number every 15 minutes when food is above 4°C (40°F) and below 60°C (140°F).

Nutrition

Practice four essential steps to prevent food contamination, as outlined by the Canadian Partnership for Consumer Food Safety Education:

1. Clean
2. Separate
3. Cook
4. Chill

1. Clean
- Always wash your hands before preparing or serving food.
- Clean and disinfect countertops, cutting boards and utensils before and after food preparation with household detergent and a mild (1:100) bleach solution: 5 mL [1 tsp.] bleach to 500 mL [2 cups] water.
- Discard cutting boards whose rough surfaces may retain germs.
- Wash all fruits and vegetables under cold, clear running water before eating or cooking. Scrub fruit and vegetables that have firm surfaces if they are not to be peeled (e.g., melons, potatoes, carrots) and cut away any damaged or bruised areas.
- Wash the tops of cans before opening them.
- Clean food-serving areas—tabletops, high chair trays—promptly after every use. Any surface where food is prepared or served should **not** be chipped or cracked.

2. Separate
- Keep your food preparation area separate from any play area.

- Try to ensure that a child care practitioner who changes diapers never handles food the same day. In settings where this does occur, follow hand-hygiene protocols meticulously.
- Have separate, clearly marked cutting boards—one for raw meats, poultry or fish and one for fruits and vegetables and other foods that will be eaten without cooking.
- Always keep food covered.
- Keep certain foods, like meats and their juices, separated from other foods during storage and preparation. To prevent juices from raw meat, poultry or seafood from dripping onto other foods or shelves in the refrigerator, place meat and fish in closed containers or sealed plastic bags on a bottom shelf.
- Never place cooked food on the same plate or cutting board that previously held raw food. Wash and sanitize all equipment used when cutting raw meat, poultry or fish promptly after use or before using it for any other purpose.
- Don't use the same knife for cooked poultry that you used for raw meat unless it has been properly washed and sanitized.
- Don't baste cooking meat, poultry or seafood with the uncooked sauce it was marinated in.
- Wash and disinfect basting brushes and use different brushes to baste raw and cooked meats.
- Teach children not to share food or utensils during meals.
- Avoid serving vegetable or fruit platters or dips to a group of children. Offer individual servings instead.
- Ensure that children eat from their own plates, not directly from a serving dish. Discard uneaten food from these plates. Avoid offering food from its original container (e.g., a baby food jar). When you do, discard any uneaten food promptly, including leftover milk or formula from an unfinished bottle.

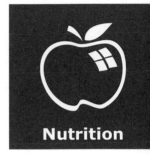

Nutrition

3. Cook

- Prepare foods quickly, cook them thoroughly, and serve them immediately. Don't let foods remain for more than 2 hours at temperatures where bacteria can grow. Bacteria grow fast in the temperature danger zone, which is between 4°C and 60°C (40°F and 140°F).
- Use a clean and sanitized food thermometer to measure the internal temperature of cooked foods:
  - ➤ Whole poultry should be cooked to 82°C (180°F),
  - ➤ Poultry pieces and ground poultry, to 74°C (165°F),
  - ➤ Food mixtures containing hazardous ingredients (e.g., eggs, meat, milk), to 74°C (165°F),
  - ➤ Pork and pork products, to 71°C (160°F),
  - ➤ Ground beef (hamburger and pork), to 71°C (160°F),
  - ➤ Fish (cooked), to 70°C (158°F),
  - ➤ Roast beef, lamb or goat, to 60°C (140°F).
- Clean and sanitize meat thermometer after every use.
- Cook eggs until the yolks and whites are firm.
- Keep soups, chili and stews hot (60°C [140°F] or higher) until just before they are served.

4. Chill

- Refrigerate or freeze perishables, prepared food and leftovers as soon as possible. Make sure your refrigerator is set at a temperature of 4°C (40°F) or colder, and keep the freezer set at -18°C (0°F). Put thermometers in your refrigerator and your freezer and check them daily.
- Marinate foods in the refrigerator, not on the counter.
- Follow guidelines about the length of time any food can be safely stored. Label food designated for one child (e.g., breast milk) with that child's name, the date opened and a discard date. Label and store lunches from home in the refrigerator until just before mealtime.
- Never defrost food at room temperature. Thaw food in the refrigerator, under cold, running water, or in the microwave if you will be cooking it immediately.
- Divide a large amount of leftovers into small, shallow containers for quicker cooling in the refrigerator. Cover or wrap leftovers promptly and try to serve them again within 24 hours.
- Reheat leftovers to a minimum internal temperature of 74°C (165°F), and to 82°C (180°F) if it's whole poultry.
- Don't overfill the refrigerator. Store food so that cold air can circulate around fridge shelves and walls.
- On field trips, make sure children's lunches are kept colder than 4°C (40°F) by using ice or cold packs in coolers, electric coolers or cold packs in individual insulated lunch bags.

Nutrition

Food storage

Food that does not require refrigeration should be stored at about 18°C (64°F) in clean, covered metal, glass or hard plastic containers that are rodent and insect proof, on racks 15 cm (6 in.) off the floor to permit air circulation. Ensure that the area stays dry and repair any holes or cracks in the walls, ceiling or floor.

When parents provide food, require that they use safe containers, such as:

- lunch boxes or cloth/nylon lunch bags,
- a thermos (vacuum bottle) for hot or cold beverages or soups,
- plastic containers for sandwiches, cheese and crackers,
- plastic cups with leak-proof lids, and
- microwave-safe containers for food to be warmed up.

> **BEST PRACTICE**
>
> Have an inventory system, so that the first foods stored are the first to be used. This rotation is known as the "FIFO" rule: First in, first out.

Microbe-prone foods

The following foods require special care when they are prepared, served and stored because they are particularly susceptible to microbial growth:

- raw and cooked meats, meat spreads, processed meats (e.g., ham),
- fish and shellfish,
- canned meats or fish (after opening),
- poultry and eggs,
- alfalfa, mung beans and radish sprouts. These can be enjoyed in a stir-fry rather than eaten raw. Even if sprouts are grown in clean conditions, salmonella can live in sprout seeds.
- leafy greens, such as spinach and lettuce. These need to be washed thoroughly—front and back of inside and outside leaves. Discard the outer leaves. **Always wash produce even if the label specifies it has been prewashed.**
- whipped cream, milk, milk products, custards, puddings, and
- dressings, mayonnaise, gravies and sauces.

Serve perishable foods immediately after preparing them or refrigerate them until mealtime. Do not serve unpasteurized milk or cheeses, or any home-canned or "preserved" foods in a child care setting. If you are cooking with children as part of an activity or if they are helping with food preparation, all the above standards apply, along with close supervision to ensure that they are met.

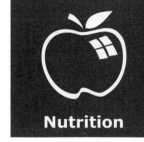

Using a microwave

A microwave oven is useful in child care settings because it allows child care practitioners to warm food quickly when children are hungry. However, because microwave ovens heat unevenly, they can cause dangerous hot spots in food. **Never use the microwave to warm bottled milk, and use extreme care when heating any food.** Cover the food, and stir and rotate it for even cooking. Use the low to medium setting for short intervals. Follow suggested standing times and check carefully for hot spots with a probe thermometer before serving. If you are heating more than one kind of food, test the temperature of each separately.

- Only heat food in containers and wraps labelled as microwave safe. Other products, such as plastic yogurt or polystyrene containers, can release toxic substances into food.
- Wipe up food spills in the microwave immediately to prevent microbial growth.

Stir and test any reheated food thoroughly before offering it to a child. Any microwaved food may be hot even though its container feels cool.

Healthy eating

Give the same care and attention to food preparation, storage and handling as you do to choosing healthy foods, and mealtimes will be as safe as they are nurturing. Offering nutritious food in a caring environment and modelling good eating habits will help the children in your care make healthier food choices as they grow.

Selected resources

Breastfeeding support

Breastfeeding Committee for Canada. 2002. The National Authority for the WHO/UNICEF Baby-Friendly Hospital Initiative in Canada, The Baby Friendly Initiative in Community Health Services. *A Canadian implementation guide*. www.breastfeedingcanada.ca

Canadian Child Care Federation. 2003. Supporting breastfeeding in child care. Resource sheet #57. www.cccf-fcsge.ca

Health Canada. 2004. *Exclusive breastfeeding duration*. www.hc-sc.gc.ca

Mohrbacher, Nancy and Julie Stock. 3rd ed., 2003. *The Breastfeeding Answer Book.* Schaumburg, IL: LaLeche League International.

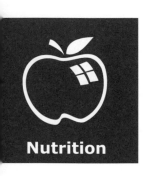

Nutrition

Resources for child care practitioners

Berman, Christine and Jacki Fromer. 3rd ed., 2006. *Meals without Squeals: Child Care Feeding Guide and Cookbook.* Boulder, CO: Bull Publishing.

———. 2001. *Teaching Children about Food: A Teaching and Activities Guide.* Boulder, CO: Bull Publishing.

Calgary Health Region, Alberta Cancer Board, Three Cheers for the Early Years. 2006. *Snacktivity box: Activities for promoting healthy eating and active living habits for young children.* www.calgaryhealthregion.ca

Canadian Child Care Federation. www.cccf-fcsge.ca

———. 2004. Connecting with your community health partners: Dietitians. Resource sheet #73.

———. 2001. Cooking and learning together. Resource sheet #22.

———. 2001. Food safety for everyone. Resource sheet #24.

———. 2000. Children's healthy eating. Resource sheet #54.

Dietitians of Canada. 2007. *Healthy Start for Life. Eating well together meal planner.* www.dietitians.ca/healthystart

Health Canada. 2007. *Eating Well with* Canada's Food Guide: *A Resource for Educators and Communicators.* www.hc-sc.gc.ca

Ontario Public Health Association. 2008. *NutriSTEP: A nutrition screening tool for every preschooler.* www.york.ca/services

Pimento, Barbara and Deborah Kernested. 4th ed., 2009. *Healthy Foundations in Early Childhood Settings.* Unit 5: Nutrition. Scarborough, Ont.: Nelson Education.

Resources for families

Best Start: Ontario's Maternal, Newborn and Early Childhood Resource Centre. 2004. *The ABC's of feeding preschoolers.* www.beststart.org

————. 2007. *Feeding your baby: From 6 months to 1 year.*

Bradshaw, Brenda and Lauren D. Bramley. 2004. *The Baby's Table: Over 100 Easy, Healthy and Homemade Recipes for the Pickiest, Most Deserving Eaters on the Planet.* Toronto, Ont.: Random House.

Canadian Paediatric Society. www.caringforkids.cps.ca

————. 2006. Feeding your baby in the first year. Brochure and parent note.

————. 2006. Iron needs of babies and children. Brochure and parent note.

Cheuy, Patricia, Eileen Campbell and Mary Sue Waisman. 2007. *Simply Great Food: 250 Quick, Easy and Delicious Recipes.* Toronto, Ont.: Robert Rose.

Government of Nova Scotia. 2006. *After year one: Food for children.* www.gov.ns.ca

Government of Saskatchewan, Healthy Living. www.health.gov.sk.ca/healthy-living

————. 2008. *Nutrition for young children.*

Health Canada. 2007. *Eating Well with* Canada's Food Guide. www.hc-sc.gc.ca

————. 2007. *Eating Well with* Canada's Food Guide: *First Nations, Inuit and Métis.*

Health Link Alberta. *Healthy eating and active living for your 1 to 5 year old.* www.health.gov.ab.ca

Inuit Tapiriit Kanatami. 2003. *Country foods: Mothers' and infants' health.* www.accel-capea.ca

Kalnins, Daina and Joanne Saab. 2001. *Better Baby Food.* Toronto, Ont.: Robert Rose/ Hospital for Sick Children.

Mendelson, Susan and Rena Mendelson. 2nd ed., 2005. *Food to Grow On: Give Your Kids a Healthy Lifestyle for Keeps.* Scarborough, Ont.: HarperCollins.

Nutrition Resource Centre, Ontario Public Health Association. 2007. *Eat right be active: A guide for parents and caregivers of preschoolers ages 3–5.* www.eatrightontario.ca

Region of Peel (Ont.) Public Health. www.peelregion.ca

————. 2005. *Cooking up some fun for parents and caregivers of young children.*

Saab, Joanne and Daina Kalnins. 2002. *Better Food for Kids: Your Essential Guide to Nutrition for All Children from Age 2 to 6.* Toronto, Ont.: Robert Rose/Hospital for Sick Children.

Satter, Ellyn. 3rd ed., 2000. *Child of Mine: Feeding with Love and Good Sense.* Boulder, CO: Bull Publishing.

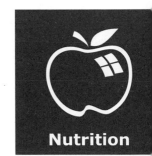

Nutrition

Sears, William, Martha Sears and Christie W. Kelly. 2002. *Eat Healthy, Feel Great.* London, U.K.: Little, Brown.

Toews, Judy and Nicole Parton. 2001. *Raising Happy, Healthy, Weight-Wise Kids.* Toronto, Ont.: Key Porter.

Food labelling

Canadian Diabetes Association/Dietitians of Canada, Nutrition Labelling Education Centre. Healthy eating is in store for you. www.healthyeatingisinstore.ca

Food safety

Canadian Partnership for Consumer Food Safety Education. www.canfightbac.org

Health Canada. 2005. Food safety. www.hc-sc.gc.ca

Region of Peel (Ont.) Public Health. 2004. *Keep on track: A health and resource guide for child care providers in Peel.* Food and drinking water safety section. Checklists for purchasing, shopping, storing, thawing, preparation, cooking and reheating, cooling, serving and leftovers. See also information on special food safety situations, allergy-safe food preparation, and picnics and outings. www.region.peel.on.ca/health/keep-on-track/pdfs/entiremanual.pdf

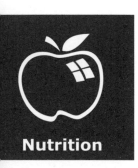

Nutrition

Special feeding issues

Canadian Society of Allergy and Clinical Immunology. 2007. *Anaphylaxis in schools and other child care settings.* www.allergysafecommunities.ca

Childhood Obesity Foundation. 2007. *What every parent should know.* www.childhoodobesity foundation.ca

Gold, Milton, ed. 2003. *The Complete Kid's Allergy and Asthma Guide.* Toronto, Ont.: Robert Rose/Hospital for Sick Children.

Manitoba Family Services and Housing. 2002. *Caring for children with anaphylaxis in a child care program: A resource manual for child care personnel who provide care to children in community programs.* www.gov.mb.ca

Neufeld, Naomi and Pete Nelson. 2004. *Kid Shape: A Practical Prescription for Helping Your Child Lose Weight, Increase Self-esteem, Establish Healthy Eating Habits, Have a More Active Lifestyle.* Nashville, TN: Thomas Nelson.

Thompson, Colleen and Ellen Shanley. 2003. *Overcoming Childhood Obesity.* Boulder, CO: Bull Publishing.

Websites

Dietitians of Canada. www.dietitians.ca

chapter

4

Dental Health

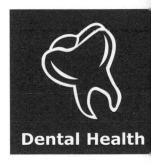

G ood nutrition, appropriate cleaning and properly timed dental visits are the three key aspects of children's dental health. Child care practitioners are often involved in the first two. Education—helping families and children learn about and practice the best ways to maintain strong, healthy teeth and gums—is also important. Child care practitioners can link families with community resources promoting oral health, and can be strong role models for good dental care, especially for children who aren't following an appropriate cleaning routine at home.

The basics

Healthy teeth are an important part of overall health, and caring for a child's teeth begins when the first tooth peeks through a baby's gums. Proper oral hygiene includes caring for the tongue and gums as well as the teeth as they grow in. Early practices—such as offering water rather than juice after a child is 6 months old, gently cleaning a baby's mouth after feeding and putting a child to bed without a bottle—help lay the groundwork for a lifetime of good oral health.

In the past, care of primary or "baby" teeth wasn't considered important because these teeth would eventually be replaced by permanent teeth. We now know that healthy primary teeth are an essential component of overall growth. They give shape to a child's face, help guide permanent teeth into the right position in the mouth and are crucial for learning to eat and to speak.

Primary teeth start forming in the womb during the first 3 months of pregnancy. A child's first primary tooth usually emerges at about 6 months of age, although appearing as early as 3 months or as late as 12 months isn't uncommon. Every child is different, but children generally have all 20 primary teeth by the age of 3. (See Figure 4.1.)

Figure 4.1: Primary teeth

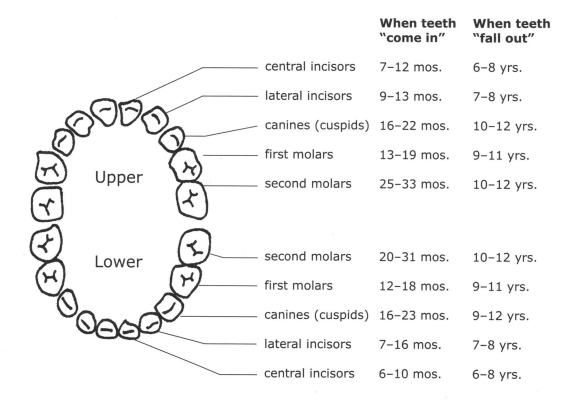

	When teeth "come in"	When teeth "fall out"
central incisors	7–12 mos.	6–8 yrs.
lateral incisors	9–13 mos.	7–8 yrs.
canines (cuspids)	16–22 mos.	10–12 yrs.
first molars	13–19 mos.	9–11 yrs.
second molars	25–33 mos.	10–12 yrs.
second molars	20–31 mos.	10–12 yrs.
first molars	12–18 mos.	9–11 yrs.
canines (cuspids)	16–23 mos.	9–12 yrs.
lateral incisors	7–16 mos.	7–8 yrs.
central incisors	6–10 mos.	6–8 yrs.

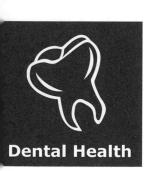

Dental Health

Primary teeth have a thinner outer enamel than permanent teeth and are particularly susceptible to decay. Plaque, which is a thick, whitish bacterial film, forms on primary teeth immediately after they appear. Bacteria in plaque can cause inflammation of the gums (gingivitis). Using the carbohydrates in a child's normal diet, plaque bacteria then produce the acids that cause cavities.

Early childhood tooth decay (ECTD), formerly called baby bottle tooth decay, is defined as tooth decay that occurs before a child is 6 years old. However, decay can begin as soon as the first tooth appears. ECTD is caused by repeated and prolonged exposure to any sweet liquid, including formula, milk, juice, soda pop and even breast milk. The most effective way of protecting against ECTD is to prevent any liquid (except water) from remaining in a child's mouth for a long time. This means **not** putting children to bed with a bottle of formula or milk or allowing them to drink juice continually from a sippy cup.

ECTD has a negative impact on children's overall health and can cause pain, making it difficult to sleep, eat or speak. Pain can also affect a child's ability to concentrate and learn. Children who develop dental decay at an early age are more likely to suffer decay throughout childhood. By making appropriate cleaning practices part of the daily routine and helping families learn about nutrition and dental hygiene, you can play an important role in preventing ECTD.

Know your local fluoride levels

Fluoride is a natural element that protects teeth from cavities. Natural water sources, such as wells and springs, may contain fluoride. In many communities, it is added to the local water supply. Fluoride is also added to toothpastes and can be applied to teeth by dentists.

In Canada, the optimum amount of fluoride in drinking water is 0.7 parts per million (ppm). This amount prevents tooth decay but does not cause a condition called fluorosis. Fluorosis occurs when a child ingests too much fluoride while teeth are forming—the period from birth to about 3 years of age. Although fluorosis is not a health problem, it can cause chalky-white or brown spots or blotches to appear on teeth.

Tap filters or "pitcher" filter systems don't usually remove significant fluoride content. If you're relying on bottled water, it is important to know the amount of fluoride it contains. Many brands have no fluoride at all.

Check with your municipality to find out how much fluoride is in your water or have your water tested. In municipalities where the level of fluoride is 0.3 ppm or less, advise parents to ask their dentist or doctor about a fluoride supplement.

Your dental care program

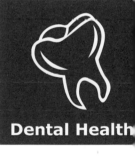

Dental Health

While parents are primarily responsible for dental care (they do most of the cleaning and arrange dental visits), child care practitioners play an important supporting role by establishing cleaning routines as part of their program.

Establishing cleaning routines

Promoting good oral hygiene and long-term dental health involves the following steps.

From birth to 12 months
- Wipe a baby's gums with a soft, clean, damp cloth twice a day—only once a day if you know that a parent is doing this too.
- As soon as the first teeth appear, clean them with a soft bristle toothbrush designed for babies. Lay the baby on a flat surface or with his head cradled in your lap to brush his teeth.
- Never leave a baby in bed with a bottle.

- After 6 months:
  - ➤ introduce a sippy cup for water and formula,
  - ➤ limit juice to no more than 120 mL (4 oz.) per day, offered in a cup rather than a bottle and only as part of a meal or snack, and
  - ➤ if a bottle is needed at nap time, offer water and not milk or juice.
- Never sweeten a soother.
- Don't give a baby teething biscuits, which usually contain sugar.

Between 1 and 3 years of age
- Advise parents to take their baby for a first dental visit at 12 months.
- Make a point of checking for ECTD once a month. Lift a child's upper lip and look for signs of decay (chalky-white or brown spots) on teeth or along the gum line. If any exist, advise parents to see a dentist as soon as possible.
- Switch to a regular cup for all drinks at 12 to 14 months.

ALERT

Don't put a soother or bottle nipple in your own mouth for any reason. This isn't good oral hygiene. Bacteria, viruses and yeast infections can be passed between adult and child in this way.

At 3 and 4 years old
- Teach children "2 for 2," which means brushing twice a day for 2 minutes each time.
- Encourage children to do some brushing, with you completing the job. Make sure that all tooth surfaces have been cleaned.
- Begin using a tiny smear of fluoride toothpaste and teach children to spit rather than swallow.
- Limit soother use to nap and bedtime only.
- Don't discourage thumb-sucking at this age. If a child continues to thumb-suck vigorously as permanent teeth begin to emerge, suggest that parents seek the advice of their doctor or dentist. (For more information on thumb-sucking, see Chapter 7, *Common Conditions*.)

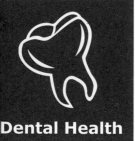

Dental Health

Preventing infection
- Ask parents to provide their child with:
  - ➤ a child-sized soft bristle toothbrush and replace it every 3 months,
  - ➤ a small (travel-sized) tube of toothpaste, so it's not too expensive to replace if the tube is dropped on the floor or otherwise contaminated.
- Label each child's toothbrush and toothpaste with their owner's name and store out of the reach of children and away from the toilet area.
- Wash your hands before and after brushing children's teeth.
- Be a role model by brushing your teeth at the same time as children do.
- Rinse toothbrushes thoroughly after brushing and ensure that each one can dry without touching others.

Healthy eating
- Between meals, quench a child's thirst with water.
- Serve fruit juice only at mealtimes.

- Limit candy, dried fruit and sugared drinks. When children do eat something sugary or sticky, clean their teeth.
- Encourage healthy snacking on fresh vegetables, fresh fruit, cheese and crackers.

Dental visits
- Be positive about trips to the dentist.
- Answer children's questions in a general way and leave detailed explanations to a dental professional, who will have special ways of describing procedures to children.
- Keep conversations upbeat and avoid negative words like "hurt" or "needle."

Community resources

Help educate children and families about oral hygiene and dental health by accessing community resources. This is particularly important in communities where children may be at risk for developing ECTD.

- Introduce games and learning tools to children and their families that teach good dental health practices. Contact your local public health agency, regional health authority or provincial/territorial dental association for good (and often free) resources to distribute in your program.
- On a family night, invite a dental hygiene student from a local college or a public health nurse to demonstrate good teeth-cleaning techniques or explain other treatments that prevent tooth decay (e.g., topical fluoride or the use of plastic sealant).
- Find out whether dental screening can be arranged for child care centres in your community.
- Inquire about access to free or affordable dental care for those in your community who qualify. Let parents know if they do.

Following basic cleaning routines and receiving timely reminders to clean teeth after eating sweets are a child's first indications that teeth are important. By sharing routines and information, providing healthy snacks and remembering out loud when it's "time to brush," you'll help bring that message home.

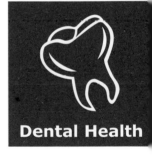

Dental Health

Selected resources

Alberta Health and Wellness. 2002. *A parent's guide: Healthy teeth for children, birth to six years*. www.health.alberta.ca

B.C. Health File, British Columbia Ministry of Health. www.bchealthguide.org, www.vch.ca/dentalhealth

———. 2007. Children and fluoride.

———. 2007. Infant dental care.

———. 2007. Dental care for toddlers.

Calgary Health Region. 2005. Promoting oral health in the early years. Powerpoint presentation. www.calgaryhealthregion.ca/programs/dental/info_az.html

Calgary Health Region. Lift the lip. Also available in traditional Chinese, Farsi/Persian, Hindi, Punjabi, Spanish, Vietnamese and Arabic, Cleaning baby's teeth, and How much fluoride toothpaste.

Canadian Child Care Federation. 2001. Seven steps to oral hygiene for children. Resource sheet #25. www.cccf-fcsge.ca

Canadian Dental Association. 2004. Dental Care for Children section contains resource sheets on each of the following topics: cleaning teeth, nutrition for children, dental development, early childhood tooth decay, your child's first visit, fluoride and your child, pacifiers and thumb-sucking, and Halloween. www.cda-adc.ca

Canadian Dental Hygienists Association. 2006. Oral health matters for you and your baby. www.cdha.ca

Canadian Paediatric Society. www.caringforkids.cps.ca

———. 2007. Healthy teeth and your child. Brochure and parent note.

———. 2006. Fluoride and healthy teeth.

Manitoba Collaborative Project for the Prevention of Early Childhood Tooth Decay. www.umanitoba.ca

———. 2004. *Prevent early childhood tooth decay: Action plan workbook and tool kit.*

———. 2005. *Healthy smile happy child: Caring for teeth and preventing early childhood tooth decay.*

Region of Peel (Ont.) Public Health. 2004. *Keep on track: A health and resource guide for child care providers in Peel.* Dental, Hearing, Vision, Speech and Language section and resources. www.region.peel.on.ca/health/keep-on-track/pdfs/entiremanual.pdf

Vancouver Coastal Health. www.vch.ca

———. 2006. Mouth care for your infant-toddler.

———. 2005. Mouth care for your 3–6 year-old.

———. 2003. Early childhood tooth decay. These resources are also available in Chinese, Punjabi, Spanish and Vietnamese.

Websites

Canadian Association of Public Health Dentistry. www.caphd-acsdp.org

Canadian Dental Association. www.cda-adc.ca

Health Canada (Healthy Living/Oral Health). www.hc-sc.gc.ca

Ontario Association for Public Health Dentistry. www.oaphd.on.ca

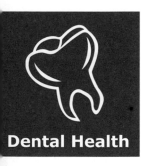

Dental Health

chapter

5

Keeping
Children Safe

Keeping children safe in child care involves providing a safe environment, preventing injury and actively supervising. Child care practitioners are responsible for all three dimensions, which often overlap. Safety is one of the most regulated aspects of the child care sector. To be licensed, both child care centres and home settings must comply with established safety standards and practices, as well as with local building and fire codes.

Providing quality child care means being thoroughly aware of provincial/territorial safety standards and being alert to changes, which are often communicated through local public health units and child care offices. Safety legislation usually involves making environments physically safe, controlling obvious product hazards and preventing common injuries. However, as with preventing infections, what child care practitioners do every day to anticipate or prevent injuries is the best protection for children in their care. Practicing preventive routines, modelling safe behaviour, taking precautions and supervising actively are the factors that determine program safety.

As with every other aspect of child care, caregivers and families need to work together. Because every child is different, communicating with parents about safety routines at

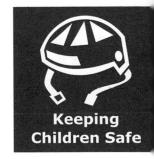

**Keeping
Children Safe**

home and understanding each child's temperament are important. However, don't assume that a cautious child will never take risks. Parents will also evaluate the safety of a program by asking questions about facility environments and their child's daily routines on and off site.

Child care practitioners face the challenge of creating a safe environment that still allows children to learn by experimenting and by developing their abilities through exploration and play. You need to provide ample opportunities for active play, but you must also recognize that no environment can be completely risk-free—minor bumps, bruises and scrapes are part of every child's development.

Types of injuries

In Canada, unintentional injuries are the leading cause of death in children over the age of 1 year. Most fatal injuries are the result of motor vehicle collisions, but deaths from fire, drowning, choking/suffocation and poisoning are still too common. A child dying from injuries sustained in connection with child care is an extremely rare occurrence, but the incidence and pattern of non-fatal injury in child care settings may be significant. Typical injuries in child care are:

- **bruises, bumps or abrasions** from colliding with other children or furniture, walls and doorways,
- **burns and scalds** caused by hot food or liquids,
- **bites**, and
- **falls**, which are the leading cause of serious injury in child care settings.

Although most falls involve play equipment, children also fall down stairs, out of windows and off furniture.

When do injuries happen?

Injuries in child care settings occur most often when practitioners are:

- distracted,
- very busy or temporarily absent,
- involved in situations that cause some confusion, such as drop-off and pick-up times.

Children are also more likely to injure themselves in the late afternoon and early evening, when they are:

- hungry or tired, or
- distracted, excited or away from their regular routines.

The situation can be complicated if you're unaware of a child's developing abilities or haven't anticipated a possible problem, or if a child is in less familiar surroundings (e.g., in a new facility or room, or on an outing or field trip), where there are unexpected hazards, supervision patterns are different, or safety rules are new or must be applied in a new way.

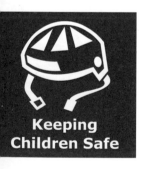

Keeping Children Safe

Injury prevention: A systematic approach

Planning effectively for children's safety is the best protection in any community setting. A systematic approach to injury prevention involves:

- active and positive supervision,
- safe space arrangement,
- developmentally appropriate programming and activities, and
- preventive policies and procedures.

Active and positive supervision means having an appropriate adult-to-child ratio for the group's size and age range. Being involved, aware and appreciative of children's behaviour means you must:

- know each child's abilities and temperament,
- set clear, simple and positive rules and reinforce them consistently,
- be aware of potential hazards,
- position yourself strategically during activities, so that you can help, remind, redirect and intervene as needed,
- scan and circulate, which can be particularly important outdoors or in a larger room. This entails looking "up and out" and moving "with the action" of a group of children.

Safe space arrangement means knowing which kind of physical layout invites children to run (e.g., a long, open hallway) and which invites a quiet game (e.g., a cozy corner), and using both appropriately. Safer spaces are often defined or set apart (e.g., using barriers, gates, fencing, doors or flooring changes). A measure of flexibility is desirable too, so that a space can be adjusted for children's activities.

Children's play times **are not** appropriate break times for child care practitioners.

Developmentally appropriate programming and activities are those in which children's ages and abilities determine play patterns and other daily routines, rather than those that require children to adjust to a fixed program. Children's physical size, strength, developmental readiness and level of concentration should be considered when you plan an outing, bring in new equipment or toys, or acquire furniture.

Finally, **preventive policies and procedures** are safety strategies that are communicated to staff, families and children—and adhered to every day. Basic policies should be set out in your program's orientation manual, and should include:

- mandatory first aid and cardiopulmonary resuscitation (CPR) training requirements,
- the distribution of trained staff on site (in larger centres),
- group size and (in larger centres) adult-to-child ratio requirements,
- safety checklists, with schedules for completion (e.g., monthly),
- the injury-reporting procedure and form,

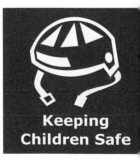

Keeping Children Safe

- basic emergency procedures, including telephone numbers, evacuation and transportation plans, children's health records and signed consents (for more about preparedness, see Chapter 11, *Emergencies*), and
- explicit policies for "no smoking" and "no weapons," including toy weapons and replicas.

The easiest and most reliable alterations are those made to equipment or the environment, rather than to the behaviour of children or adults.

Staff responsibilities

Preventing injury requires education, shared experience, and the regular review and reinforcement of safe practices. Injury prevention courses and safety workshops are key components of the early childhood education curriculum, and recognizing potential hazards and taking precautions should be intrinsic to program routines. When an injury does occur, a child care practitioner must document the incident and the events surrounding it on an *Injury report* (Appendix 5.1). This report is carefully reviewed to identify what went wrong and prevent a recurrence. Corrective measures are then communicated to staff. When required, the report is submitted promptly to local licensing or other authorities.

Risk assessment

Assessing situations for potential risk of injury usually involves both physical and psycho-social considerations. Evaluating the safety of a piece of play equipment, for example, includes the basic questions set out in Table 5.1.

TABLE 5.1

Considerations in risk assessment of play equipment

Staff training	Do all staff know, understand and follow the rules for using this equipment?
Type and level of supervision	Who is supervising, and how? Are there enough adults present for the age group and the activity? Are staff actively supervising?
Meaningful rules	Are the rules for using this equipment simple, clear and appropriate for the ages and stages of the children present?
The equipment	Does this play equipment meet current CSA* standards, and is it an age-appropriate size for the children present?
Children's cognitive and physical abilities	Can this group follow the rules for safe use? Are they developmentally ready to play safely on this equipment?
The physical environment	Does the protective surfacing underneath this equipment meet current CSA standards?
The social context	Can these children take turns? Is the equipment positioned with the recommended "safety zone" around it, so children won't collide while using it?

* CSA = Canadian Standards Association. See *Children's Playspaces and Equipment*, 2007.

Keeping these questions in mind when planning/equipping play areas helps to eliminate potential hazards in advance.

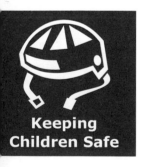

Keeping Children Safe

When an injury occurs, proper reporting, review and precautions can prevent a recurrence. Factors to consider and possible solutions are set out in Table 5.2.

TABLE 5.2

Factors involved and possible solutions in incident reporting

Factors involved	Possible solutions
What happened? *Outline critical steps in the sequence of events.*	
The level and type of supervision (ratio, proximity, ability to react)	• Change the type or level of supervision. • Provide additional staff training.
The condition of the equipment or toy	• Repair, replace or eliminate hazardous equipment or toys.
The environment	• Redesign the physical space. • Ensure that both equipment and surfacing meet current safety standards.
Children's behaviour/actions	• Re-evaluate the rules for an activity. • Set precise limits for children, if needed.

Reports usually confirm that the injury was completely preventable, as most injuries are.

Regular safety inspections

The provincial/territorial laws governing safety in regulated child care settings cover the basics: physical environment, equipment, adult-to-child ratios and some practices (e.g., food preparation and handling.) They also provide for regular safety inspections by local authorities. Child care practitioners should also develop checklists geared to the specific needs and characteristics of their own facility, and inspect their premises weekly, monthly, seasonally and annually, as needed. The safety checklists beginning on page 63 can be adapted or expanded to suit any facility and may be especially helpful for home settings. They cover:

- safety modifications for stairways, halls and entranceways, windows, floors and doors,
- precautions to take in each room, and
- basic specifications for toys, equipment and accessories common in child care.

Caregivers operating child care programs in home settings need to be as vigilant about conducting regular and thorough safety inspections as those in centre settings. (See Appendix 5.2, pages 100–07, for safety inspection schedules and checklists.) Consider risk potential and update safety checklists whenever:

- new equipment or materials are introduced, including toys and craft materials,
- renovations or repairs have been made, or
- a new activity or a field trip is being planned.

REMEMBER

Health Canada develops and enforces regulations for consumer products and is a vital source of information on the safe use of household products. Check for product advisories, recalls and product safety information at www.hc-sc.gc.ca.

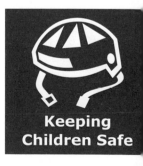

Keeping Children Safe

Safety rules to teach children

Modelling safe behaviours and teaching basic safety rules are essential aspects of quality child care. Toddlers can be introduced to basic safety rules, and preschoolers can be taught to follow simple and concrete rules and identify some obvious hazards in their environment. However, young children also require repeated explanation, consistent application and positive reinforcement of simple rules. Encourage young children to follow these basic safety rules:

- "Stop, look and listen" when their name is called. Listening and following your instructions are the first steps toward participating in safe behaviour. "No" means "Stop and look at me." "Okay" means "Go." The "Stop, look and listen" rule is especially important around traffic, in the playground, on outings and during water play.
- Pick up toys after play to prevent tripping and falling.
- Keep stairs and hallway floors free of toys, shoes and clothing.
- Use hand rails when climbing up and down stairs.
- Learn the difference between hot and cold water faucets, and turn on the cold water first.
- Know danger symbols marked on hazardous products or places and do not touch anything with these symbols.

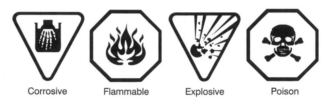

Corrosive   Flammable   Explosive   Poison

- Keep small objects and toys (anything small enough to fit inside an empty toilet roll) away from children under 3 years of age.
- Bring any toy that is broken or dirty straight to an adult.

Be consistent about stating and applying safety rules, using positive guidance as you would for other forms of behaviour. When children behave safely, give them verbal reinforcement. Children who are not following the rules need a gentle reminder, a simple explanation and—if an unsafe behaviour persists—removal from the activity. If children are doing something physically dangerous, a warning is not enough. Stop the activity immediately and explain later.

To work, a rule needs to be consistent and appropriate for a child's age and stage of development. A rule should be expressed clearly and positively, without frightening a child or discouraging him from an activity. ("We climb up the ladder and come down the slide." "Our toys stay on the ground when we climb.") Communicating with families about your safety rules can have the extra benefit of encouraging safer environments and behaviour in children's homes.

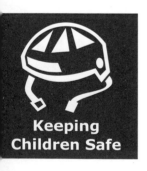

Keeping Children Safe

Indoors

All provinces and territories regulate physical spaces for child care, although specifications vary widely in scope and detail by jurisdiction. Regulated home and centre settings must meet basic requirements for cleanliness, safety and accessibility, but other physical specifications (e.g., the amount of space allotted per child, how well a setting is organized, furnished or equipped) are far from standardized. They are not regulated in unlicensed home settings. Good home child care environments come in all shapes and sizes, but adapting your home for child care involves some key safety steps.

The first step is to define play spaces, such as areas for active and quiet play, and individual and group play. These may be separate rooms or well-defined or enclosed spaces within a larger room that is kept free of hazardous accessories or furniture, such as exercise equipment or chairs that rotate or recline. In home settings, one main play area often accommodates children of different ages, and organizing spaces (e.g., grouping toys and activities that are age-appropriate) is essential. Ideally, there are separate play areas for children under and over 3 years of age, to reduce the risk of small children being stepped on, tripped over or pushed by older children, and to minimize access to older children's toys, which may pose a choking or other hazard.

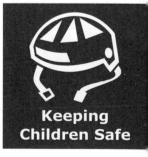

Keeping Children Safe

After defining and organizing indoor spaces, ensure the safety of indoor equipment and accessories. Remember, accessories such as a bouncy chair, baby swing or stationary activity centre might provide a few minutes of "hands-free" time for you, but they are potentially hazardous. They should be used only for a short time, and only while you are in the same room with a child who is using one. Children also outgrow these items very quickly, at which point using them is dangerous. Follow weight and height guidelines for equipment and accessories. Check consumer product safety information at the Health Canada website (www.hc-sc.gc.ca) regularly to make sure that no children's product you have is under recall.

Indoor play structures

No safety standards exist for indoor play structures or protective surfacing. Falls from indoor and outdoor climbing structures are the most common and severe cause of injury in child care settings. These structures are dangerous when they:

- are too high,
- tip over, or
- don't have sufficient protective surfacing to cushion a child's fall.

Because toddlers have difficulty changing from a standing to a sitting position on play equipment, they can easily lose their balance and fall. A few precautions can make play structures safer, but **there is no substitute for active supervision** during any climbing activity.

For children younger than 2 years of age, play structures should be low to the ground, with a maximum platform height of 60 cm (2 ft.). They should be stable, placed on a flat surface at least 1.8 m (6 ft.) away from all furniture and walls, and have no sharp edges or corners. Make sure that:

- age and height restrictions are followed at all times.
- older children do not play on a structure intended for younger ones. Their extra weight can damage the structure or cause it to tip.
- the surface under the structure includes a 1.8 m (6 ft.) fall zone, measured in all directions from the structure. This area must be kept clear of furniture, large toys and other equipment.
- surfacing is sufficient. Carpet, one layer of safety floor tiles or resting mats are **not** thick enough to cushion a child's fall, even from 30 cm (1 ft.) off the floor. Dense foam mats at least 3 cm (1¼ in.) thick or two layers of dense interlocking foam tiles, each at least 1.5 cm (5/8 in.) thick, provide some protection. Gymnastic mats 10 to 15 cm (4 to 6 in.) thick will cushion falls, but they create an unstable surface for indoor play structures and shouldn't be used. Hire a certified playground inspector to test whether the surface you've provided is sufficient.
- the space between the top rung of a play gym ladder and the platform is **at least** 22.9 cm (9 in.) wide, or less than 9 cm (3.5 in.). Spaces that measure between 9 and 22.9 cm can trap a child's head and cause strangulation.
- children are not permitted to eat or drink while climbing.
- the structure is checked regularly for loose or broken parts.

Plastic gyms are easier to take outside in good weather but shouldn't be used outside in winter.

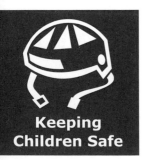

Keeping Children Safe

Toys

Children in your care should have access only to toys that are safe and developmentally appropriate for their age and stage. While Canadian toy safety legislation doesn't require toys to be labelled for age appropriateness or to have warning labels for choking or other hazards, safety labelling is strongly encouraged. Common alerts include small parts warnings ("Toy parts may present a choking hazard"), age recommendations and warnings ("Recommended for ages 6+" or "Not suitable for children under age 3"), and an indication that the toy has been safety tested.

Toys for children over 3 years old are **not** appropriate for children under 3. They often have small parts that are choking hazards for younger children. In a program attended by children of different ages, preschoolers' toys **must** be stored separately in areas that are inaccessible to younger children. If possible, store toys on open shelves at different heights instead of in toy boxes or chests. Shelves limit breakage and make toy selection easier. But if keeping toys separate and less accessible is an issue, storing them in a plastic bin with a lid or in a laundry basket off the floor also works. Keep toys and craft items intended for older children (e.g., scissors) off the floor and out of the reach of babies and toddlers at all times. Teach preschoolers to give only "baby" toys to younger children.

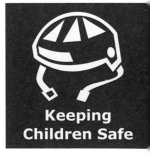

Keeping Children Safe

Toy guidelines

Choosing toys

- Always check the manufacturer's label for age and safety recommendations. Adhere to age-related toy warning labels closely and keep these and toy instructions on file for future reference.
- Provide quality toys to reduce the risk of toxins (e.g., lead in cheap plastic or painted products or play jewellery).
- Choose well-constructed, durable toys with covered hinges and joints, to prevent pinching.
- Make sure toys have **no** loose or detachable parts, sharp edges or cords longer than 20 cm (8 in.).
- Check that all cloth books, soft dolls or toys have sturdy seams and are machine-washable.

Children discover the defects of any toy very quickly. Watch them handle any new object or toy to make sure that it is safe to play with.

Toys to avoid

- **Magnetic toys**: Product recalls, design problems and the hazards connected with ingesting magnets indicate that **no magnetic toy is appropriate in a child care setting**.
- **Battery-operated and electric toys**: Batteries are a choking **and** poisoning hazard, and electric toys can cause a shock or burn if the wire is split, damp or mouthed by a young child.
- **Latex balloons**: These types of balloons are the second most common cause of death by choking in young children (food is the most common) and should not be used in child care. Children can inhale a balloon while playing or trying to blow it up, or inhale and swallow a piece of broken balloon. Foil or mylar balloons filled with helium are safer for all ages, though they should be discarded as soon as they deflate because they also pose a suffocation hazard.
- **Propellant toys**: These include toys such as rockets or dart guns.
- **Mouth instruments**: These are likely to be shared and can spread germs.

Table 5.3 lists basic age-appropriate toys for child care settings.

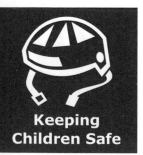

Keeping Children Safe

TABLE 5.3

Age-appropriate toys for child care settings

Age	Appropriate toys
Infants 0 to 6 months old ...	like colourful toys that are interesting to touch and hear, but **not** loud: • cloth, vinyl or board books • soft plastic or fabric blocks • a shatterproof mirror • rattles • soft washable animals or dolls (with sewn—not button—eyes) • stacking or nesting cups or rings • bright cloth or rubber balls • squeeze toys (with non-removable squeakers)
Babies 6 to 12 months old ...	see anything within reach as a potential toy. They enjoy all of the above toys, plus: • cups, little pails and other unbreakable containers • large building blocks • large plastic balls • shape sorters • push-pull toys (with short pull cords) • soft plastic toys small enough to handle
Toddlers 1 to 2 years old ...	become more interested in toys as their skill in handling them grows. The simplest ones—blocks, floating bath toys, your own pots and pans or empty plastic containers—are often the safest. Babies and toddlers don't need expensive or complicated toys. Toys that are safe and appealing include all of the above, plus: • blocks, wooden threading beads or snap-together beads (all larger than 4 cm [1.5 in.] in diameter) • simple dolls or animals that can be dressed (no buttons or small parts: choose Velcro closures) • a peg bench • musical instruments designed for children under 3, such as tambourines, xylophones, shakers and drums • toy telephones (with short cords) • large crayons or non-toxic, washable markers (with active supervision) • puzzles with knobs and a few large pieces • steerable, age-appropriate riding toys • large soft balls to kick and throw • dress-up clothes • sand and water toys, such as buckets, shovels, rakes and sieves
Preschoolers 2 to 4 years old ...	enjoy using their imagination at play and like a challenge. Toys that are safe and appealing for preschoolers include all of the above, plus: • puzzles with more large pieces • size-shape matching toys and games • board books with short stories • soft, non-toxic modelling clay (with close supervision) • finger or non-toxic, water-based liquid paints • construction sets with large pieces • puppets

For information about cleaning and disinfecting toys, see Chapter 8, *Preventing Infections*.

For arts and crafts, use only materials that are labelled as intended and safe for use by children. A "non-toxic" label can be misleading. While there may be no acute or immediate poison risk, the product may still cause harm to certain children under certain circumstances. Screen non-toxic materials as cautiously as you would any chemical product, and be aware of local regulations about the use of potentially hazardous art supplies (e.g., epoxy, instant glues, or any solvent-based glue, or permanent markers) on child care premises.

Table 5.4 identifies arts and crafts materials to be avoided and lists safer substitutes.

TABLE 5.4

Materials for arts and crafts

Avoid	Use
Powdered clay. It is easily inhaled and contains silica and possibly asbestos. Do not sand dry clay pieces or engage in other dust-producing activities.	Talc-free, pre-mixed clay. After using clay, wet mop or sponge surfaces thoroughly.
Ceramic glazes or copper enamels.	Water-based paints instead of glazes. An adult may waterproof pieces with shellac or varnish.
Cold-water, fibre-reactive dyes or other chemical-based commercial dyes.	Vegetable and plant dyes, such as onion skins or tea, as well as food dyes.
Instant papier mâchés, which create inhalable dust and may contain lead or asbestos.	Papier mâché made from black and white newspapers and library or white paste.
Powdered tempera paints, which create inhalable dust and may contain toxic pigments.	Liquid tempera paints or paints pre-mixed by an adult.
Pastels, chalks or dry markers that create dust.	Oil pastels, crayons or dustless chalks.
Solvents such as turpentine, toluene and rubber cement thinner. Also avoid solvent-containing materials such as solvent-based inks, alkyd paints and rubber cement.	Water-based products only.
Aerosol sprays.	Water-based paints with brushes or spatter techniques.
Epoxy, instant glue, airplane glue or other solvent-based adhesives.	Water-based white glue or library paste.
Permanent felt-tip markers, which may contain toxic solvents.	Water-based markers only.
Casting plaster. Besides creating dust, casting body parts can result in serious burns.	Plaster mixed by an adult in a ventilated area or outdoors for sand-casting and other safe projects.

Source: Canadian Child Care Federation, *Safety in the Arts* (Resource sheet #21). Adapted with permission.

Here are a few additional tips:

- Never use objects that are small enough to lodge in a child's ear or nose (e.g., buttons, dried macaroni) in craft activities for children under 3 years of age.
- Use only large beads (more than 4 cm [1.5 in.] across) for stringing—anything smaller is a choking hazard.
- Don't allow children to eat or drink while working on arts and crafts projects.

Children need to be closely supervised when doing any art or craft activity.

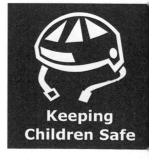

Keeping Children Safe

Outdoors

Playing outside is an important part of every child's day. Being able to run, make noise, play games, socialize spontaneously and explore in the open air is the best outlet for children's natural energy. As long as children are properly dressed and actively supervised, they should have outside play to experience and look forward to every day, in almost any weather. (For more about development, games and play, see Chapter 2, *Healthy Activities*.)

Specifications for the size, location and layout of outdoor play areas are regulated for child care services, but vary widely according to the program setting and jurisdiction. Research indicates that the best-practice size for an outdoor play space is about 6 m² (6.5 sq. yd.) per child. The optimal location for an outdoor play area is on site and directly accessible from indoors. An optimal layout encourages movement, supports safety and development, is comfortable, and enhances both children's and staff's sense of control.

When adapting your home to accommodate a child care program, take these preventive measures:

- Make sure that any gate is self-closing and self-latching, and that a fence separates the children's play space from the driveway and garage areas.
- Install stair gates at entrances to porches, decks and balconies. Make sure these areas have railings with vertical rungs that are 10 cm (4 in.) apart or less, and that furniture is kept well away from railings to prevent climbing-related falls.
- Learn the names of plants around the yard. Some common plants are toxic enough to cause a rash or stomach upset, and others may be fatal if ingested. (See Appendix 5.3.) Consider removing poisonous plants, but if that isn't possible, take these precautions:
  - ➤ Store bulbs and seeds out of sight and reach.
  - ➤ Discourage children from putting plant parts (leaves, stems, seeds, berries) in their mouths.
  - ➤ Let children know that plants eaten by birds and animals might not be safe for humans.
  - ➤ Teach preschoolers what poison ivy looks like ("Three leaves in a group, and they droop"), and tell them to stay far away.
- Make sure children can't wander into standing water, such as garden ponds, ditches, dugouts, or water that collects after a spring thaw or heavy rains (5 cm [2 in.] or deeper). These are all drowning hazards. Fence them off, and keep children well away.
- Keep all yard and power tools locked in a shed or garage. Never use them when children are playing in the yard.
- Keep children away from the barbeque at all times.

Play equipment and surfacing

Consult the Canadian Standards Association's (CSA) *Children's Playspaces and Equipment* when selecting or evaluating outdoor play equipment and protective surfacing. Complying with current requirements and being aware of local regulations or bylaws that may apply

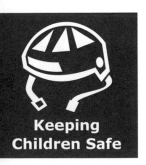

Keeping Children Safe

in your jurisdiction are essential to quality child care. Facility directors can usually obtain this information through the local school board, licensing authority or parks and recreation office. Young children may ingest leachable chemicals from wood and playground surfacing, so find out all you can about the presence or use of pressure-treated wood and sealants for play equipment at your local playground.

Follow the manufacturer's instructions for installing/ assembling play equipment and contact them or the dealer if their instructions aren't absolutely clear. Keep any instruction sheets for future reference and remember that modifying equipment can make it less safe. Take these additional steps when assembling play equipment:

- Anchor outdoor play equipment securely to the ground, as directed by the manufacturer.
- Make sure that all nuts and bolts are tight. Any bolt that extends beyond a nut should be covered with an acorn nut or plastic cap.
- Remove or file down any sharp points or edges.
- Make sure that all tent pegs or stabilizer bars at ground level are easy to see, so that children won't trip.
- Adjust the height of swings to ensure children can get on and off safely, while leaving enough space for children's legs and feet to move freely while swinging.
- Purchase plastic covers for swing chains to prevent children's fingers from catching in the loops.

BEST PRACTICE

If you are designing a play area or installing play equipment on site, hire a certified playground inspector to conduct a full assessment of your program's play spaces— both indoors and out. An inspector will make sure they conform to standards and can recommend a schedule for maintenance and follow-up inspections. For details, go to the Canadian Playground Safety Institute website at www.cpra.ca.

Maintaining play equipment is as important as proper assembly. Plastics take a beating when left out in all weather, so check any parts that are intended to hold a child's weight regularly and carefully for brittleness or "fatigue." You can often buy replacement parts, such as swing seats, slide tops, ladder rungs and tube end-covers, from the manufacturer or a local dealer.

Whether you are creating a play space or evaluating the safety of a local park or playground, make sure that:

- there is sufficient space for your group to play safely,
- play equipment is age-appropriate,
- surfacing is sufficient,
- there is active supervision, and
- rules are followed.

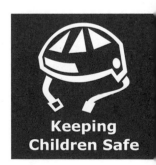

Keeping Children Safe

Sufficient space: There should be at least 1.8 m (6 ft.) between any two pieces of equipment or between equipment and a fence or other backyard structure. Swings and slides require even more space. The "encroachment area" refers to the ground space underneath and surrounding a piece of play equipment, and is regulated to include an additional "safety zone." Traffic paths are also specified in the CSA standards. They lie beyond this safety zone to reduce the risk of children colliding while playing on and around play equipment.

Age-appropriateness: While one set of CSA requirements applies to equipment intended for use by children 18 months to 5 years of age, there is no Canadian standard for home use, indoor use or equipment designed for children younger than 18 months old. However, an ASTM (American Society for Testing and Materials) standard has been developed for children 6 to 23 months of age, with these specifications:

- For children under 2 years of age, platform height should be less than 80 cm (32 in.).
- Play equipment for children 2 to 5 years of age should have platforms no higher than 1.2 m (4 ft.).

A play structure must have a permanently attached label to indicate the age group for which it has been designed. When assessing the safety of any playground structure, be aware of:

- points that may catch on children's clothing, especially at the top of slides, S-hooks on swings, joints in climbing structures, and nearby fencing.
- spaces that measure between 9 and 22.9 cm (3.5 and 9 in.)—such as the spaces between ladder rungs. These can trap a child's head and cause strangulation.
- swing seats. They should be made of soft material, such as rubber or canvas, rather than metal or wood. Back supports and safety bars are needed for very young children or those with a disability.
- seesaws. They should have wooden blocks or rubber tires placed on the underside of the seats to prevent children's feet from getting caught.

A child is much more likely to be injured on equipment that she cannot reach or use without help.

Review CSA standards before selecting play equipment for your facility. Hire a certified playground inspector to ensure that play equipment and protective surfacing at your facility meet standards.

Sufficient surfacing: Grass is not soft enough to cushion a child's fall. Play equipment must be positioned over one of the following surfaces: sand, wood fibre, synthetic surfacing or pea gravel. Each type of surfacing has advantages and disadvantages, depending on the age of the children, availability and cost, climate conditions and geography. The depth recommendation for the most common "loose fill" surfaces (e.g., sand, pea gravel, wood/bark mulch or engineered wood fibre) is at least 30 cm (12 in.). Test playground surfacing periodically using a portable accelerometer to make sure that surfaces under all play equipment meet standards. The maintenance of surfaces is also regulated. Be sure to:

- check daily for any glass, litter, animal feces or small, hazardous objects that toddlers might put in their mouths.
- rake weekly and ensure that surfacing material is soft and evenly distributed around equipment. Top it up regularly. A child only needs to fall 1 m (3 ft.) to a hard surface to suffer a fatal head injury.

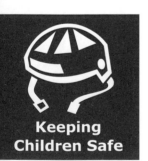

Keeping Children Safe

Active supervision: Actively supervising and staying within arm's reach of children who are on play equipment or a climbing structure are essential to avoid playground injuries. The number of staff needed to supervise will depend on the number of children at play, their ages, and the risk associated with particular activities. Extra staff members may be required to supervise swings, slides and elevated equipment. Young children will try to use playground equipment intended for older children and need to be closely monitored. It is especially important to stay within arm's length of toddlers playing on elevated equipment.

Before allowing children on a play structure, make sure of the following:

- Their clothing has no drawstrings or cords that might catch on climbing or other play equipment. In winter, make sure they are wearing a neck warmer rather than a scarf, and mitten clips instead of strings.
- No ropes or cords are tied to the play structure.
- The children have removed their helmets before starting to climb.

Rules: Enforce simple, age-appropriate safety rules in any outdoor play space or local playground. You can introduce these basic safety rules:

- Always take off your helmet in the playground. A helmet can catch on playground equipment.
- Keep your shoes on.
- Don't push or shove around play equipment. Wait your turn.

Basic rules for **swings**:

- Keep away from moving swings.
- Sit in the middle of the swing seat. Don't stand or kneel, and hold on with both hands while swinging.
- Don't jump off a moving swing.
- Only one person on a swing at a time.
- Don't push empty swings.
- Don't twist a swing with a child in it to make it twirl.

Basic rules for **slides**:

- Wait your turn at the foot of the ladder.
- Slide feet first.
- Don't slide lying down.
- Leave the slide quickly once you reach the bottom.

Basic rules for **climbing structures**:

- Only one person on one rung or bar at a time.
- Use both hands to climb and a "lock grip"—fingers and thumb.
- Drop with your knees bent, landing on both feet.
- Stay off the climbing structure when it's wet.

ALERT

- Never help children climb to unsafe heights.
- Never allow a child with a skipping rope to climb a play structure.

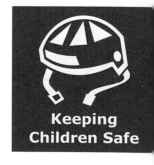

Keeping Children Safe

Basic rules for **seesaws** (for children 4 years of age and older):

- Sit up straight and face your partner.
- Hold on tight with both hands.
- Keep your feet out from under the board.
- Tell your partner when you want to get off, and get off carefully.

Trampolines

Trampolines are not recommended for use—indoors or outdoors—in any child care setting. They can cause serious injuries, including fractures of the spine and spinal cord, even when children are closely supervised. Young children's muscles are not strong enough for them to bounce correctly or safely, and more injuries occur while children are playing on a trampoline than from falling off it. Neither the kind of trampoline (e.g., mini or full-size) nor precautions for use (e.g., setting the trampoline at ground level or using padding) are effective in preventing trampoline-related injuries, which have nearly doubled since 1990.

Ride-on toys and tricycles

Ride-on toys and tricycles are hazardous when children are too old or too young to be using them. If a child is too big for a ride-on toy, it will be unstable; if a child is too small, the toy becomes more difficult to control. If your play space and budget permit, have ride-on toys or tricycles of various sizes available for toddlers and preschoolers.

Children under 1 year of age are too young for ride-on toys. A child may be ready to straddle a ride-on toy and push with her feet once she can walk with some steadiness. She may learn to alternate feet when using this toy, but she is still too young to pedal or steer. For children 12 to 18 months old, make sure that a ride-on toy has four (or more) recessed wheels or castors. It will be more stable than a two- or three-wheeled model and less likely to bang against a child's feet or legs. In general, a riding toy that a child sits inside and propels with her feet is harder to steer and manoeuvre than a straddled model.

With all ride-on toys, including tricycles, take the following precautions:

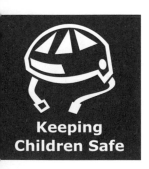

Keeping Children Safe

- Make sure children wear helmets.
- Follow age, weight and height specifications for any model. To be safe, wheeled toys must be appropriate to the age and developmental stage of children in your care.
- Make sure a child can put both feet flat on the ground when sitting in the seat.
- Some models tip easily. Test stability by placing your weight directly on the handlebars or rear of the ride-on toy to see if it flips forward or backward. Models with a seat close to the ground and a long wheelbase are usually more stable.
- Wheeled toys have been involved in serious falls. Keep them away from stairways, decks, porches or swimming pools and off the driveway or street.

- A child on a wheeled toy can move very quickly. Remove furniture that the child might collide with or pull down in passing.

Children start learning to pedal at 2 years of age but are not yet able to steer. This skill becomes easier at around age 3, which paves the way for riding a tricycle or even a small two-wheeled bicycle with training wheels. With tricycles, follow these additional guidelines. A tricycle should have:

- a low centre of gravity,
- widely spaced rear wheels,
- padded handlebars,
- non-slip pedals and handgrips,
- rubber tires (30 to 33 cm [12 to 13 in.] high for a child 3 years of age), and
- hubcap wheel covers, not spokes, which can catch fingers or clothing.

Check tricycles regularly for missing or damaged pedals and handgrips, loose handlebars and seats, or any other broken parts. Storing them inside helps reduce wear and tear.

Reinforce helmet use every time children use a tricycle or riding toy. The right bicycle helmet is age-appropriate for the child wearing it and certified by the CSA. Never use a hockey helmet as a substitute for a proper bicycle helmet: they are designed for different kinds of impacts. A helmet fits properly when:

- there are two finger-widths between the eyebrow and the helmet brim,
- side straps lie flat and form a "V-shape" under the ears,
- there is space for only one finger between the chin and chin strap,
- the helmet stays in place if the child shakes his head with the helmet unstrapped. If the helmet moves, insert foam padding that comes with the helmet.

Replace helmets that have been in a collision or are 5 years old. Make sure children remove their helmets before using play equipment.

Children on tricycles or ride-on toys must be supervised by an adult at all times. If they are riding outside the fenced area of a child care centre or home setting, the ratio should be 1:2 for slow riders and 1:1 for speedy toddlers. Teach children basic rules for tricycle riding:

- Always wear your helmet.
- Never go on the road.
- Don't allow passengers.
- Remember that going downhill is dangerous.
- Don't ride down a step or curb.
- Keep your hands and feet away from the wheels.

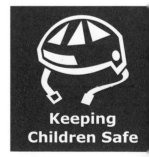

Keeping Children Safe

Bicycles with training wheels must have foot brakes because preschoolers are not strong enough to control hand brakes. While some children between 4 and 5 years of age have the balance and coordination to ride a bicycle without training wheels, they remain at high risk of falling and can't anticipate the dangers of riding near traffic or pedestrians. Constant adult supervision is essential. When a child is learning to ride a bicycle, you need to stay close and be able to intervene when necessary.

Water safety

Children under 5 years of age are at much greater risk of drowning than older children. Drowning is the second most common cause of death for children this age (after motor vehicle collisions). One-third of these tragedies happen in backyard pools, nearly always in pools with inadequate safety gates.

Taking the following essential precautions around water will help protect children in your care:

ALERT

- A baby or toddler can drown silently and in a matter of seconds, in as little as 5 cm (2 in.) of water. Never leave a child unattended near water.
- About 70 per cent of Canadian children 1 to 4 years of age go swimming, mostly in parent-and-tot classes. But remember: even if children are swimming early, **swimming lessons do not protect preschoolers from drowning**.

- Make sure that swimming pools—whether in- or above-ground—are fenced in on four sides. That means **not** having access to a pool from the deck, patio or back door (i.e., the house doesn't count as a "side"). The fence should be climbing-resistant and at least 1.2 m (4 ft.) high. Any gate to the pool area should be self-closing and self-latching.
- Make sure that hot tubs and spas not contained within the fenced pool area have a locking hard cover or are located in an area that can be closed and locked.
- Actively supervise children and stay within arm's reach whenever they are in or near water. The Lifesaving Society recommends a supervision ratio of at least one adult for every two young children and one adult for every baby.
- Make sure that supervisors know water rescue techniques and CPR. Keep a charged cell phone nearby.
- Have children wear a life jacket or personal flotation device (PFD) that fits properly—i.e., is appropriate for the height and weight of the child—and make sure it stays buckled up. Keep all safety straps fastened, including the crotch strap.
- Remember that water wings, bathing suits with flotation devices in them, inflatable rings and other swim toys **are not** safety devices. There are no life jackets for babies weighing less than 9 kg (20 lbs.).
- Make sure that a child who cannot swim does not use an inflatable toy in water any higher than waist-deep.
- Only use a slide or play equipment that is specifically designed for pool use.
- Use diapers designed for use in water. They don't get as heavy as regular diapers and are less likely to unbalance a child in a wading pool.
- Be sure to empty buckets and pails, ice chests with melted ice, or bathtubs immediately after use. Do not keep a container filled with water (e.g., a rain barrel) around a home setting. Empty your portable wading pool and turn it upside-down when not in use. These precautions also discourage mosquito breeding and reduce the risk of West Nile virus.

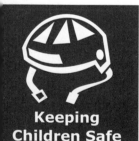

Keeping Children Safe

- Keep children away from ponds and streams at any time of year, unless you are with them.

Teach children the following important pool rules and adhere to them at all times:

- No swimming without an adult.
- No running or pushing.
- No food or drinks.
- No riding toys.

When children are playing under a sprinkler on a hot summer day, watch for pools of water collecting on the ground. These can be slippery, so move the sprinkler regularly or stop the activity until the water has drained. Use the sprinkler on a grassy surface only, and make sure the play area is free of obstacles and debris. A backyard water slide should be used with caution. Set it up on a soft, grassy slope, free of bumps and well away from trees or shrubs. Teach children to slide in a sitting position. A wet water slide is extremely slippery, so don't allow children to walk or run on it, or to slide lying down.

Sun safety

Protecting children from getting too much sun is important, whether they are playing outdoors or are with you on an errand. A child can sunburn easily, even on a cloudy day. When it comes to sun safety, these simple steps are essential:

- Make sure favourite play areas have a shady spot or take along a sun umbrella. Teach children the "shadow rule": They should play in shady places or indoors when their shadow is shorter than they are. This occurs when UV rays are most intense—between 10 a.m. and 2 p.m. Help children to identify shady places or different ways to have fun in the shade. If possible, schedule outdoor activities before 10 a.m. or after 2 p.m.
- At least 30 minutes before heading outside, apply a sunscreen with a sun protection factor (SPF) of at least 30. Apply enough so that the skin appears wet. Reapply it every few hours and after swimming or vigorous play. Don't forget to protect a child's ears, nose, backs of neck and legs, and tops of feet. Use an SPF 15 lip balm as well.

Sunscreen should **not** be used on infants under 6 months old, who can rub it into their eyes and mouth.

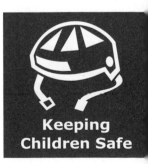

Keeping Children Safe

- Make sure all children, even infants, wear a sun hat with a wide brim and a flap or "tail" to protect the back of the neck—and sunscreen—every day, from the beginning of April to the end of September. For strong sunlight, encourage parents to provide their child with sunglasses that screen out all UV rays ("broad spectrum") and are CSA-approved. Label these items with the child's name and keep them in her cubby.
- To prevent overheating, dress children for warm weather in light loose clothing, in layers that can be put on or taken off easily.
- If a child in a wheelchair is wearing shorts, be careful that his thighs don't get sunburned. Use a light cloth or towel for protection, and watch that the vinyl and metal of the wheelchair don't get too hot.

- To prevent dehydration, offer plenty of water to children over 6 months old before, during and after outdoor play. Children won't necessarily feel thirsty while they play.
- Teach children the "Slip, slap, slop" rule:
  ➤ Slip on a shirt.
  ➤ Slap on a hat.
  ➤ Slop on some sunscreen.
- Teach by example. Model the above precautions and wear a hat, sunglasses and sunscreen every sunny or hazy day.

Be alert for signs that a child is experiencing heat illness and needs to come inside. Signs include thirst, fatigue, leg or stomach cramps, and cool, moist skin, which can be a sign of heat exhaustion. Bring the child inside or into a cool, shady area, and offer frequent, small sips of water. Removing extra clothing and fanning can help the child cool down slowly. If you suspect heat stroke, lay the child down, raise his legs about 20 cm (8 in.) off the ground, and offer comfort and reassurance. Encourage full and regular breathing. **Seek medical attention immediately.**

Protection against insect bites

Children enjoy picnics, and eating any meal outdoors can be fun if you take a few precautions against insects.

- Be careful when serving sweet foods (e.g., juices, fruit) that tend to attract stinging insects. Wipe up spills and keep children's hands clean.
- Have a fly swatter handy.
- Remind children that getting too excited or trying to kill an insect can increase the likelihood of a sting. Keeping calm and still is safer.
- Keep garbage bins or containers well sealed, away from outdoor play areas.

Insect repellents (bug sprays) provide protection, but they can irritate the skin, eyes and mouth if improperly applied. They should not be used in enclosed spaces, such as a tent. Use bug sprays sparingly and carefully, and follow these guidelines:

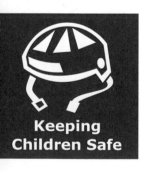

Keeping Children Safe

- Don't use insect repellents on children under 6 months of age.
- For children 6 months to 2 years of age, use an insect repellent with the least concentration of N,N-diethyl-m-toluamide or DEET (10% or less), only once a day. For children between 2 and 12 years old, use a product containing no more than 10% DEET, no more than 3 times a day. Avoid products containing citronella or lavender oil, which can cause an allergic reaction.
- Spray repellent sparingly on children's clothing and exposed skin. Don't apply it directly to a child's face or hands.
- Be careful where you spray. Repellents containing less than 10% DEET can be sprayed on cotton, wool and nylon but may damage spandex, rayon, vinyl and plastic (e.g., sunglasses).
- Be careful not to get spray in children's eyes. If that happens, rinse immediately with water.
- Don't spray irritated or sunburned skin.

- If you think a child is having an allergic reaction to a repellent, bathe the area and get medical help. Take the spray with you.
- Advise parents to wash off bug spray at the end of the day.

At the beginning of the summer, let parents know that bug spray might be used during outdoor play, and obtain their written permission to apply it if needed, using the *Medication consent form and record sheet* (see page 139–40). Children can use bug spray and sunscreen at the same time, provided all instructions for proper application are followed. Apply sunscreen first, then bug spray.

Safety around pets and other animals

Families must be informed at the time of enrolment if a pet is present in a child care setting. Besides issues of cleanliness, risk of infection and allergies, there are basic safety factors to consider when children and pets share living space. Dog and cat bites or scratches can happen at any time. These injuries can be serious if they become infected. Dog attacks, though rare, can have tragic consequences. If your dog stays outside your home setting throughout the day, it must be kept in an area that is inaccessible to the children's outdoor play spaces.

When a young child and any household pet are together, you need to provide constant supervision. Even the friendliest dog or cat may bite or scratch a baby or toddler who grabs its tail. Teach children to be gentle around and with animals. They should not disturb an animal that is sleeping, eating or caring for its young. Children should not try to take a toy, stick or food away from a dog.

Animals that are never appropriate in a child care setting include reptiles (e.g., turtles, snakes, lizards), amphibious or aquarium animals (e.g., frogs, toads, newts), and wild or exotic animals (e.g., rabbits, ferrets, monkeys, parrots). If one of these animals is on the premises, it must be kept in a room that children cannot access.

Take precautions around animals in playgrounds, parks or petting zoos. Teach older children some basic rules:

- Do not touch or hand-feed wild animals, such as squirrels or chipmunks.
- Keep away from any animal that looks sick, hurt or scared.
- Never try to stop an animal fight.
- Do not approach a dog you don't know. Even if an adult says it's safe, always let the dog make the first move.

If a strange or hostile animal is in your path:

- Keep still, with arms at your sides, and start to back away.
- Drop any food you're carrying and move away from the food.
- If you must pass the animal, move slowly, speak soothingly and keep your distance.

Remind children to wash their hands after touching pets or animals. For more about pets in child care settings, see Chapter 8, *Preventing Infections*.

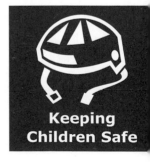

Keeping Children Safe

Winter safety

Outdoor play is as beneficial for children in the winter as it is in the summer, provided they are properly dressed for the season. Usually, if children's feet and hands are warm, what they are wearing is appropriate. If children are dressed too heavily, they are likely to sweat and feel colder when they stop playing. Ask families to take a few important precautions:

- Remove any drawstrings or cords from children's clothing that might catch on climbing or other play equipment. Velcro closures, snaps and zippers are the safest fasteners for winter wear. Also make sure children are wearing neck warmers rather than scarves, and mitten clips instead of strings. Scarves and mitten strings can catch on a climbing structure and strangle a child.
- Dress children in layers of clothing that can be put on and taken off easily.
- Provide children with a warm hat and a hood that covers the ears. Most body heat is lost through the head, and ears can be easily frostbitten.
- Provide warm, waterproof boots that are roomy enough for an extra pair of socks and for toes to wiggle comfortably.

Active games, making snow angels and building snowmen help keep children warm. Teach children a few important rules to go along with winter play:

- No snowball fights, which can cause an eye injury. Snowballs are more hazardous if the snow is hard-packed or icy.
- Don't build snow forts or tunnels. These structures can collapse and suffocate you.
- Don't play in or on roadside snow banks. The driver of a snowplow or other vehicle may not see you.
- Don't mouth metal objects in cold weather. Your lips or tongue can freeze to the metal and cause a painful injury.
- Don't eat snow, which may contain contaminants.

When taking children sledding, choose a slope that is gentle, free of trees, fences or other obstacles, not too crowded, and well away from roads or parking lots.

- When sledding, children should wear a ski or hockey helmet at all times. A bicycle helmet is no substitute for a ski or hockey helmet because it must be replaced after one crash and is only tested up to -10°C (14°F).
- There should be no sharp or jagged edges on the sled, and handholds must be fastened securely.
- Children should sit up or kneel on the sled—lying down and/or going down "head first" increases the risk of head, spine and abdominal injuries.

Teach children to slide down the middle of the hill and climb up the sides, to watch out for other sledders, and to move quickly to one side once they reach the bottom.

When taking children skating, try to choose a public indoor or outdoor rink. Never assume that it is safe to skate on a lake or pond, and always confirm with local authorities that pond or lake ice is at least 10 cm (4 in.) thick before taking children out on it. Obey all signs posted on or near ice and never walk on ice near moving water.

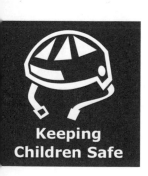

Keeping Children Safe

- Make sure children wear a properly fitting hockey or ski helmet while skating.
- Closely supervise them at all times.

Never send children outside in extreme weather conditions, such as a snowstorm, and keep them indoors whenever the temperature falls below -25°C (-13°F), regardless of wind chill. Also keep children indoors, regardless of temperature, when the wind chill factor is reported to be -28°C (-15°F) or lower, the point at which exposed skin begins to freeze. Know and follow provincial/territorial child care regulations for your jurisdiction if they differ from these recommendations. (For information about treating frostbite and hypothermia, see Chapter 11, *Emergencies*.)

Young children have less muscle mass, generate less body heat, and get cold more quickly than adults. Check often that children are staying warm and dry while playing outside in the winter, and offer a warm drink when they come in from the cold.

Safe routines

Preventing common injuries often involves recognizing a potential physical hazard and taking steps to eliminate it. However, establishing supportive routines and sharing them with the children in your care is the best way to keep them from harm. Children can be injured in an apparently safe environment if they are left unattended or undersupervised, if basic rules aren't reinforced, or if you have few protective routines.

Meals and snacks

Meals are an opportunity for social bonding and should be experienced as relaxed, regular and comfortable routines. It's no coincidence that the basics of eating safely are also good table manners. Manners matter because choking on food is a common hazard for toddlers and preschoolers. Teach children to:

- stay seated while eating,
- be calm and not to speak with food in their mouths,
- chew well before swallowing, and
- avoid feeding other children.

The safest eating utensils for children are either metal or hard plastic. Polystyrene or styrofoam cups and soft plastic utensils should **not** be used because they are easily broken and children can choke on the pieces. After frozen treats on wooden or plastic sticks are eaten, collect and discard the sticks immediately. Do not use corn-on-the-cob holders or offer food on cocktail or fondue skewers, or on toothpicks. Eating meals and snacks with the children in your care is the best (and most enjoyable) precaution of all. (For more about safe feeding, see Chapter 3, *Nutrition*.)

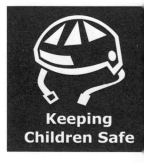

Keeping Children Safe

Safe sleep

Nap times are a daily routine in child care. Their timing, length and location will depend on the type of facility and the ages and individual needs of children in your care. Sleep areas need to be supervised. In child care centres, regular checks at a window overlooking the sleep area is the usual method of monitoring. Having a baby monitor in addition to your regular checks is useful in home settings.

Place infants on their back to sleep—the safest sleep position for healthy babies. Cribs must meet current safety standards. For crib safety specifications, see pages 89–90. Take these important steps to ensure safe sleep:

- Maintain a normal, comfortable room temperature.
- Cover babies with just a light blanket or dress them in a sleeper. An overheated baby is at increased risk of sudden infant death syndrome (SIDS).
- Never put a baby to sleep on any soft surface, such as a pillow, comforter or waterbed, sofa or chair.
- Don't smoke, and keep smokers out of your facility. Babies exposed to second-hand cigarette smoke are at increased risk of SIDS.
- Don't lull a baby to sleep in his crib with a feeding bottle.
- Never use sleeping devices such as hammocks, bassinets or cradles. These are not safe alternatives to a crib.

Babies who sleep on their back tend to turn their head to one side and may develop a flat spot. Changing the sleep position in the crib each day (i.e., placing the baby's head toward the head of the crib one day and toward the foot the next) and having daily supervised "tummy time" will help prevent a flat spot from developing.

A playpen is not a safe alternative to a crib for unsupervised sleep. Babies have died as a result of a playpen collapsing or from getting trapped between a playpen rail and an accessory when left unattended. In a child care setting where you remain in the same room, a playpen can be used for supervised napping.

For playpen safety specifications, see the checklist on page 91.

ALERT

A child should **never** be left unattended or asleep in a bouncy chair, baby carrier or swing.

Infant/baby seats and carriers, swings, bassinets or cradles, sofas and adult beds are **not** safe sleep alternatives to a crib.

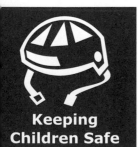

Keeping Children Safe

For toddlers and preschoolers, many child care settings use sleeping mats or cots on the floor for nap times. If your facility provides after-hours or overnight care, cots, mattresses of a specified thickness or toddler beds on site may be required. Check child care regulations for your jurisdiction. Do not use pillows on beds for children under 2 years of age. For all types of children's beds:

- Rails that are part of the bed structure must have a space between the vertical bars that is no wider than 6 cm (2-3/8 in.).
- The mattress must fit snugly inside the bed frame. A toddler can get trapped between the rail and the mattress if the mattress is too small.

- Mattress cross-supports, such as wood slats, should be permanently nailed or screwed on. This prevents the mattress from becoming dislodged when children are playing on or under the bed.

(For more about naps, see Chapter 12, *Children's Emotional Well-Being*. For more about cleaning bed linens, see Chapter 8, *Preventing Infections*.)

Junior or toddler beds with portable (removable) side rails and bunk beds are **not** safe for sleeping. They should not be used in a child care setting.

Baths

Child care settings that offer after-hours or overnight services need to provide some bathing facilities and routines appropriate to the ages and stages of the children in their care. Although there are few regulations or bathing guidelines available, the following points apply for all young children, all the time:

- **Never leave a child unattended in a bath**, even with a sibling or older child.
- Don't force the issue of bathing. Children don't need a bath every day. If a child seems to resist, a warm washcloth will keep her clean between baths at home.
- Make sure the bathroom is warm.
- Remove any jewellery that might scratch a child during a bath.
- Avoid scalding by:
    - ➤ ensuring that the hot water heater's temperature is set to 49°C (120°F),
    - ➤ running the cold water first, then hot, when filling the bathtub,
    - ➤ not placing the child in the bathtub while the water is running,
    - ➤ testing the temperature carefully, and
    - ➤ keeping the child away from the faucet end of the bathtub.
- Don't fill the bathtub more than a few inches deep. Baths don't need to be deep to be fun.
- **Never use a baby bath seat or ring**—these are not safety devices and can give a false sense of security. Babies have drowned in the bath while using a bath seat or ring.
- Use a rubber mat to prevent slipping and encourage children to stay seated in the bathtub.
- Bubble bath can irritate children's skin and isn't recommended. Use mild, unscented soap and a "no tears" shampoo, and be sure to rinse well with clean water.
- Help children out of the bathtub and have towels ready to wrap them in.

Safety checklists

Providing children with a safe environment, protective routines and active supervision are essential elements of quality child care. Training helps child care practitioners recognize and respond to potential risks, but systematic safety checks are a key determinant of safety in any child care setting.

If you are adapting your home to accommodate a child care program, make the following important modifications.

Keeping Children Safe

Facility-wide

❑ Install a carbon monoxide detector **and** a smoke detector on each level of your home. There should also be a smoke detector near each sleeping area. Test smoke alarms monthly. Change the batteries every 6 months or use a "long-life" battery, which may last up to 10 years. Replace alarms that are more than 10 years old. If your facility is in a newer home, one or more alarms may be hard-wired into the house wiring and connected to a private alarm-monitoring service.

❑ Use only a ground-fault interrupter (GFI) type of electrical outlet near water, such as in the bathroom, kitchen or outdoors, to decrease the risk of shock if a plugged-in appliance comes into contact with water.

❑ Cover all unused electrical outlets with protective safety covers, whether they are in the wall, on a power bar or on an extension cord.

❑ Avoid using extension cords. If you must use one, make sure it's the single-receptacle type and cover the empty outlet with a safety cover. Run an extension cord behind furniture so that children won't trip or find it easily. **Never nail an extension cord to a wall or run it under rugs**.

❑ Test your hot water temperature at the tap to ensure the temperature runs no higher than 49°C (120°F). Contact your local utility company, public health office, landlord or local water heater manufacturer about the best way to reduce water temperature. Options include using anti-scald devices, installing in-line plumbing valves that regulate the temperature or reducing the temperature setting on your hot water heater. Anti-scald devices are available at plumbing, hardware and home-improvement stores.

❑ Install a safety guard in front of gas and wood-burning fireplaces and a barrier around wood stoves to prevent a child falling against them. Barriers should be at least 56 cm (22 in.) high and made of non-combustible materials. Choose space heaters that are cool to the touch and have an automatic shut-off. Keep them away from fabrics such as bedding and curtains, and furniture.

❑ Check paint finishes in older homes and facilities for lead content. Lead paint, especially if it is peeling or chipped, poses a hazard to children if ingested. Test kits are sold in paint, hardware and home-improvement stores. Some contractors also have special equipment to test for lead content.

❑ Use anchors, L-shaped angle brackets or furniture straps to bolt cubbies, shelves, dressers, bookshelves, entertainment units/TV stands and cabinets securely to the wall. Even low furniture can fall forward or be pulled over by a child.

❑ Choose furniture with rounded edges or put corner cushions on furniture or structures that a toddler might fall against (e.g., a coffee table or fireplace mantle).

❑ Remove any houseplants that are poisonous. (See Appendix 5.3 for a list of poisonous plants.)

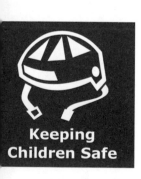

Keeping Children Safe

Stairways

❑ Install hardware-mounted safety gates at the top and bottom of all open stairways. These should be fixed securely to the wall or door frame using the hardware provided. To block access to rooms, use pressure gates, which are kept in position by a pressure bar. Install these gates with the pressure bar on the side away from children to discourage climbing.

- Do not use any gate made before 1990, an accordion-style expandable gate, or a gate with an opening that could trap a child's head or neck.
- Use only a hardware-mounted gate at the top of a stairway. An eager or anxious child leaning on a pressure gate can dislodge it, resulting in a fall down the stairs.
- Make sure there is no more than 5 cm (2 in.) between the bottom of the gate and the floor, so a child can't slip underneath.

❑ Make sure stair railings are designed to prevent climbing and are less than 10 cm (4 in.) apart.

❑ Keep stairways well lit and clear of toys, clothes or any other items that pose a tripping hazard.

❑ Consider installing handrails at a child's height (15 cm [6 in.] below the adult handrail) on both sides of stairways that are more than 10 m (4 ft.) wide.

Halls and entranceways

❑ Keep halls and entranceways well lit and free of toys, boxes or any other items that pose a tripping hazard. Keep boots and shoes from getting underfoot by lining them up on mats or putting them in a basket.

❑ Provide safe storage out of the reach of children for purses, knapsacks and diaper bags.

Windows

Blind or curtain cords can strangle a child whose head gets caught in a dangling loop or cord that wraps around his neck. Never leave cords hanging.

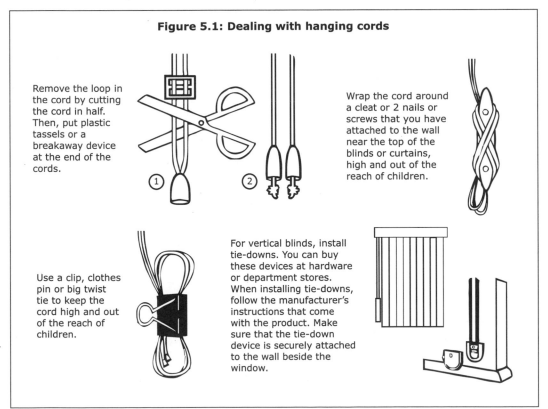

Figure 5.1: Dealing with hanging cords

① Remove the loop in the cord by cutting the cord in half. Then, put plastic tassels or a breakaway device at the end of the cords.

②

Wrap the cord around a cleat or 2 nails or screws that you have attached to the wall near the top of the blinds or curtains, high and out of the reach of children.

Use a clip, clothes pin or big twist tie to keep the cord high and out of the reach of children.

For vertical blinds, install tie-downs. You can buy these devices at hardware or department stores. When installing tie-downs, follow the manufacturer's instructions that come with the product. Make sure that the tie-down device is securely attached to the wall beside the window.

Source: Health Canada, 2005. *Danger! Children can strangle on blind and curtain cords*. Adapted with permission.

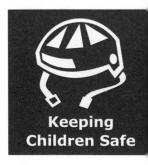

Keeping Children Safe

❏ Cut the cords short when blinds are fully down or when curtains are fully closed.

❏ Whether the blind is up or down, make sure children can't reach the cords. Tie them out of reach. There are special fastenings available for this.

❏ Place furniture well away from windows, to prevent children from climbing up to reach a blind or curtain cord or falling from a window.

❏ Ensure that windows above the first floor cannot open more than 10 cm (4 in.) or install window guards.

Screens do not prevent falls from windows.

Check local building and fire codes to make sure that you do not block fire escape routes when limiting children's access to windows.

Floors

Floors should not be highly polished but maintained to prevent cracks and splinters.

❏ Clean up spills promptly to keep floors dry and slip-resistant.

❏ Put a non-slip backing or double-sided tape under throw or area rugs, to prevent trips and falls.

Doors

When children are not allowed access to another floor or room in your home or facility, the area must remain locked, blocked or gated.

❏ Use elevated or child-resistant doorknobs to prevent toddlers from accessing stairways, rooms with hazards, front and back doors.

❏ Use latches at adult height to keep doors open or closed as necessary.

❏ Install locks or guards on patio and balcony doors.

Pinch injuries from closing doors are common in settings where there is more than one child.

❏ Install hinge guards to protect little fingers.

❏ Equip doors with devices that prevent them from closing quickly.

❏ Keep sliding and folding doors latched open or closed—these are pinching hazards.

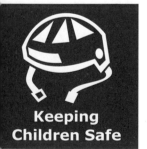

Keeping Children Safe

Kitchens

Children are not allowed into the kitchen area in some child care centres. However, in home settings—with meal and snack preparation, mealtimes and cleaning up—child care practitioners can spend a lot of time in the kitchen. While it's probably unrealistic for them to keep children out, there are essential precautions and safe behaviours to protect the children from harm.

Never leave children unsupervised in the kitchen.

- ❏ Keep a baby behind a safety gate or secure in a high chair when you're cleaning, cooking or making hot drinks.
- ❏ Keep a fire extinguisher in the kitchen and check the test window monthly.
- ❏ Cook on the stove's back burners and keep pot handles turned in. Use a microwave to warm food when this is the safest option.
- ❏ Remove front- or top-mounted stove knobs between cooking times, especially on a gas stove.
- ❏ Keep the oven and dishwasher doors closed. Keep children out of the kitchen when the dishwasher is running.
- ❏ Keep appliances or gadgets at the back of the counter when they're not in use and be sure appliance cords are not left dangling or accessible to children.
- ❏ Keep hot food and drinks away from table and counter edges.
- ❏ Use placemats instead of a tablecloth.

Make sure the following everyday household items are stored both out of sight and beyond the reach of children, preferably in a latched drawer or cupboard:

- ❏ cleaning supplies and all corrosive/poisonous household products,
- ❏ scissors, skewers, knives or other sharp kitchen utensils,
- ❏ plastic bags, which should also be tied in a knot,
- ❏ kitchen garbage can and compost container.

Make sure a pet's food and water dishes are kept off the floor when children are present or in an area that children can't access.

Even before a baby in your care starts eating solid food, you may be using a high chair to keep her in sight and out from underfoot while you work in the kitchen. However, high chair-related injuries occur all too often. Whether a high chair is new or second-hand, take these precautions:

- ❏ Follow the manufacturer's weight, height and age guidelines at all times.
- ❏ Make sure your high chair has a wide and stable base. The base on many older high chairs is too narrow, making them easy to tip over.
- ❏ If the chair folds, be sure it is locked securely in its upright position.
- ❏ Always use the safety straps—including the waist and crotch belt—to keep a baby from sliding out the bottom of the chair.
- ❏ Keep the high chair away from counters or tables—anything that a child could push or pull on and tip the chair over—and well away from appliances and window blind and curtain cords.
- ❏ Be careful not to pinch fingers when removing or replacing the tray.
- ❏ **Never let a child stand up in a high chair.** Once a child is trying to climb out, it's time to switch to a regular chair.
- ❏ Do not permit children to climb or play on a high chair.

> REMEMBER
>
> **Never** leave a child unattended in a high chair.

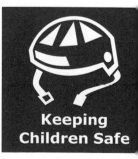

Keeping Children Safe

Using a hook-on chair allows a baby to eat at a table with other children. The child's weight helps to hold the chair in place when it hooks onto a table surface.

❑ Make sure the chair has locks or clamps that tighten securely.
❑ Never use these chairs on a table that may tip.
❑ Always use the safety straps—including the waist and crotch belt—to keep a child from sliding forward and out of the chair.

Bathrooms

Between washing hands and cleaning teeth, toilet learning and bathing (in programs with after-hours care), children can spend a lot of time in the bathroom. They need your active supervision to be protected from drowning, scalds and poisoning. Take these steps to make your bathroom a safer place:

❑ Install a hook-and-eye latch on the outside of the door so it's always closed when not in use. Install the latch at the top of the door so that preschoolers cannot reach it.
❑ Keep all bathroom cleaning products, medications, personal care products (e.g., shampoo and make-up) and devices (e.g., hairdryer, curling iron and shaving equipment) up high, out of children's reach. Lock one or more cabinets for safe storage, if possible.
❑ Roll up any electrical cords to prevent them dangling over the counter edge.
❑ Keep the diaper pail tightly closed, preferably inside a latched cupboard.
❑ Keep the toilet seat down and latched when not in use.
❑ Ensure that platforms or stools used by children to reach the sink are stable and have a non-slip surface and base.
❑ Teach preschoolers to run cold water before turning on the hot water tap.

Diaper change area

Because even a very young infant is sufficiently active to fall from a change table or other raised surface, always keep one hand on a baby as you change his diaper. Put him in a safe place, preferably a crib, while you are cleaning up the area after a diaper change. These precautions will make the nursery or other change area safer:

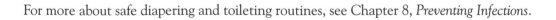

> **REMEMBER**
>
> No child should be left unattended on a change table or other raised surface.

❑ Anchor nursery shelving and heavy furniture, like the change table or dresser, securely to the wall.
❑ Use only a change table that has a guard rail and restraining strap and use them every time you change a baby's diaper.
❑ Store everything you need for changing diapers—wipes and washcloths, ointment and diapers—within easy reach, so you never have to turn away.
❑ Keep safety pins for cloth diapers and diaper cream containers closed and out of children's reach.
❑ Do not use products such as baby powder, talc or cornstarch. They can damage a child's lungs if inhaled.

For more about safe diapering and toileting routines, see Chapter 8, *Preventing Infections*.

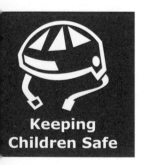

Keeping Children Safe

Equipment and accessories

Cribs

A crib is the safest place for a baby while you go to the bathroom, clean up a mess or do a task where you can't be present to supervise for a **very brief period**.

Never use a crib that was made before government safety regulations changed in 1986. Any crib you use should have a permanent label with the manufacturer's name, the model number or name, the date of manufacture, instructions for assembly, and a warning statement about mattress size and proper crib use. **Never use a crib that is missing this label or a crib that is homemade or has been modified.** Here are some basic safety specifications for cribs:

- ❏ Crib bars should be no more than 6 cm (2-3/8 in.) apart. Make sure that none are missing or loose.
- ❏ The mattress should fit tightly within the crib frame. If there is more than 3 cm (1-3/16 in., or two finger-widths) between the mattress and crib side when you push the mattress toward the other side, it is too small. A baby can become trapped in that space and suffocate.
- ❏ Corner posts should be either no higher than 3 mm (1/8 in.) above the top of the end panels—such as four-poster cribs—or too high to catch on clothing.
- ❏ There should be no cut-out designs in the head or footboards or openings between the corner post and top rail—a baby's clothing or limbs can catch on an edge.
- ❏ The crib's drop-side latches should be securely in place when the rail is raised. Always raise and lock this rail in its highest position when a child is in the crib.
- ❏ The mattress support hangers should be secured with the bolts or closed hooks supplied by the manufacturer. These fixtures should all be tight and strong. Don't use a crib where these hooks are Z- or S-shaped.
- ❏ You should use only the original hardware. Contact the manufacturer to obtain missing hardware.

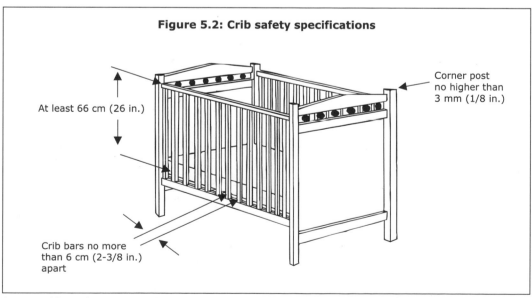

Figure 5.2: Crib safety specifications

At least 66 cm (26 in.)

Corner post no higher than 3 mm (1/8 in.)

Crib bars no more than 6 cm (2-3/8 in.) apart

Source: Health Canada, 2003. *Crib Safety*. Adapted with permission.

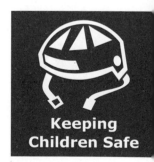

Keeping Children Safe

Safe placement and use are as important as the crib's structure:

❑ Place the crib away from windows, window coverings and blind cords. No strings or cords should dangle in or near the crib. Make sure there are no wall hangings, lamps, pictures or furniture near enough for a child to grab them from inside the crib.

❑ Make sure the mattress is firm, flat and covered with a fitted crib sheet. **Never use removable plastic wrapping, dry-cleaning bags or garbage bags as mattress covers.**

❑ Keep soft items like bumper pads, pillows, lambskins, quilts, stuffed toys and comforters out of the crib. They prevent proper air circulation around the face and can cause overheating, suffocation and sudden infant death syndrome (SIDS). Also, older babies can use these items to climb out of the crib.

❑ Check the overall condition of a crib regularly, especially if it has been moved.

❑ Set the crib mattress at its lowest level. Once a child starts trying to climb out of the crib or is 90 cm (35 in.) tall, she is ready to switch to a toddler bed. You may put the crib mattress on the floor as a transitioning step.

❑ Hang mobiles out of reach, fastened solidly to the crib. Remove them as soon as a baby is 4 months old or can push up on hands and knees. Don't tie toys or anything else across the crib.

Playpens

A playpen can be a safe place for a baby or very young child for a short time, while you fix a meal or attend to another child. The playpen should be positioned in such a way that you and the child can watch one another and interact as you do a task or take a phone call.

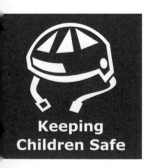

Keeping Children Safe

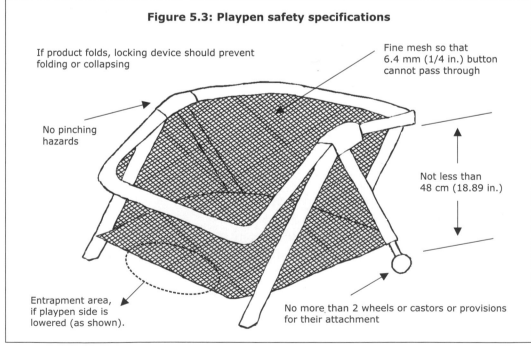

Figure 5.3: Playpen safety specifications

If product folds, locking device should prevent folding or collapsing

Fine mesh so that 6.4 mm (1/4 in.) button cannot pass through

No pinching hazards

Not less than 48 cm (18.89 in.)

Entrapment area, if playpen side is lowered (as shown).

No more than 2 wheels or castors or provisions for their attachment

Source: Health Canada. 2003. *Information to dealers of second-hand children's products.* Adapted with permission.

Here are some basic safety specifications for playpens:

❑ Make sure the playpen has a permanent label stating that it complies with federal playpen regulations and listing the manufacturer's name, the model number or name, and the date of manufacture. The instruction booklet must be kept with the playpen. Follow the instructions for assembly and adhere to the weight and height limits at all times.

❑ Ensure that the model you are using has not been recalled. Check for product advisories and recalls at Health Canada's website (www.hc-sc.gc.ca). **Never use a playpen that has been recalled.**

❑ Make sure the playpen has sides made of a fine mesh with holes less than 6.4 mm (¼ in.) across and well-padded surfaces. It should be stable and sturdy. No items (e.g., a mobile or play gym) should be attached to playpen sides.

❑ Ensure there are no exposed joints or sharp edges. These can cause a pinch or scrape.

❑ Make sure the top rails and sides are locked and secured whenever the playpen is set up. **Never leave a baby in a playpen with a lowered side** (as in Figure 5.3).

❑ Follow weight and/or age guidelines for playpen accessories (e.g., a change table, bassinet). **Do not leave these accessories in place when a child is using the playpen.** There have been fatal injuries due to strangulation when a child has been trapped between a playpen's rail and an accessory.

❑ Check regularly for tears in the vinyl rail covering, in the mattress pad and in the mesh. A baby can choke on small pieces of vinyl or strangle if a button becomes caught in a tear.

❑ Never leave an object or toy a child might climb on in a playpen.

Bouncy chairs or infant/baby carriers

Never leave a baby unattended in a **bouncy chair** or **infant/ baby carrier**. Always take the following precautions:

❑ Make sure the safety harness is holding a baby securely in place. Always use the crotch strap to keep her from sliding forward. The crotch strap also prevents strangulation in the harness if a baby slips under the waist strap.

❑ **Put the chair or carrier on the floor near you,** and well away from high-activity areas in a room. **Never set a bouncy chair or infant carrier on a washer/dryer, kitchen counter, table or any other raised surface.** Babies have rocked themselves right off the top of furniture and countertops, and another child can push the chair over an edge very quickly.

❑ Place the chair or carrier well away from dangling cords or hazards (e.g., a plant or small object) that may be within a baby's reach.

❑ Stop using the chair or carrier as soon as a baby has outgrown the manufacturer's age/weight limits.

REMEMBER

Supervised tummy time, several times a day, is better for babies than being in a bouncy chair or carrier. Not only does time on the tummy help prevent a flat spot on a baby's head, but it is very important for development.

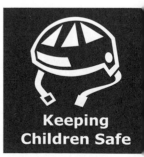

Keeping Children Safe

Baby swings

A baby swing can sometimes lull a baby to sleep or calm a fussy child. Most swings are portable and freestanding, with a mechanized (crank) or battery-operated mechanism that allows them to swing for a set period of time. **Never leave a child unattended in a swing. Don't let a baby swing for more than 20 minutes.** If she falls asleep, take her out of the swing and place her in a crib. Always take the following precautions:

❑ Make sure you have an instruction manual that includes weight or age limits. Follow all instructions for use.
❑ **Do not use a swing that has a carrier or cradle bed.** This attachment is used in place of the swing seat, allowing the baby to lie down while swinging. A baby can slide forward against the side of the carrier and suffocate.
❑ Let the swing rock gently and not too quickly.
❑ Make sure the swing has a strong and stable base.
❑ Always use the seat belt **and** crotch strap. Some models have a crotch pillar attached to the tray or seat. Secure the harness snugly to keep the baby safely in place.
❑ Prop a baby up so that her head doesn't roll forward and get trapped between the backrest and the bars the seat hangs from. A rolled receiving blanket can help support her head.
❑ When moving a baby into or out of an infant swing, be careful not to pinch fingers in the swing's tray or buckles.

Stationary activity centres

Stationary activity centres have a seat in the middle of a surrounding tray or play surface with toys or other objects within a baby's reach. While the seat may allow a baby to turn around, the centre itself does not move. A stationary activity centre is not to be confused with a baby walker, which has wheels. **Baby walkers are banned in Canada, which means it is illegal to advertise, buy or sell a new or used one. Baby walkers are very dangerous and must never be used.**

Never leave a baby unattended in an activity centre. Be sure to take these precautions:

❑ Do not put babies under 4 months of age in an activity centre. They do not have enough head control and neck strength to play in an activity centre.
❑ Do not leave a child in an activity centre for more than 30 minutes.
❑ Follow the weight and height guidelines carefully. If the activity centre moves or tips over, a baby can suffer a head injury, get trapped or fall down stairs. If you notice that a child is able to move a stationary activity centre, stop using it.
❑ Keep the activity centre well away from stairways, plants, bookshelves, blind or curtain cords, and hot surfaces such as stoves, fireplaces and heaters. A child in an activity centre can reach out or up, and pull things down on top of himself.
❑ Clean activity centres after use. When cleaning, check the toys to make sure they are not broken or loose. Small pieces can be inhaled or ingested and cause choking.

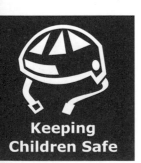

Keeping Children Safe

Selected resources

General

B.C. Health Planning. 2003. Preventing injury in child care settings. www.health.govbc.ca/health

Calgary Health Region, Injury prevention and control, Childhood injury prevention resources. www.calgaryhealthregion.ca

Health Canada, Consumer Product Safety. www.hc-sc.gc.ca

Public Health Agency of Canada, Injury Prevention. www.phac-aspc.gc.ca

Region of Peel (Ont.) Public Health. 2004. *Keep on track: A health and resource guide for child care providers in Peel*. Section 9: Health and safety—mind and body: Creating a safe environment, Air quality, Scalds and burns, Pets and wild animals, Sun safety information to prevent heat-related Illnesses, Bicycling and scooter safety, Playground safety, Setting the environment, Evaluation of hazards, Sandboxes, Frequently asked questions about chromated copper arsenate (CCA) wood, What helmet for what activity? www.region.peel.ca/health/keep-on-track/pdfs/entiremanual.pdf

Indoor spaces and equipment

Canadian Child Care Federation. Healthy spaces. www.cccf-fcsge.ca/healthy-spaces

Canadian Paediatric Society. 2007. Keep your baby safe. Also available as a brochure. www.caringforkids.cps.ca

Health Canada. Consumer product safety, Children's products, Child care equipment and children's furniture. www.hc-sc.gc.ca

————. 2007. Be careful with lighters and matches. Fact sheet.

————. 2006. Is your child safe? Booklet.

————. 2006. Safer homes for children: A guide for communities.

————. 2005. Danger! Children can strangle on blind and curtain cords. Pamphlet.

————. 2005. Do you know what these symbols mean? Fact sheet.

————. 2004. Baby's stationary activity centre. Fact sheet.

————. 2003, 2004. Crib safety. Booklet, fact sheet.

Safe Kids Canada. Poisoning, Product safety, Home safety. www.sickkids.ca/safekidscanada

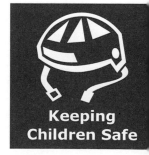

Outdoor spaces and environments

Canadian Cancer Society, Prevention, Use SunSense. Information on UV index, sunscreen and sun safety and children. www.cancer.ca

————. 2005. *Made in the shade: Sun protection*.

Canadian Child Care Federation. www.cccf-fcsge.ca

——. 2003. Toxic plant list. Resource sheet #29.

——. 2003. Children at play in the great outdoors. Resource sheet #68.

——. 2001. Sunshine—Approach with caution. Resource sheet #20.

——. 2001. Water safety. Resource sheet #28.

——. 2001. When Jack Frost comes nipping. Resource sheet #18.

Canadian Dermatology Association. Tips for daycares: Teaching preschoolers sun safe play, every day. Fact sheet. www.dermatology.ca

The Canadian Paediatric Society's website for parents and caregivers, Caring for Kids, has information on seasonal and safety topics included in this chapter. Documents can be downloaded at www.caringforkids.cps.ca, reproduced and shared with families.

——. 2008. West Nile virus: What parents should know.

——. 2007. Frostbite.

——. 2007. Sun safety.

——. 2006. Insect repellents for children.

——. 2002. Winter safety: Advice for parents and kids. Also available as a brochure.

——. 2001. Halloween safety: Tips for parents and kids. Also available as a brochure.

Capital Health (Edmonton), Kidsafe Connection. 2003. "Get the Facts" series of brochures on topics such as child pedestrian safety, sledding safety, home safety, backyard safety, playground safety, cold weather/ice safety, bicycle safety. www.capitalhealth.ca

Environment Canada. 2002. Wind chill fact sheet. www.msc.ec.gc.ca

Health Canada. www.hc-sc.gc.ca

——. 2006. Safe summer fun. Fact sheet.

——. 2003. Swimming pool safety. Fact sheet.

——. 2003. Winter sports safety. Fact sheet.

Region of Peel (Ont.) Public Health. 2007. *Hot weather guidelines: Child care centres*. www.peelregion.ca/health/heat/child-care-guidelines.htm

——. 2007. *West Nile virus: Information for children attending camps, schools and daycares.* www.peel-bugbite.ca

Safe Kids Canada. www.sickkids.ca/safekidscanada

——. 2008. Pedestrian safety.

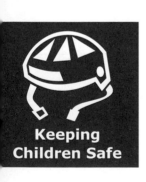

Keeping Children Safe

Safe Kids Canada. 2004. Making it happen: Pedestrian safety.

———. 2005. Make it a Safe Kid summer. Booklet.

Playground safety and environment

Canadian Child Care Federation. 2001. Playground safety. Resource sheet #32. www.cccf-fcsge.ca

Canadian Paediatric Society. 2007. Playground safety. Also available as a brochure. www.caringforkids.cps.ca

Canadian Standards Association. 2007. *Children's Playspaces and Equipment: Z614.* www.csa.ca. Also available for purchase at www.cccf-fcsge.ca

Evergreen Learning Grounds Program. www.evergreen.ca

Health Canada. 2005. Playground—danger of strangulation. Fact sheet. www.hc-sc.gc.ca

Safe Kids Canada. Playground safety. www.sickkids.ca/safekidscanada

———. 2006. CSA standards, inspections and liability, Kids under 5, Play value and accessibility, Protective surfacing, Playground safety tips, Pressure-treated wood.

Toys and materials

Canadian Child Care Federation. www.cccf-fcsge.ca

———. 2003. Polyvinyl chloride toys. Resource sheet #47.

———. 2001. Safety in the arts. Resource sheet #21.

———. 2001. Toy safety. Resource sheet #26.

Canadian Paediatric Society. 2007. Are home trampolines safe? www.caringforkids.cps.ca

Consumer Product Safety Commission (U.S.). 2002. Age determination guidelines: Relating children's ages to toy characteristics and play behaviour. www.cpsc.gov

Health Canada. 2006. Industry guide to Canadian safety requirements for children's toys and related products. www.hc-sc.gc.ca

Wheeled toys

Ontario Ministry of Transportation. 2000. Young cyclist's guide. Booklet. www.mto.gov.on.ca

Safe Kids Canada, Wheeled activities. www.sickkids.ca/safekidscanada

———. 2002. Got wheels? Get a helmet! Flyer.

Websites

Canada Safety Council. www.safety-council.org

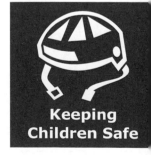

Keeping
Children Safe

Canadian Playground Safety Institute. www.cpra.ca

Child Safety Link. www.childsafetylink.ca

Consumer Product Safety Commission (U.S.). www.cpsc.gov

Lifesaving Society. www.lifesaving.ca

National Resource Center for Health and Safety in Child Care and Early Education (U.S.). www.nrc.uchsc.edu

Ontario Injury Prevention Resource Centre. www.oninjury.resources.ca

Ontario Poison Centre. www.sickkids.ca/ontariopoisoncentre.ca

Plan-it-Safe, Child and Youth Injury Prevention Centre. www.plan-itsafe.com

Safe Start (B.C.'s Children's Hospital). www.bcchildrens.ca

Smart Risk. www.smartrisk.ca

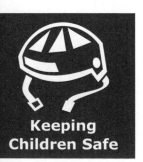

**Keeping
Children Safe**

Appendix 5.1: Injury report

Child's name: _____ Date of birth: _____

Date of injury: _____ Time: ❑ a.m. ❑ p.m.

Parents notified: _____ Time: ❑ a.m. ❑ p.m.

When was the facility director (if applicable) notified of the injury? _____

Date: _____ Time: _____

Name(s) of child care practitioner(s) who were on site: _____

_____

_____

Names of staff who witnessed the injury: _____

_____

_____

Where did the injury occur?_____

What was the staff-to-child ratio when the injury occurred?_____

Describe the injury (type, extent). If appropriate, use the line drawings to indicate where the injury was located on the child's body:

_____   _____

_____

_____

Describe how the injury occurred (include sequence of events, group size and age mix, your proximity and ability to react, and the child's behaviour or actions):

_____

_____

_____

If the environment (e.g., surfacing), a piece of equipment or a product was involved, describe how:

_____

_____

_____

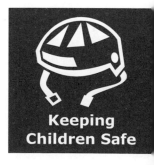

Keeping Children Safe

Was first aid administered? ❑ No ❑ Yes (If yes, specify what was done, and by whom):

_____

_____

_____

Was further action taken (e.g., child taken to hospital, taken home)?

_____

_____

_____

Doctor's contact information, if one was consulted:

_____

_____

If the child remained at the facility, what was the child's level of participation?

_____

_____

_____

Other comments:

_____

_____

_____

_____

_____

_____

What corrective action should be taken to prevent further injuries of this type? Consider:

- the type or level of supervision,
- the need for additional staff training,
- the repair, replacement or elimination of equipment or toys,
- the reorganization of space or furniture, and
- the reinforcement of rules or limits.

_____

_____

_____

_____

_____

_____

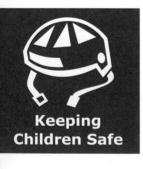

Keeping Children Safe

Signature of reporting child care practitoner: _____ Date: _____

Signature of facility director or co-worker: _____ Date:_____
(if applicable)

Signature of parent/guardian: _____ Date:_____

Name of child: _____ Date: _____

Indicate site of injury with an "x"

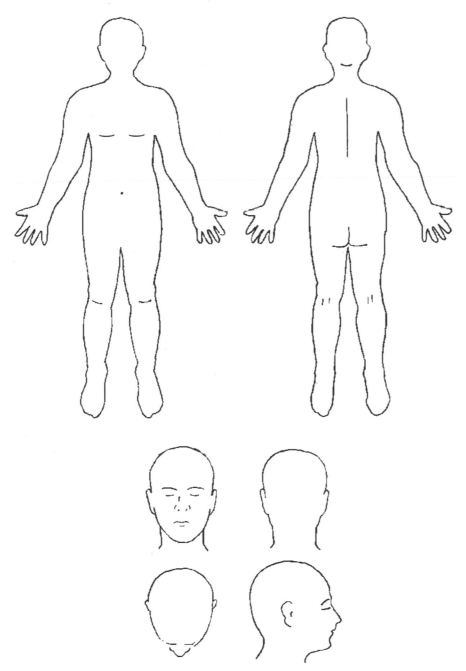

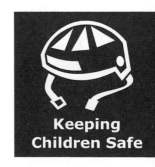

Keeping Children Safe

 Give a signed copy of this form to the child's parent/guardian and keep the original readily accessible in the child's personal file.

Appendix 5.2: Safety checklist schedules

Weekly safety checklist

Name of person doing inspection: _____ Date: _____

Indoors	Okay	Action required	Specify action	Date completed	Comments
Facility-wide					
Strict "no smoking" and "no weapons" policies are in force.	❏	❏			
Entranceways and exits are free of obstacles or clutter.	❏	❏			
Doors can be easily opened by adults, but not by children.	❏	❏			
Staff and visitors can store their purses, backpacks and other personal belongings out of the sight and reach of children.	❏	❏			
Diaper/laundry bags that are to be sent home are hung out of the sight and reach of children.	❏	❏			
Telephones are easily accessible by staff, and a list of numbers for emergency services is posted next to every phone.	❏	❏			
All unused electrical outlets have protective safety covers.	❏	❏			
Single-receptacle extension cords are inaccessible by children and have not been nailed to a wall or run under rugs. ❏ The empty outlet has a protective safety cover.	❏	❏			
Garbage containers are foot-activated, plastic-lined, and have tightly fitting lids.	❏	❏			
Throw or area rugs do not slide or buckle.	❏	❏			
Pet food bowls and litter boxes are not accessible to children.	❏	❏			
All blind and curtain cords are tied up and secured with safety hooks.	❏	❏			
Window guards prevent windows from opening wider than 10 cm (4 in.).	❏	❏			
Halls and stairways are well lit and free of obstacles and clutter.	❏	❏			
Hardware-mounted safety gates are installed at the top and bottom of stairways, and pressure gates are used to prevent access to hazardous areas, as appropriate.	❏	❏			
Floors are vacuumed every day and as needed.	❏	❏			
Furniture					
Cribs, playpens and high chairs have intact, readable labels bearing the manufacturer's name, product name and model number. ❏ They meet all current safety standards. ❏ Specifications for safe use, including height, age and weight limits, are known and adhered to.	❏	❏			
The height, age and weight limits for accessories (e.g., a baby swing or a stationary activity centre) are known and adhered to.	❏	❏			

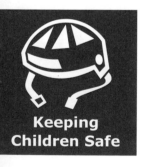

Keeping Children Safe

Indoors	Okay	Action required	Specify action	Date completed	Comments
No infant under 4 months of age is put into a stationary activity centre.	❏	❏			
A stationary activity centre is positioned away from stairways, plants, hot surfaces, or any object that can be reached for and pulled over.	❏	❏			
Furniture is positioned away from windows.	❏	❏			
There are no wall hangings, lamps or pictures within reach of a crib.	❏	❏			
Crib mobiles are removed if a child using the crib is 4 months old or can push up on hands and knees.	❏	❏			
Potentially hazardous items (e.g., a rotating chair, chairs that pull out, retract or recline, or exercise equipment) are not accessible by children.	❏	❏			
Cubbies, bookcases, change tables, dressers and entertainment units are well constructed, stable and anchored to the wall.	❏	❏			
Other heavy objects (e.g., a TV) are anchored securely to the wall to prevent toppling.	❏	❏			

Play areas, toys and indoor play structures					
Play areas for children under and over 3 years of age are separated, to minimize the risk of injuy to younger children during play, as well as their access to inappropriate toys.	❏	❏			
Toys are age-appropriate and suited to the abilities of the children playing with them.	❏	❏			
Toys for different age groups are stored separately.	❏	❏			
No toy small enough to fit inside an empty toilet roll is accessible by babies and toddlers.	❏	❏			
Toy labels with age-related and small parts warnings and instructions for safe use are known and adhered to.	❏	❏			
Toy instructions or manuals are kept on file.	❏	❏			
Age-appropriate, non-toxic, non-edible arts and crafts materials are stored in labelled containers out of the reach of children.	❏	❏			
No toy has a pull cord or string longer than 20 cm (8 in.).	❏	❏			
Indoor play structures are safely positioned, away from windows and other furniture, with ❏ a proper fall zone, and ❏ sufficient surfacing to cushion a fall.	❏	❏			
Wheeled toys (e.g., ride-on toys) are appropriate for the age and stage of children using them. ❏ Their height, age and weight specifications are known and adhered to.	❏	❏			
Children wear a certified helmet when using wheeled toys.	❏	❏			

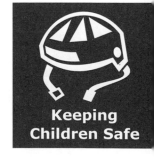

Keeping Children Safe

Indoors	Okay	Action required	Specify action	Date completed	Comments
Kitchen and eating areas					
The kitchen is equipped with a working fire extinguisher that staff have access to and know how to use.	☐	☐			
Hot water faucets have a scald guard, and ☐ the water heater's temperature setting is no higher than 49°C (120°F).	☐	☐			
A safety gate is installed in the kitchen doorway to prevent toddlers from entering the room at unsafe times (e.g., when the dishwasher is running).	☐	☐			
There are no dangling appliance cords.	☐	☐			
Sharp objects (e.g., knives, scissors) and plastic bags are inaccessible by children.	☐	☐			
Medications (including vitamins) are stored out of the sight and reach of children (in a locked cupboard or sealed container in the fridge).	☐	☐			
The high chair is positioned away from furniture or appliances that a child might reach for.	☐	☐			
Placemats rather than a tablecloth are used at the table.	☐	☐			✓
Stove knobs at child height are removed when not in use.	☐	☐			
The garbage can and compost container are inaccessible to children.	☐	☐			
Foods that pose a choking risk are inaccessible to children.	☐	☐			
Bathroom, washroom, diapering area					
The bathroom door is locked with a hook-and-eye latch when not in use, and cannot be locked by a child from inside.	☐	☐			
Non-slip step stools are provided for sinks and toilets, as needed.	☐	☐			
All household cleaning agents are stored in their original containers, ☐ out of the sight and reach of children, and ☐ preferably in a locked cupboard.	☐	☐			
Bleach solutions are properly labelled (e.g., 1:10, 1:100), and ☐ are inaccessible to children.	☐	☐			
The diaper pail is inaccessible to children, preferably in a latched cupboard.	☐	☐			
Soiled cloth diapers are disposed of in securely tied plastic bags.	☐	☐			
Soiled diapers and plastic bags are inaccessible to children.	☐	☐			
Medications and personal care products (e.g., mouthwash, cosmetics) are stored out of the sight and reach of children.	☐	☐			
Faucets have a scald guard.	☐	☐			
Items such as hairdryers are unplugged when not in use and inaccessible to children (e.g., no dangling cords).	☐	☐			

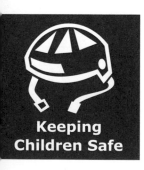

Keeping Children Safe

Outdoors	Okay	Action required	Specify action	Date completed	Comments
Transition and storage areas					
A "no idling" policy is in force at drop-off and pick-up times.	❏	❏			
The fence separating the children's play area from the driveway or garage is at least 1.2 m (4 ft.) high, ❏ climbing resistant, and ❏ in good repair.	❏	❏			
Gates work properly (e.g., they self-close and self-latch).	❏	❏			
Stair gates on the porch, deck or balcony are properly installed, and always used when children are present.	❏	❏			
Porch and deck rails are no more than 10 cm (4 in.) apart, and in good repair.	❏	❏			
Garbage storage areas and bins are away from play areas, and inaccessible to children.	❏	❏			
Lawn machines and power tools are inaccessible by children, and never used when children are playing in the yard.	❏	❏			
The garage is inaccessible to children.	❏	❏			
The barbeque is inaccessible to children.	❏	❏			
Play area					
Play equipment is checked for rusting, new pinch- or catch-points, and other signs of wear and tear.	❏	❏			
Surfacing under play equipment is checked daily for litter and sharp or foreign objects, and ❏ raked weekly to maintain depth, softness and an even distribution around play equipment.	❏	❏			
Plants known to be toxic and mushrooms are removed.	❏	❏			
No new pool of water more than 5 cm (2 in.) deep is accessible to children (e.g., rain run-off).	❏	❏			
The facility vehicle					
The vehicle is insured, in good repair, and equipped with age-appropriate child seats, or a seat belt, for every child and staff member to be transported.	❏	❏			
Car seats have a CMVSS label and meet current safety standards. ❏ They are installed correctly, using UAS/LATCH or seat belt, and ❏ installed securely (e.g., they do not move more than 2.5 cm (1 in.) forward or from side to side).	❏	❏			
The height, age and weight specifications for each car seat are known and adhered to.	❏	❏			
Copies of the manufacturer's instructions for all car seats and the vehicle owner's manual are kept in the vehicle.	❏	❏			
Loose items are stowed so that they will not fly in case of a sudden stop.	❏	❏			
The vehicle is equipped with a first aid kit.	❏	❏			

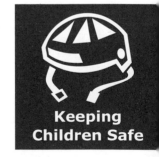

Keeping Children Safe

Monthly safety checklist

Name of person doing inspection: _____ Date: _____

Indoors	Okay	Action required	Specify action	Date completed	Comments
Facility-wide					
Health Canada's website at www.hc-sc.gc.ca (consumer product safety) has been checked for product advisories, recalls and product safety information that might affect the facility.	☐	☐			
All smoke detectors are tested and working, and the test window on all fire extinguishers has been checked.	☐	☐			
Ceilings and walls have no cracked or broken plaster. There is no peeling or badly chipped paint.	☐	☐			
All lights are in good working order (e.g., bulbs and wires are checked if lights flicker or buzz).	☐	☐			
Outlets near water (e.g., kitchen, bathroom, outside) are protected by ground-fault interrupter circuitry, and have been tested.	☐	☐			
Ceilings, walls and window frames are checked for "soft" or damp spots that may indicate a leak or mould growth.	☐	☐			
Window screens are secure and in good repair.	☐	☐			
Plants known to be poisonous have been removed.	☐	☐			
There are no cracks or splinters in the flooring.	☐	☐			
Shelves are securely anchored to walls, and ☐ heavy or breakable items are well back from shelf edges.	☐	☐			
Furniture					
Cribs, playpens and change tables are checked carefully for pinch- or catch-points, exposed joints, loose parts, tears, or any other signs of wear and tear.	☐	☐			
Play areas, toys and indoor play structures					
All toys are checked for loose or broken parts, tears, and any signs of wear that might pose a choking or other hazard.	☐	☐			
Bathroom, washroom, diapering area					
The bathtub and surrounding tiles are checked for loose grout or caulking.	☐	☐			
Non-skid or other decals in the tub are not lifting or loose.	☐	☐			
Pets and animals					
There are no inappropriate animals on facility premises.	☐	☐			

Keeping Children Safe

Indoors	Okay	Action required	Specify action	Date completed	Comments
House pets are fully immunized and are fed and exercised in areas inaccessible to children.	❏	❏			
There is no contact between children and pets without active supervision by staff.	❏	❏			

Outdoors	Okay	Action required	Specify action	Date completed	Comments
Play area					
Each piece of play equipment is checked to ensure that: ❏ bolts, screws and other fastenings are covered with an acorn nut or plastic cap, or are well recessed, ❏ all nuts and bolts are tight, ❏ there is no rust or chipped paint on metal surfaces, ❏ there are no broken parts, or sharp edges that need filing down, and ❏ there are no uprooted or exposed footings that could be a tripping hazard.	❏	❏			
Ride-on toys and tricycles are in good repair and stored inside when not in use.	❏	❏			
There are enough properly certified helmets for children using wheeled toys at the same time.	❏	❏			
No helmet has been in a collision or is more than 5 years old.	❏	❏			
Shaded play areas are accessible, ❏ clean and dry, and ❏ free of plants known to be poisonous.	❏	❏			
The facility vehicle					
The vehicle is equipped with basic tools (e.g., for a tire change), and an emergency kit (e.g., blankets, candles) in case of a breakdown.	❏	❏			
All height, age and weight specifications for car seats are known and adhered to.	❏	❏			
Every potential driver of the facility vehicle is fully licensed and insured.	❏	❏			

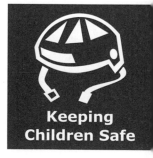

Keeping Children Safe

Seasonal safety checklist

Name of person doing inspection: _____ Date: _____

Outdoors	Okay	Action required	Specify action	Date completed	Comments
Pools, hot tubs and spas, whether on site or neighbouring the facility, are inaccessible to children. ❑ They are fenced in on all four sides, with a self-locking gate. ❑ Fences are at least 1.2 m (4 ft.) high and climbing-resistant.	❑	❑			
Wading pools are emptied and turned upside-down when not in use.	❑	❑			
Surfacing material under play equipment is topped up to prevent it from becoming too compact or hard.	❑	❑			
Indoor play gyms are not used outside in the winter.	❑	❑			
Sand or salt is put down on walkways to prevent falls in cold weather.	❑	❑			
The facility is equipped for extreme weather with basic emergency supplies (flashlights and candles, bottled water, non-perishable food, extra blankets, etc.).	❑	❑			

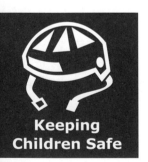

Keeping Children Safe

Annual safety checklist

Name of person doing inspection: _____ Date: _____

Indoors	Okay	Action required	Specify action	Date completed	Comments
Facility-wide					
The provincial/territorial child care office or local public health unit has been consulted for changes to building and fire codes that might affect the facility.	❏	❏			
All children's furniture, equipment and accessories have been checked for product recalls, and eliminated or replaced as necessary.	❏	❏			
A certified playground inspector has checked play areas (**indoors and out**) and all play equipment for safety, proper placement and surfacing. ❏ There is a schedule for maintenance and follow-up inspections.	❏	❏			
There is a firmly anchored mat or non-slip floor covering at each entrance.	❏	❏			
Floors are in good condition, clean, and have non-slip surfaces.	❏	❏			

Outdoors	Okay	Action required	Specify action	Date completed	Comments
Play area					
Active play areas (e.g., for ride-on toys, running) are clearly delineated from areas for quiet activities (e.g., a sandbox).	❏	❏			
The local school board, licensing authority or parks and recreation office has been consulted for changes to local by-laws governing play equipment that might affect the facility.	❏	❏			
All play equipment conforms to current CSA safety standards, and ❏ is age-appropriate.	❏	❏			
Play equipment is properly installed, ❏ is safely positioned away from other play apparatus or fencing, and ❏ is properly anchored.	❏	❏			
Each piece of play equipment higher than 30 cm (12 in.) above the ground has at least 25 to 30 cm (10 to 12 in.) of cushioning material beneath it (more if it is higher).	❏	❏			
Surfacing material extends 1.8 m (6 ft.) beyond each apparatus.	❏	❏			
Surfacing material meets current CSA safety standards, and ❏ is age-appropriate for the children who have access to it (e.g., pea gravel is a choking hazard for babies and toddlers).	❏	❏			
There are no head entrapment areas on play equipment (spaces measuring between 9 and 22.9 cm [3.5 and 9 in.]).	❏	❏			

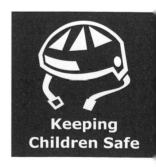

Keeping Children Safe

Appendix 5.3: Plant safety

If a child in your care eats or touches a plant, berry, seed, bulb or wild mushroom that you think may be poisonous, call your local poison centre for advice. This emergency number should be posted by all phones in your facility. When you call, be prepared to answer the following questions:

- Are there any signs of illness?
- What is the name of the plant (if known)? The person you will speak to is a specialist in poison information, not plants. A plant cannot be identified over the phone.
- How much and what parts were eaten?
- How recently was it eaten or touched?
- How old is the child?

You will be advised what to do and what symptoms to watch for. Children can react differently to the same plant.

Here are some helpful hints to avoid plant poisoning:

- Where possible, keep plants, berries, seeds and bulbs out of the reach of young children.
- Teach children to stay away from plants you're not sure of and to avoid eating non-food items.
- Know the names of plants and trees inside and outside your home, just in case.
- Leave the tags on all items you bring home from a plant nursery. If you don't know a plant's name, an expert from a plant nursery may be able to help you identify the plant and give you a tag to place near it.

Be careful:

- Don't assume that a plant is safe for people just because birds or wildlife eat it.
- Be aware that jewellery, craft items and maracas, especially those purchased outside of Canada, may contain poisonous seeds.
- Don't encourage children to suck nectar from flowers.
- Keep cactus plants away from children.

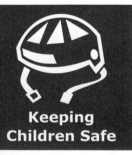

Keeping Children Safe

Poisonous plants

- Some of the plants in the following list will not cause serious poisoning unless a large amount is eaten.
- Seeds or pits from apples, apricots, cherries, nectarines and peaches are poisonous, but only if eaten in large amounts.
- Accidentally swallowing a few seeds will not cause illness.
- Remember that a young child may choke on any plant.
- This is not a complete list of all poisonous plants.

The following plants are known to be poisonous to humans. If any of these poisonous plants are eaten, call your provincial/territorial poison centre immediately:

Amaryllis
Angel's Trumpet
Arrowhead Vine
Autumn Crocus
Azalea
Bittersweet
Black Locust
Boston Ivy
Caladium
Calla Lily
Castor Bean
Chinese Lantern Plant
Clematis
Cotoneaster
Croton
Cyclamen
Daffodil
Daisy (Chrysanthemum)
Delphinium
Dieffenbachia (Dumb Cane)
Elephant's Ear
English Ivy
Eucalyptus

Euonymus
Foxglove
Gladiola
Holly
Horse Chestnut
Hyacinth
Hydrangea
Iris
Jack-in-the-Pulpit
Jequirity Bean
Jerusalem Cherry
Jimson Weed
Larkspur
Lily-of-the-Valley
Lobelia
Lupine
Marijuana
Milkweed
Mistletoe
Monkshood
Morning Glory
Mother-in-law's Tongue
Narcissus

Nightshade
Oleander
Peony
Periwinkle (Vinca)
Philodendron
Poison Ivy
Poison Oak
Pokeweed
Potato (all green parts)
Pothos
Rhododendron
Rhubarb Leaves
Rosary Bean
Snake Berry
Snow on the Mountain
Star of Bethlehem
St. John's Wort
Tobacco
Tomato (plant & unripe fruit)
Virginia Creeper
Water Hemlock
Wisteria
Yew

Non-poisonous plants

The following plants are considered non-poisonous to humans.

- A person is unlikely to get ill from these plants, but certain people may have an unusual reaction.
- Remember that a young child may choke on any plant.
- This is not a complete list of all non-poisonous plants.

Although the following plants are non-poisonous to humans, the ones marked with one asterisk(*) may cause skin irritation. A plant marked with two asterisks(**) may also cause nausea or vomiting.

African Violet
Alyssum
Asparagus Fern
Astilbe
Baby's Breath*
Baby's Tears
Bachelor's Buttons
Black-eyed Susan*
Boston Fern
Chinese Evergreen
Christmas Cactus
Coleus*
Coral Bells
Cosmos
Crocus (spring-blooming only)
Dahlia*
Dandelion
Daylily*
Dracaena
Easter Lily
Evening Primrose

Ficus Benjamina*
Freesia
Fuchsia
Gardenia*
Gloxinia
Grape Hyacinth
Hens and Chicks
Hibiscus*
Hollyhock
Honey Locust
Hoya
Impatiens
Jade Plant
Maple (seeds and young leaves)
Marigold*
Money Plant
Mountain Ash
Mulberry
Peperomia
Persian Violet
Petunia

Phlox
Poinsettia**
Polka-Dot Plant
Portulaca
Prayer Plant
Primrose*
Purple Coneflower
Rose*
Rubber Plant*
Schefflera*
Snapdragon
Spider Plant
Spiraea
Statice*
Tulip*
Wandering Jew*
Weeping Fig*
Weigela
Yucca
Zinnia

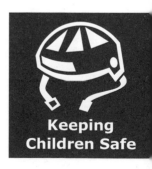

Keeping Children Safe

First aid

If a child is choking, unconscious, or having trouble breathing or swallowing:

- **Call 911** immediately (or emergency services where 911 service is unavailable).

If the child appears well:

Poison Ivy

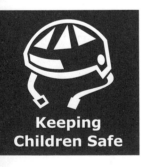

- Look for pieces of the plant in the mouth and remove any pieces you find.
- Give small sips of water.
- Do not try to make the child vomit.
- Call your local poison centre for advice.

Some plants may cause skin irritation, itching, a rash or blisters. If a child **touches** a poisonous plant:

- Remove any clothing touched by the plant or its sap.
- Wash the skin immediately with lots of soap and lukewarm water.
- Call your local poison centre for advice.

Mushroom safety

Poisonous and non-poisonous mushrooms grow side by side. Only a mushroom expert can tell the difference. It is dangerous to eat any mushroom that you find outdoors. Cooking wild mushrooms does **not** make them safe to eat.

Please note:

- Eating even small parts of some mushrooms can cause sickness and death.
- After eating a poisonous mushroom, a person may not become ill for many hours.
- Do not wait until a child feels sick before calling your local poison centre for advice.

Helpful hints to prevent mushroom poisoning:

- Remove and throw away all mushrooms growing near your facility.
- Check the lawn for mushrooms before children go outdoors to play, especially after a rainfall.

Source: Ontario Poison Centre, 2008. Adapted from the Hospital for Sick Children's "Plant Safety" brochure. For more information on poison prevention, visit www.sickkids.ca/ontariopoisoncentre.ca.

Keeping Children Safe

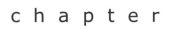

c h a p t e r

6

Transportation Safety

Transporting children, whether in a private vehicle or on public transportation, involves some risk. In fact, motor vehicle collisions and traffic injuries are the leading cause of death among children under 6 years of age; this toll includes child passengers, pedestrians and cyclists. Child care practitioners should avoid transporting children whenever possible. If your program does take on this responsibility, you must:

- comply with all current laws for transporting children,
- determine safe transportation policies and procedures for staff, children and parents, and
- be prepared to respond if an emergency occurs.

Transportation policy

Every child care facility should have a transportation policy that specifies when child care practitioners may transport children, the rules to follow when transporting them, the responsibilities of staff members who are driving or accompanying children, and emergency procedures. Share this policy with parents at the time of enrolment and with all staff. It should include:

- a clear statement of when and how the facility will transport children in its care, and
- a sample permission letter to be signed by parents, detailing the facility's transportation responsibilities.

Drop-off and pick-up procedures

Your transportation policy should also include the following minimum guidelines:

Enforce a "no idling" policy outside your facility, for safety as well as for environmental health reasons. Drivers must make a full stop and switch off their ignition at drop-off and pick-up times.

- Parents or other designated caregivers must come into the facility at drop-off and pick-up times, to hand off children to (or receive them from) a staff member.
- Children should never be unaccompanied during these busy transition times.
- Vehicles should try to park on the same side of the street as their destination—or pick-up point—to load and off-load children.
- Children should get in or out of a vehicle on the curb-side only.
- Parents should assist children who are in car seats or booster seats on the driver (traffic) side of the car, and accompany them to the sidewalk.

Transportation services

All transportation services offered by your facility must be fully compliant with federal, provincial and municipal laws and regulations governing the transportation of children. In addition:

- **A minimum of two staff members from your child care facility must travel with even one child.** At least one adult (not the driver) must be designated as being responsible for the care of the children being transported.
- Your facility's motor vehicle must be equipped to accommodate the number and type of car seats for the number, ages, weights and heights of the children being transported.
- Staff must be aware of and follow Transport Canada's guidelines for securing children in car seats, booster seats and seat belts. All children must be seated in the back seat when travelling.
- Your facility must have adequate insurance coverage to transport children.
- Every vehicle should be equipped with a first aid kit, a copy of each child's emergency record, a fire extinguisher, a cell phone and emergency numbers, and emergency supplies. These items should be checked regularly to ensure that they are complete, up-to-date and functioning properly. **A driver should not use a cell phone unless the car is parked.**
- Each vehicle must be well maintained and serviced according to the manufacturer's recommendations.
- Vehicles associated with your program should be locked at all times and the keys kept out of sight and out of reach of children.

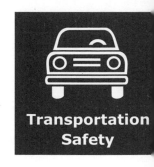
- A child must never be left alone in a car. Heat, cold or lack of supervision can result in injury.
- Emergency drills for vehicle evacuation must be conducted periodically. This drill should include unbuckling children from their car seats.
- Smoking must not be permitted in any vehicle transporting children.
- Drivers must be trained to eliminate distractions (e.g., no eating, no using the radio or CD player, no cell phone or headphone use).
- Trips must be planned so that travelling times are less than 1 hour in each direction (optimally 20 to 30 minutes or less).

Legal requirements

Vehicles

Children can be transported only in vehicles that have been registered and insured, and that meet all provincial requirements under the Motor Vehicle/Highway Traffic Acts and local child care regulations. All provinces and territories require the use of restraint systems (child seats) for children up to about 4 years old, as well as seat belts for older children, youth and adults. However, laws vary among jurisdictions as to age, height and weight limits for child restraint systems and for booster seat use. Review these regulations periodically to ensure your child/booster seats conform to best practice and are fully compliant with the law.

ALERT

Fifteen-passenger vans do not meet the same safety standards as school buses and are at much higher risk of rolling over or going out of control than other vehicles. They are not recommended for use in child care.

Drivers

The driver of any vehicle is responsible for passenger safety. All drivers must have a valid driver's licence for the class of vehicle being driven.

Transportation rules

1. Secure each child in his own car seat or booster seat. Never secure two or more children with the same belt.
2. Transport preschoolers in the rear seat only. Don't allow a child under 13 years of age to sit in the front seat of a vehicle.
3. Before every trip, conduct a safety check of the vehicle to make sure it's working well and contains nothing that could harm a child. This includes ensuring good tread and pressure on all tires, checking that lights and signals are in working order, and making sure the gas tank is full.
4. Before getting in the driver's seat, walk around the vehicle to look for children. Backing up is particularly risky around toddlers.
5. Stay alert to any changes in a vehicle while driving. Unusual odours, sounds or vibrations can be warning signals of a possible breakdown.

6. Never transport a child in the cargo area of a station wagon, van or pick-up truck.
7. Never leave a child alone inside or near a vehicle.
8. Keep sharp, hard or heavy objects (e.g., lunch boxes, water bottles and backpacks) in the trunk. They can become deadly projectiles in a sudden stop or collision.
9. If a child is travelling with a toy, make sure it isn't hard or sharp. A held toy can injure a child in a sudden stop.
10. Do not give children food or drink in a moving vehicle. In a collision, a child can choke on food and a container can become a dangerous flying object.
11. Load and off-load children at the curb-side or in a driveway, and only into the care of an authorized adult.
12. If the vehicle has childproof locks on rear car doors, use them. Windows near a toddler's car seat should open only part way. (A car dealer can adjust them so they won't open wider.)
13. Never allow children to put their arms or head out of the window.
14. Ensure that all hands and feet are inside before closing doors.
15. Teach children to behave responsibly when riding in a vehicle. If behaviour is inappropriate, find a safe place to pull over before dealing with the situation.

Consistent rules about how to behave in a vehicle—learned early and modelled by child care practitioners—help toddlers understand that safety must come first.

- Make sure everyone is buckled in properly before starting the vehicle.
- If a toddler is helping to buckle up her own harness, she's more likely to try unbuckling as well. It's best to secure children in their car seats yourself. If a child undoes her chest-clip or harness buckle, pull over and stop the vehicle right away.
- Don't compromise about car seat rules—even for the shortest trips.
- Don't permit behaviour that distracts the driver. Pull over and stop if children fight, throw things or move around the vehicle.

Stay calm and consistent about rules. Modelling all car rules yourself teaches children to follow them too.

Infant and child safety systems

Certified car seats are labelled with the letters "CMVSS" (Canadian Motor Vehicle Safety Standard) and have the national safety mark indicating that they have been tested by the manufacturer and found to comply with all safety standards set by Transport Canada. It's illegal to use a car seat bought outside of Canada because devices sold elsewhere may not conform to Canada's stringent safety standards.

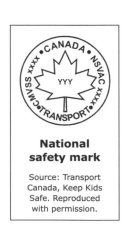

**National
safety mark**

Source: Transport Canada, Keep Kids Safe. Reproduced with permission.

Check car seats periodically to make sure they haven't been cited under a product recall. Mailing in the registration card promptly after purchase allows the manufacturer to contact you immediately if there's a recall or safety notice issued. Check for recalls on the Transport Canada website at www.tc.gc.ca.

Surveys suggest that improper use of car seats in Canada is as high as 80 to 90 per cent. Properly used, child restraint devices are highly effective in preventing death and injury. Having a Universal Anchorage System (UAS) or LATCH (Lower Anchors and Tethers for Children) system is the law for all new vehicles, and essential to car seat safety.

Share these general guidelines with families, and adhere to them at all times.

- Read both the car seat's instruction manual and the vehicle owner's manual before installing or using a child restraint system.
- Keep the original instruction manual with the car seat (there's usually a pocket or slot for this). Make an extra copy and keep it at your facility.
- Educate all staff and volunteers in the proper installation and use of the car/booster seats required by your facility. Practice periodically and before every field trip.

You'll also need to clean the car seat cover, harness straps and other parts periodically. Follow the manufacturer's instructions for how to clean each part.

Infants up to 1 year of age

For at least the first year, a baby must travel in a **rear-facing infant car seat** that fits correctly. Transport Canada recommends a rear-facing car seat until a child weighs 10 kg (22 lbs.). When installing an infant car seat in your facility's vehicle, make sure you do the following:

- Ensure the car seat label indicates that the car seat will fit the baby's weight and height. If additional information is needed, your local public health unit or Transport Canada can help.
- Ensure that the car seat fits properly in the rear seat, preferably in the middle and never in front of an active air bag. Install it according to the instructions, then make sure the seat cannot be moved more than 2.5 cm (1 in.) forward or from side to side.
- When installing, push down on the car seat with your knee at the same time as you tighten the seat belt or UAS/LATCH strap.
- Secure the car seat, routing the UAS/LATCH strap **or** the vehicle seat belt correctly. Some lap/shoulder combination seat belts require a special **locking clip**.

Follow the vehicle **and** car seat instruction manuals.

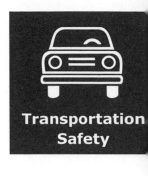

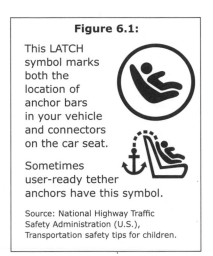

Figure 6.1:

This LATCH symbol marks both the location of anchor bars in your vehicle and connectors on the car seat.

Sometimes user-ready tether anchors have this symbol.

Source: National Highway Traffic Safety Administration (U.S.), Transportation safety tips for children.

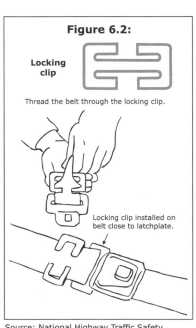

Figure 6.2:

Locking clip

Thread the belt through the locking clip.

Locking clip installed on belt close to latchplate.

Source: National Highway Traffic Safety Administration (U.S.), Transportation safety tips for children.

A baby's position in the car seat is important:

- Harness straps must be snug, and threaded at or just below the shoulders. Position the chest clip at armpit level. If you can put more than one finger between the harness straps and a baby's collarbone, the harness is too loose.

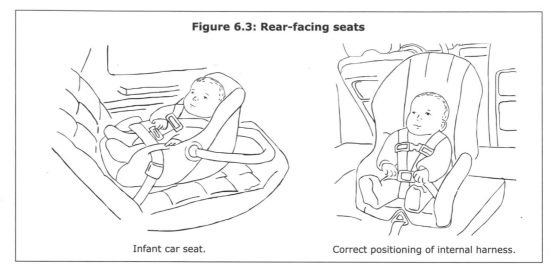

Figure 6.3: Rear-facing seats

Infant car seat.   Correct positioning of internal harness.

- Using a bunting bag with a car seat is not recommended because it can interfere with the car seat's harness system. If it's chilly, lay a blanket over the baby after securing him in the car seat.

Toddlers

Don't be in a hurry to switch a child from a rear-facing to a forward-facing child car seat in your facility's vehicle. The longer you use a rear-facing seat that fits correctly (is appropriate for the weight and height guidelines specified on the label), the safer children will be during a sudden stop or collision. **All babies under 1 year of age should be rear-facing.**

Forward-facing car seats are designed to spread the forces of a sudden stop or collision over the strongest parts of a child's body. It is essential to use a seat that fits the child's weight and height. Before installing a forward-facing child seat:

- Weigh the toddler and measure his height.
- Check the car seat's label to be sure the seat is designed for his weight and height.
- Make sure the child seat fits securely in the back of the facility's vehicle.

ALERT

- **Never** put a car seat with a baby in it on an elevated surface, such as a table or counter.
- **Do not** leave a baby in a car seat to sleep.
- **Do not** use a second-hand car seat.

The seat must be properly installed and used for every trip. A toddler's car seat should be installed in the rear seat of the facility's vehicle, preferably in the middle and never in front of an active air bag. Read the instructions for the car seat and the vehicle owner's manual for proper installation using a tether strap and the seat belt **or** a tether strap and the UAS/LATCH.

REMEMBER	• A top tether strap **must** be used on all forward-facing child seats.
	• The tether strap hook must be attached to a tether anchor.
	• You will need one tether anchor for each child seat used in the vehicle.
	• If your facility's vehicle does not have enough tether anchors, ask a dealer to install additional ones.

Installing with a seat belt

- Route the vehicle seat belt through the child seat, as shown in the car seat instructions.
- Buckle the seat belt and make sure it's tight. Use a locking clip when required.
- When installing, push down on the car seat with your knee at the same time as you tighten the vehicle seat belt.
- Attach the tether strap to the proper vehicle tether anchor to hold the top of the child seat in place, and then tighten the strap.
- The child seat should not move more than 2.5 cm (1 in.) forward or from side to side.

Installing with UAS/LATCH

Car seats manufactured after September 1, 2002 have connectors that attach to lower anchor bars in a vehicle's rear seats (second and third rows). Check your vehicle owner's manual for the seating positions that are equipped with UAS/LATCH.

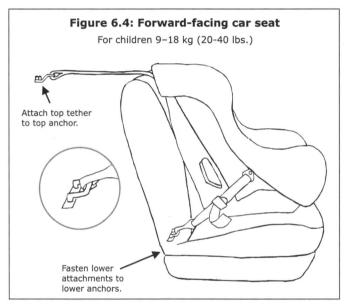

Figure 6.4: Forward-facing car seat
For children 9–18 kg (20-40 lbs.)

Attach top tether to top anchor.

Fasten lower attachments to lower anchors.

Source: National Highway Traffic Safety Administration (U.S.), The simple facts about LATCH.

- Attach the two UAS connectors on the car seat to the UAS anchor bars in the vehicle and tighten the strap. **Never fasten more than one car seat to an anchor.**
- When installing, push down on the car seat with your knee at the same time as you tighten the strap.
- Attach the tether strap holding the top of the child seat in place and tighten.
- The child seat should not move more than 2.5 cm (1 in.) forward or from side to side.

To secure a toddler in a forward-facing child seat:

- Adjust the harness straps to the slot positions that are at or slightly above the shoulders.
- Make sure the child is seated in an upright position with her back flat against the back of the car seat.

- Ensure that the harness straps are fastened tightly. "Tightly" means only one finger fits between the harness strap and the child's chest.
- The chest clip should be positioned at armpit level to hold the harness straps in place.

Additional car seat safety tips

Do not use add-on features for car seats that the seat manufacturer does not provide, such as a head-hugger, tray or comfort strap. These may interfere with the safety of the seat and can be dangerous in a collision.

- Metal buckles and plastic or vinyl coverings left in the sun can cause a serious burn. Seats not in use should be covered with a blanket or towel. Check the temperature of metal pieces before putting a child into a car seat.
- Make sure to fill out and mail the registration card that comes with any new car seat. If there's a recall, the company will be able to contact you. For recall information, check with Transport Canada at 1-800-333-0371 or visit www.tc.gc.ca.
- Replacement parts such as chest clips can be obtained from the seat manufacturer and some specialty car seat stores. Always use parts specifically designed for the model of car seat.

Preschoolers

Once a child weighs at least 18 kg (40 lbs.), he may be ready for a combination car/booster seat. Most children reach this weight by the time they are about 4½ years of age. However, some children grow too tall for a forward-facing car seat before they reach 18 kg (40 lbs.). A child is too big for his seat as soon as he has outgrown the specified height or weight limit for the car seat. Transport Canada recently increased the maximum weight limits for forward-facing seats. Newer models with higher weight limits may accommodate older children.

Children between 4 and 8 years of age are often "graduated" to seat belts too soon, greatly increasing their risk of injury, disability or death in a collision. Before age 8, most children are too small to use a regular seat belt in the correct position. A combination car/booster seat raises a child enough to correctly position the lap belt over the hips and the shoulder belt across the shoulder and chest. Unless they still meet the weight and height limits of their forward-facing car seat, children between 18 kg (40 lbs.) and 36 kg (80 lbs.) should be properly secured in a booster seat in the rear seat of a vehicle when travelling.

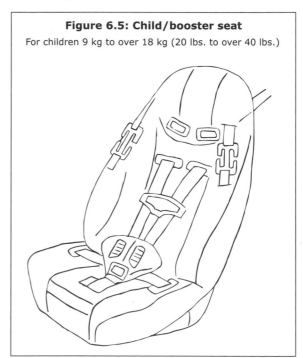

Figure 6.5: Child/booster seat
For children 9 kg to over 18 kg (20 lbs. to over 40 lbs.)

Source: Alberta Infrastructure and Transportation, Child safety seats. Reproduced with permission.

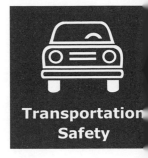

- Choose a booster seat that fits both the child and your facility's vehicle.
- Read the vehicle owner's manual and the instructions for the booster seat to ensure it is properly installed and used.

When to replace a car seat

- Any car seat that has been in a collision should be replaced, even if a child was not riding in the seat at the time.
- If the car seat has reached the expiry date, it needs to be replaced. If there's no expiry date, call the manufacturer. Replace the seat if there are signs of wear and tear.

All children who have outgrown the height and weight limits of their forward-facing car seat (when they weigh at least 18 kg [40 lbs.] and are about 4 years of age) should use a booster seat.

Children should use a booster seat until they are big enough to wear a seat belt safely, usually once they are 145 cm (4 ft. 9 in.) tall, 8 to 9 years old and weigh 36 kg (80 lbs.). Follow the law for your province or territory.

Safety education

Children

Teach children in your care these four rules for being safe passengers:

1. Always ride in your car seat or booster seat.
2. Buckle up properly—no matter how short the trip.
3. Ride in the back seat—it's the safest place to be.
4. Ride quietly.

Good modelling means that the driver and adult passengers must all wear their seat belts. Position the lap belt across the hips, not the stomach.

Parents and caregivers

Inform parents at the time of enrolment that the four rules above will be strictly enforced and enlist their support in teaching children proper transportation safety. When a new family joins the program, share your facility's transportation policy. Provide new parents with information and guidelines on safe transportation, especially the proper selection, installation and use of car seats. Consider holding a car seat clinic at your facility but be sure to have certified child restraint technicians to check seats and provide advice. Many free resources on car seats and other road safety topics are available through Transport Canada, provincial/territorial highway authorities or your local public health unit.

Field trip safety

Pre-trip planning

- Find out which amenities are available at the destination, including phones, washrooms, clean drinking water, shaded rest areas, and accessibility for strollers and/or wheelchairs, and plan accordingly.

Transportation Safety

- Notify parents **at least** 24 hours in advance, giving details of the trip, and obtain signed parental consent.
- Make sure the parental consent form includes the method of transportation, the time of departure and return, contact information for the destination, and the purpose of the field trip. Parents should note any special requirements for their child, along with the date and their signature.
- Calculate the staff-to-child ratio needed. Because the children will be in an unfamiliar, non-childproofed space among strangers, providing a higher than usual staff-to-child ratio is often essential. Don't count volunteer parents in your ratio: they aren't trained as supervisors in unfamiliar settings. If the destination is an environment designed for young children, with a trained facilitator on site, fewer extra staff may be needed.
- Make sure that all drivers, including parent volunteers, have a valid driver's licence and that any private vehicles to be used are equipped with appropriate car seats and are registered and insured. Obtain copies of these documents for your files. Review the centre's insurance policy to ensure that all stipulations are met.
- Make an identification tag for every child to attach to a jacket or shirt. The tag should have the name, address and telephone number of your child care facility. (Do not put children's names on their tags. This prevents strangers from calling a child by name.)
- Ensure that the children's emergency medical records are up-to-date and that parents' contact information is current and correct. Make an extra copy to take along on the trip.
- Discuss rules for safety and appropriate conduct with the children.
- Inform people at the destination of your estimated time of arrival and other staff and parents of your estimated time of return.
- For longer or out-of-town trips, establish your route to and from the destination and leave a copy of directions with staff and/or parents.
- Have at least one fully charged cell phone and sufficient cash/coins for pay phones.
- Ensure that at least one child care practitioner travelling with the children has first aid training. Make sure you know the location of the nearest hospital and the best route to get there from your destination.
- Have a plug-in cooler or ice packs ready to transport food if a meal or snacks aren't being provided on site. (For more about safe food handling, see Chapter 3, *Nutrition*.)
- Plan for emergencies, especially in winter. Allow extra driving time and ensure that the vehicle is equipped with blankets, winter candles, waterproof matches, flares and any other equipment recommended by Public Safety Canada (www.getprepared.ca).
- Consider installing in-vehicle communications technology as a safety feature. By operating from a central control facility, problems such as critical assistance, direction finding and vehicle malfunctions can be more quickly reported and resolved in some locations.
- The parking lots at your destination and at rest stops are particularly risky places for toddlers. Ensure that each child is held by the hand (for smaller groups), or walked in a line with an adult leading, a spotter, and an end-of-line monitor (for larger groups).

The day of the trip

- Take attendance.
- Pack a copy of your centre's attendance forms so that there is a record of all children and adults on the trip.
- Pack a copy of the emergency medical records with the first aid kit. Carry all required medications that may be needed for any children with chronic conditions (e.g., EpiPen, Twinject, asthma inhaler).
- Assign children to supervising adults according to provincial/territorial child care regulations for group size/ratios on field trips or as specified by the destination (e.g., at a local wading pool, the adult-to-child ratio may be set at 1:2 and 1:1 for babies and children with special needs).
- Give adults a written list of the names of children in their group (ideally with photos of the children they are responsible for).
- Pair up children age 4 and older as "buddies," so they can watch out for each other. Practice buddy checks beforehand and do regular buddy checks during the trip.
- Review rules for safety and appropriate conduct with the children.
- Make sure all children are wearing their identification tags. For outings involving several groups, colour code these tags to help adult supervisors identify and track the children for whom they're responsible.
- Ensure that all necessary items are packed: extra clothing, diapers, sunscreen, water, alcohol-based hand rubs, hand-wipes, extra snacks and bottled baby food, as needed. Make sure no one has forgotten their lunch, and keep perishable food in a cooler.
- Explain to preschoolers what to do if they get lost or separated from their group. Decide on a central and recognizable meeting spot. Remind children to ask for help (from a guide, security officer or other designated adult) and to go to the meeting spot or stay in one place until an adult from the group finds them.

Transportation Safety

Using public transportation

When using a public bus, trolley or light rail, follow these guidelines:

- Maintain an appropriate adult-to-child ratio.
- Assign one adult supervisor to lead the group on and off the vehicle, a second to help children board and disembark, and a third to remain with the group waiting in line.
- Have tickets/fares/payment ready for the driver beforehand.
- If possible, keep children 5 giant steps (3 m or 10 ft.) back from where the vehicle is to pick them up.
- Watch for book bags with straps or dangling objects that can get caught on vehicle handrails or doors.
- Do a head count as soon as the group has boarded and upon disembarking to make sure no one is missing.
- Ensure that children are safely seated before the vehicle moves and that they remain seated for the entire journey.

Transportation Safety

- Remind children to follow these rules when using public transportation:
  - ➤ Face forward in your seat and don't slide around.
  - ➤ Obey the driver.
  - ➤ Speak in a quiet voice.
  - ➤ Don't dangle arms or objects out of windows.

Using a school bus

Follow all the guidelines for using public transportation above, plus:

- Know the number of passengers the vehicle is licenced to transport and make sure it isn't exceeded.
- Verify that the driver has a valid driver's licence for that class of vehicle.
- Wait until the bus stops, the door is open and the driver says it's okay, before boarding.

All newly built school buses are required to have a minimum number of seating positions equipped with lower and tether anchorages for installing appropriate car seats. This number varies according to bus size. Children weighing more than 18 kg (40 lbs.), who would use a booster seat in a car, are considered to be sufficiently protected by normal seating in a school bus.

BEST PRACTICE

Transport Canada recommends that children under the age of 4½ and/or weighing less than 18 kg (40 lbs.) be transported in an appropriate child restraint system while on a school bus.

Taking children on walks and errands

Your facility's orientation booklet should specify that short, unscheduled outings are part of the regular program, so parents know spontaneous walks will be part of their child's day. Walking around the neighbourhood, going to the playground or shopping can be opportunities for learning and exploration. Minimize the risks that come with stepping out of familiar surroundings by being organized (e.g., packing snacks and water in advance) and prepared for minor mishaps (e.g., taking bandages and alcohol-based hand-rub). Maintain an appropriate supervision ratio—a minimum of two adults should be present even when children are harnessed in a multi-seat stroller. One adult can retrieve a wandering child or attend to an ill or injured child while another stays with the stroller's other occupants. Take these steps:

- Notify other staff (or leave a note at your home setting) as to which children are on the walk, your destination and route, time of departure and estimated time of return. A standardized form or notepad can be used for this purpose.
- Take an emergency bag—containing a first aid kit and children's emergency medical records—along with water, cups, snacks, sunscreen, etc.
- Choose a route with sidewalks and avoid high traffic areas.
- Take a fully charged cell phone and sufficient cash/coins for a pay phone.
- Consider using a walking rope for toddlers and having each child hold on.

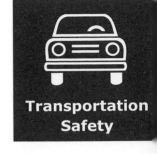
- Assign one adult to the front of the line and another to the back. Other staff may accompany children on either side, according to the appropriate adult-to-child ratio.
- Pair up children 4 years of age and older as "buddies." Practice buddy checks before the outing and do regular buddy checks during your walk.
- Take attendance periodically.
- Obey all traffic signs and cross streets only at crosswalks or traffic lights.
- Accompany children to public washrooms.

If you plan to walk with children in a **wagon** or **stroller**, check that brakes, wheels and handles are in good working order before each outing. Stroller-related injuries are all too common and usually happen because the lap belt was not in use or a child was left unattended. Before you use a stroller:

- Ensure that the stroller is sturdy and appropriate for the age, height and weight of the child.
- Make sure the stroller has a permanent label with the manufacturer's name, model number or name, date of manufacture and a warning to use the safety harness and crotch strap. Adhere to the age, height and weight specifications and the instructions for safe use at all times.
- Check that the stroller has a 5-point harness system, with belts that come down over both shoulders, two that connect at the waist, and a crotch strap.
- Make sure the harness is solidly attached to the seat or frame of the stroller. The seat should not pull away from the frame, even when you pull sharply on the lap belt.
- Make sure the wheels are fixed tightly, and that the brakes work and are easy to use.
- Make sure there are no sharp edges or tears in the upholstery, "pinch" points or sharp corners.

Carriage strollers are best for infants under 4 months old, who need to be in a reclined (almost flat) position. Do not use folding "umbrella" strollers for children this age. They don't give young infants sufficient head or neck support or recline far enough.

Any stroller made before safety regulations changed in 1985 is **not** safe.

Here are some tips for using strollers safely:

- **Never** leave a child unattended in a stroller.
- **Always** use the safety harness and crotch strap.
- **Always** use the brake when putting a child into the stroller or taking her out.
- **Never** park a stroller on a sloping surface, such as a driveway or hill.
- Before adjusting the stroller (e.g., reversing the handle), make sure a child's hands and feet are clear.
- Do not carry more than one child unless the stroller is specifically designed for it.
- Some strollers have baskets underneath for extra storage. Follow the manufacturer's guidelines for maximum weight.
- Do not hang bags or other items from a stroller. The extra weight can cause it to tip over.

- Make sure children don't overheat inside a stroller with a canopy and sides. If your facility's multi-seat stroller has no sun canopy, choose a shady route and have children wear their sun hats. Consider purchasing a sun canopy for a multi-seat stroller, provided it is made by the same manufacturer.
- Remove the child before carrying a stroller up or down stairs and when using an escalator.
- Don't tip the stroller backward and prop the handles (e.g., on a chair) to create a napping spot. A serious head injury can occur.
- Don't use pillows, folded quilts or blankets to cushion a carriage or stroller.
- Don't allow other children to play with or on a stroller.

Check your facility's stroller periodically to make sure the harness remains solidly attached and that all stroller parts are working and in good repair. (For information about walking with children who are riding tricycles or mobility toys, see Chapter 5, *Keeping Children Safe*.)

A **front baby carrier**, which keeps an infant snuggled close to your chest or stomach, may be an appropriate alternative for taking infants along on an errand or outing as long as:

- you are not using one and pushing a stroller at the same time,
- you are able to put the carrier on and take it off by yourself, and
- the carrier has shoulder and head support for the infant, as well as leg openings that are small enough to prevent the child from slipping out.

A baby must be at least 6 months old and have good head control before you can switch to a **back carrier**. Make sure that:

- the frame is padded near the baby's face,
- leg openings are small enough to prevent a baby from slipping out but big enough to prevent chafing, and
- the carrier has strong stitching and large, heavy-duty closures to prevent unintended release, and proper safety and anchor straps. These should fit snugly, not loosely.

ALERT

A back carrier is not safe for a sleeping baby, who should be moved to a crib to sleep as soon as possible.

If you are shopping with children, be aware of the dangers of **shopping carts.** Take these precautions:

- Choose a cart with a safety strap, to keep a child sitting down in the seat.
- Do not let a child ride in the basket part—it's too easy to climb on a grocery item and fall out.
- Do not allow another child to ride on the outside of a cart—it's more likely to hit something or tip over.
- Allow only one child to ride in a shopping cart unless multiple seating positions are provided.
- **Never** allow a child to stand on the seat.
- **Never** leave a child unattended in, or with, a shopping cart.

For physical and developmental reasons, children are particularly at risk as pedestrians. First, because children are small, it's harder for them to see oncoming cars and for drivers to see them. Second, they have more restricted peripheral vision than adults and are therefore less likely to notice a car approaching from the left or right. Third, young children don't yet have the ability to judge a car's speed and distance, which is required to cross the street safely. Children are also more likely to be impulsive (dashing off the sidewalk after a toy), to use intuitive logic (thinking that if they can see the driver of a car, then the driver can see them) and to act out of curiosity.

Transportation Safety

When you're out walking, remind children of these simple **road rules**, and model them yourself at all times:

- Look left-right-left for traffic at every intersection. Preschoolers can be taught to look ALL WAYS.
- Cross only when the street is clear of traffic and the signal says it's time to go.
- Keep looking for cars as you're crossing the street.
- Do not walk between parked cars.

Constant supervision in and around motor vehicles and roadways and meticulous use of appropriate child restraints are the best protections you can provide while transporting children in your care. Being a good model yourself and sharing information with parents will also help to instill a lifetime's worth of safe behaviours.

Selected resources

Aird, Laura Dutil. 2007. Moving kids safely in child care: A refresher course. *Exchange: The Early Leaders' Magazine*. www.ChildCareExchange.com

Alberta Infrastructure and Transportation. 2003. Child safety seats. www.saferoads.com

Canada Safety Council. www.safety-council.org

———. 2006. Backing up: Toddler danger.

———. 2006. Buckle up basics.

———. Hot car warning.

Canadian Child Care Federation. 2001. *Car travel with preschoolers*. Resource sheet #4. www.cccf-fcsge.ca

Health Canada. www.hc-sc.gc.ca. Consumer product safety: Children's products.

Public Health Agency of Canada. www.phac-aspc.gc.ca. Safe Healthy Environments: Safe Transport.

Public Safety Canada. www.getprepared.ca

Region of Peel (Ont.) Public Health. 2004. *Keep on track: A health and resource guide for child care providers in Peel*. Car seat safety, Turn it off: Idling gets you nowhere. www.region.peel.on.ca/health/keep-on-track/pdfs/entiremanual.pdf

Transportation Safety

Safe Kids Canada. 2004. www.safekidscanada.ca
Child passenger safety, Pedestrian safety, Product safety (Baby carriers, Strollers), Car seat and vehicle manufacturers, Rear-facing car seat, Forward-facing car seat, Booster seat; Summer—kids in hot cars; Why kids lack good judgement about traffic.

——. 2007. Kids that click; Kids that click booster seat. Brochure and DVD formats.

Transport Canada. www.tc.gc.ca

——. 2003. Infant seats are not cribs: Questions and answers.

——. 2006. Keep kids safe: Car Time, stage 1: Safe travel in a rear-facing infant seat; stage 2: Safe travel in a forward-facing child seat; stage 3: Safe travel in a booster seat; Child restraint and booster cushion notices.

——. 2006. How to protect children in vehicles with side air bags. Fact sheet.

——. 2007. Child seats on school buses.

Common Conditions

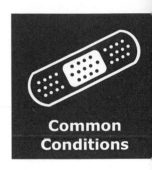

**Common
Conditions**

Each condition described in this chapter occurs frequently among babies and toddlers, either because it is a normal part of every child's development (e.g., teething) or because it is experienced by many children (e.g., colic, orthopedic conditions). Some conditions are behavioural (e.g., thumb-sucking), while others, such as diarrhea, may be a sign of infection. What these conditions have in common is that they are rarely serious and usually do not last long, but they do require appropriate management in any child care setting. It is much easier to keep children comfortable and maintain consistency in their day-to-day routines when parents and child care practitioners share information and methods of care. Here is basic information about these conditions and also some guidelines for responding to and caring for children who have them.

Colic

For an infant, crying is one form of normal self-expression that is usually—but not always—associated with hunger, fatigue or discomfort. All babies cry, and some healthy babies cry much more than others. While most infants have a fussy period once a day, commonly in the evening or early morning, some cry inconsolably for hours at a time. An infant who is fed, changed and cuddled but still cries long and hard (without a break) is considered to be "colicky." A period of longer, stronger, unexplained crying typically begins when infants are about 3 weeks old, peaks in intensity at around 6 to 8 weeks, and tends to decrease at the age of 3 to 4 months, although it can last longer. Only about 10 per cent of infants are colicky.

Although colic signals an infant's distress, it seldom indicates pain and isn't caused by parental or caregiver stress—although it can cause stress. A very small percentage of babies who cry excessively may have an underlying illness or other medical condition. There is little evidence that prolonged crying is caused by gas, wind or sensitivity to cow's milk protein. In fact, crying causes infants to swallow air, which can look like a digestive problem when they burp or pass wind.

It is stressful being responsible for a baby who cannot be comforted, especially when there are other children needing your care.

What you can do

While dealing with colic is always demanding, adopting and maintaining a routine for prolonged crying episodes can make life easier for all concerned. Discuss coping techniques with the baby's parents to find out what, if anything, works for them. After ruling out other causes for a baby's crying, such as hunger or a soiled diaper, there are some soothing techniques you can both try:

- Respond quickly to the infant's cries. Pick her up and rock her gently. Although movement can be an effective means to soothe a baby, too much handling, patting or passing the baby from person to person can have the opposite effect.
- Try placing the baby face-down along your arm, with a steadying hand between her legs and her head at your elbow. Hold her in place with your other hand and rock her gently.
- Wrap the infant snugly in a blanket and cradle her comfortably.
- In general, the more a baby is carried and held, the less she cries. Try using an infant carrier or sling.
- Try the steady, smooth motion of a rocking chair and lower light levels, which can be soothing.
- Try putting her in a stroller, going for a walk outdoors or using a gentle back-and-forth motion indoors.
- Distract her with soft music or white noise (e.g., an air cleaner, running water, static or a gentle "shushing" noise), which sometimes has a calming effect.

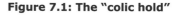
Figure 7.1: The "colic hold"

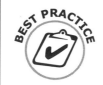

- During periods of intense crying, take turns soothing a colicky infant with another child care practitioner. Spelling one another off can help.

- If you are working alone in a home setting, place the infant in her crib for short intervals. Reading to other children or doing a quiet activity within sight of the crib may be calming.

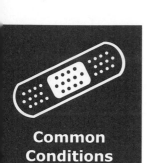

Common Conditions

Constipation

A baby or child is constipated when stools are hard, infrequent, or difficult or painful to pass. Having infrequent bowel movements alone doesn't indicate constipation. Stool patterns vary widely from infant to infant and vary even more if a child is breastfed rather than formula-fed. Breastfed infants may have a bowel movement following every feeding in the first few weeks of life and only once every 5 days when they get older. Both patterns are normal. Formula-fed infants tend to pass stools less often, usually once a day. Constipation is rare in infants and isn't caused by the iron levels in baby formula.

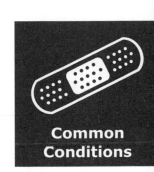

Common Conditions

Many young infants appear to have difficulty with bowel movements. They grunt and groan, raise their legs, cry, turn red and push hard, but nothing may come for a while. This behaviour usually isn't a sign of constipation, but a learning process involving a baby's reflex actions and control of developing intestinal and abdominal muscles. An infant is constipated only if his stool is hard and dry.

Older children's bowel movements also vary widely in number and type from day to day, and going a few days without having one can be normal for many children. The main cause of constipation in older children relates to diet. A baby or toddler who is drinking more milk than recommended may not be eating enough fibre to help keep bowels functioning well. Occasionally, a toddler or preschooler will become constipated from withholding stool. He might do this because he is having difficulty learning to use the toilet or because he has anal pain either from passing a large stool or from a fissure or tear. Withholding stool can lead to chronic constipation.

While constipation is not dangerous and is only rarely a sign of a medical problem, it can cause discomfort either from abdominal cramping or from anal pain when passing a large stool. Chronic constipation, which occurs in about one in six children, may also persist into adulthood.

What you can do

Your role is to help prevent constipation. By paying attention to changes in a child's bowel movements, you can also help detect constipation early. Report any signs of discomfort, straining or hard stools to a child's parents and review his diet together. Common dietary contributors to constipation are:

- not enough dietary fibre,
- not enough water,
- too much milk.

If you adjust for these factors and constipation persists, advise parents to visit their doctor or consult a nutritionist, who will usually recommend adding strained vegetables and fruits (for babies) and offering more raw fruit and vegetables (for older children) to encourage softer stools. Diet can often be improved by increasing fibre and water intake and by limiting juice and milk products to recommended portions. Prune, apple and pear juices contain sorbitol, which sometimes helps to increase stool frequency. Avoid adding foods to (or removing foods from) any child's diet without consulting parents first. For a time, keeping an "at home" and "in care" record of the child's bowel movements, as well as what he is eating and drinking, will help monitor improvement.

If constipation develops while a child is learning to use the toilet, the cause may be more behavioural than dietary. You and the child's parents should revisit approaches to toilet learning. Make sure you aren't rushing the child, and that he is given regular, unhurried opportunities to go to the bathroom, and a comfortable potty that allows him to place his feet on the floor to push. (For more about toilet learning, see page 298.)

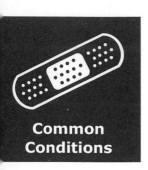

Common Conditions

If you see blood spotting on toilet tissue after wiping and suspect that a child has an anal fissure, ask parents to consult their doctor. A stool softener and/or an ointment to decrease pain and promote healing may be prescribed. Chronic constipation may be treated with medication. Never administer a laxative unless it is:

- recommended in writing by a doctor,
- consented to in writing by parents, and
- given in strict accordance with instructions.

(See Appendix 7.1 for a sample *Medication consent form and record sheet*.)

Cradle cap

Cradle cap, which occurs only in infants, is a layer of thick, greasy or flaky scales on the baby's scalp. It's the result of normal changes in an infant's skin and doesn't indicate lack of care. Cradle cap will go away on its own and does not need to be treated. You may also notice redness on other parts of an infant's body, such as in neck creases, armpits, behind the ears, on the face or in the diaper area. This is called seborrheic dermatitis, a condition that, like cradle cap, usually disappears on its own.

What you can do
In child care, it's best to leave cradle cap alone and not attempt to remove scales. Parents can choose to treat it with mineral oil followed by a gentle shampoo, but over-bathing or shampooing often aggravates cradle cap. If a baby has seborrheic dermatitis, a doctor may recommend treatment with a mild (0.5–1.0%) corticosteroid cream. Be sure to obtain the requisite parental permission and follow specific instructions if this treatment needs to be applied while the infant is in your care. (See Appendix 7.1 for a sample *Medication consent form and record sheet*.)

Diaper rash

Diaper rash, also called diaper dermatitis, is caused by the reaction of a baby's skin to wet or soiled diapers. It also occurs when organisms in urine or stool in the diaper irritate a baby's skin, making it inflamed, tender and red. Soap residues can further irritate this condition. Some babies have very sensitive skin and will quickly develop a tender rash, while other babies never do.

Diaper rash can also be caused by *Candida*, a type of yeast that is naturally present in the intestines without causing illness. When *Candida* causes diaper rash, it tends to be in the deepest creases of a baby's groin or buttocks. The rash is usually very red, with small red spots close to large, defined patches. When this yeast infection occurs in a child's mouth, it's called thrush. *Candida* skin infections need to be treated with an antifungal medication prescribed by a doctor and applied to the skin. Be sure to obtain the requisite parental permission and follow specific instructions if this treatment is to be applied while the child is in your care. (For more about thrush and *Candida* diaper rash, see Chapter 9, *Managing Infections*.)

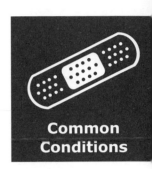

Common Conditions

What you can do

To prevent a rash, change a baby's diaper often. Be particularly vigilant when a child has diarrhea. The stools associated with diarrhea can be acidic and burn the skin, making it more prone to irritation.

When a baby develops a diaper rash, you can help with treatment:

- When changing diapers, wash the baby's bottom with mild soap and warm water (just water if there is no stool), rinse and pat dry thoroughly, especially after a bowel movement.
- Ask parents about using an unscented barrier ointment, such as petroleum jelly or a cream with zinc oxide, to protect and lubricate the area after each diaper change. If using a cream, remove it thoroughly with soap and water after each change. Creams and ointments should **not** be shared among children.
- Using wipes can dry out a baby's tender skin. Suggest to parents that wipes should be alcohol-free.
- Do not use baby powder or talc.
- If possible, keep the baby's diaper off for short periods to expose skin to the open air. This may ease inflammation, help the child feel better and speed healing.

If a diaper rash is severe, a doctor may prescribe a mild (0.5–1.0%) corticosteroid cream. Be sure to obtain the requisite parental permission and follow specific instructions if this treatment needs to be applied while the infant is in your care. (See Appendix 7.1 for a sample *Medication consent form and record sheet*.)

Diarrhea

A child has diarrhea when there are more bowel movements **and** the stools are more liquid and watery than usual. Diarrhea is usually mild and brief, lasting less than a week. Mild diarrhea, with a few loose stools on a single day, may be caused by a dietary change or a high intake of fluids, especially fruit juice (so-called "toddler's diarrhea"). It can also be a side effect of some antibiotics. However, infectious diarrhea can strike rapidly in child care settings and needs careful management.

What you can do

If a child's diarrhea is accompanied by other signs of illness, such as fever or vomiting, notify parents for an early pick-up and start giving an oral rehydration (electrolyte) solution (ORS) to prevent dehydration as soon as possible. Although these solutions are usually available as frozen pops, ready-to-serve preparations or powders, they are considered medications and parental consent is needed before you can give them. (See Appendix 7.1 for a sample *Medication consent form and record sheet*.)

Mild to moderate dehydration can be managed with ORS in combination with a child's normal food intake, including breast milk. However, **an ill child with diarrhea and/or vomiting should be taken home as soon as possible, while all hand hygiene, diapering, toileting and food preparation routines are reviewed and reinforced with staff.** Advise parents to consult their doctor or to go to hospital if diarrhea is severe, persists for longer than a week, seems to contain blood, or if vomiting persists over a period of 4 to 6 hours in spite of giving ORS. (See also Chapter 9, *Managing Infections*.)

BEST PRACTICE

- **Do not offer** over-the-counter medications to stop diarrhea. These can mask symptoms and even prevent the body from getting rid of infection.

- **Do not offer** sugary drinks, fruit juice, pop, gelatin, sweet tea, broth, rice water or any other home-made rehydration solution. These liquids can make diarrhea worse.

Drooling

Babies drool because they haven't yet developed the ability to swallow the saliva they produce. Sucking stimulates saliva production, and babies who suck a lot on their fist or thumb tend to drool more than others. Sometimes a baby gets a rash around the mouth or chin from saliva, if drool remains in contact with the skin for a prolonged period (e.g., during sleep). Babies also tend to drool more heavily when they are teething. A baby holding her mouth open frequently or for longer than usual because of a sore mouth, throat or other infection will drool more heavily. Drooling rarely signals a problem, although it can help spread certain infections in a child care setting. (See Chapter 9, *Managing Infections*.) New drooling might indicate that something has become lodged in a child's throat.

What you can do

Pat—don't rub—a baby's face to wipe away drool. If a child develops a rash, ask parents about applying a barrier cream to the affected area.

REMEMBER

Put on disposable gloves:

- before you clean the face of a child with cold sores who is drooling,

- if you have a lesion on your own hands that might come into contact with the drool of a child who has an infection.

Encourage kissing on the cheek, not on the mouth.

Eczema

Eczema is a common childhood skin disorder that shows up as a red, patchy, scaly rash or as tiny red bumps that can blister, ooze or become infected if scratched. In babies, eczema

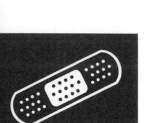

Common Conditions

usually appears on the forehead, cheeks or scalp, although it can spread to the arms, legs, chest or other parts of the body. In older children, it tends to localize in the creases of the elbows and knees, on the neck and behind the ears. The rash may be moist and weepy or dry and scaly, and is usually very itchy. Often, though not always, eczema occurs in children who have other allergic conditions, such as asthma or hay fever, or where there's a family history of allergy or eczema. In a small proportion of children, eczema can be aggravated by certain foods or environmental factors, including the weather. While there is no cure for eczema, it can usually be controlled and often will go away after several months. Half of children with eczema will outgrow this condition by adulthood.

What you can do

Alert the child's parents to any sign of rash and ask them to see their doctor for a diagnosis. Together, you and the family can take steps to protect the child's skin from irritants that tend to aggravate eczema and provoke more itching and scratching. Help parents take the following preventive measures:

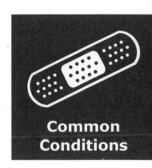

**Common
Conditions**

- Avoid wool or synthetic clothing—loose cotton layers breathe better.
- Take care not to overdress the child—sweating can irritate eczema.
- Use only mild soaps, and avoid bleach, harsh detergents or fabric softeners when laundering children's clothing or bed linens.
- Keep the air in your child care facility's sleeping area slightly cool.
- Don't bath too frequently or too long (more than 10 minutes). If you do bath children in your care, add non-allergenic oil to the bathwater. Afterward, apply a thin coating of petroleum jelly all over a baby's body. Apply a gentle, unscented moisturizing cream all over a toddler's or preschooler's body while the skin is still moist.
- Apply a non-perfumed hydrating cream or lotion daily, or as needed.

A doctor may prescribe an anti-inflammatory ointment or cream, usually a corticosteroid, to treat eczema. For older children, taking an antihistamine to relieve itching may also be recommended. Be sure to obtain the requisite parental permissions to give these medications and follow all instructions. (See Appendix 7.1 for a sample *Medication consent form and record sheet*.)

Enuresis

Enuresis is involuntary urination. This condition is called "nocturnal enuresis" when a child wets the bed at night while asleep and "diurnal enuresis" when a child wets while awake during the day. Although most children become "dry" and are able to use the toilet between 2 and 4 years of age, approximately 20 per cent still wet the bed at night at age 4. Bladder control in children develops at different rates, just as the ability to crawl or walk does. **Let parents know that nocturnal enuresis tends to run in families and doesn't mean there is something wrong with their child.**

When a child who has been dry for at least 6 months begins to wet again, it's called "secondary enuresis." This is often the result of a new stress in that child's life, such as the birth of a sibling, a family death or divorce. "Secondary enuresis" almost always occurs at night and usually stops by itself with time. If the loss of control of urine starts to occur during the day, it could be the signal of an underlying illness, such as a urinary tract infection.

What you can do

Alert a child's parents to any new daytime wetting. Often, this happens because the child holds in urine for too long. A child 4 years of age or older who wets on most days should see a doctor. A child who has been dry for 6 months but begins wetting again should see a doctor regardless of age. Here are some strategies for dealing with daytime wetting:

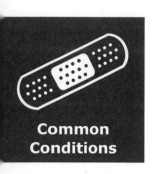

Common Conditions

- Offer lots of opportunities for using the bathroom and encourage children to say they "need to go," even in the middle of an activity.
- Pay attention to how often a child uses the toilet and encourage him not to wait too long between visits.
- Don't offer water just before bedtime, and have him try to use the bathroom before a nap.
- Require that parents keep you supplied with one or two complete changes of clothes.
- When a child does wet, quickly help him change his clothes. Respect his right to privacy, and let him know you understand and that he isn't at fault.
- Teach the other children in your care to be understanding and don't allow any teasing.
- For sleeping, use a hospital-strength plastic mattress cover and mattress and place a large towel underneath the sheet for extra absorption.

If the child is old enough, involve him in cleaning up after an "accident." This can help him feel more in control.

Gastroesophageal reflux

Gastroesophageal reflux (GER), regurgitation or "spitting up" is one of the most common infant conditions: all babies spit up to some extent. Reflux happens because the ring of muscle surrounding an infant's esophagus as it enters the stomach is still "immature" in the first months of life. When infants burp up swallowed air, breast milk or formula escapes at the same time because this muscle is weak. Spitting up may go on for hours after a feeding. It usually decreases as an infant gets older and this muscle ring gets stronger.

In rare cases, a baby has gastroesophageal reflux disease or GERD, which occurs when additional stomach contents leak back, or reflux, into the esophagus. GERD can cause repeated vomiting, excessive irritability, coughing and other respiratory problems. GERD is caused by an immature digestive system. Most babies grow out of the condition by the time they are 1 year of age.

Spitting up is rarely an indication that a baby has an allergy or intolerance to any food, breast milk or formula. Only rarely will an infant bring up enough milk or formula to reduce caloric intake and slow normal weight gain. Parents will need to discuss severe spitting up with a doctor if it persists past a child's first birthday, if their child resists normal feeding or if the reflux is green in colour.

What you can do

When you are bottle-feeding an infant, burp him every 3 to 5 minutes. Avoid laying him down immediately after a feeding. Avoid putting a baby into a seat or swing right after a feeding—it increases the likelihood of spitting up because of pressure on the stomach. Be sure to consult with parents before adjusting the child's feeding routine.

Hiccups

Hiccupping is caused by a sudden spasm of the diaphragm. Almost all healthy infants and children get hiccups. They are completely harmless and are not caused by indigestion, gas or any physical problem. They seldom upset the child.

What you can do

Usually, absolutely nothing. If hiccups are interfering with infant feeding, take a break and try burping her. If a toddler or preschooler has hiccups and seems uncomfortable, tricks like holding her breath or drinking from the back rim of a cup sometimes help.

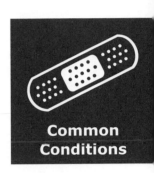

Common Conditions

Orthopedic conditions

Some children are born with a mild orthopedic condition or develop one as they grow.

- A **club foot** is diagnosed at birth. It is usually an isolated condition but may also be associated with a neuromuscular disorder.
- **Developmental dysplasia** of the hip, which causes an unstable hip joint, is also usually detected at birth.

Both conditions need to be cared for by an orthopedic surgeon and normally require treatment with casts, splints and, occasionally, surgery.

Other orthopedic conditions may develop as children grow:

- **Toe-walking**: A child's tendency to walk toward the front of the foot often happens when the heel cord (Achilles tendon) is abnormally tight, as in the case of children with cerebral palsy or spinal cord problems. They are usually in a doctor's care and treated accordingly. If toe-walking seems more habitual than physical, advise parents to consult their doctor.
- **Flat feet**: Children under 3 years of age normally have a fat pad under the arch of each foot, making their feet look flat. Most children with mild or moderate flat feet don't need treatment. Older children may need to wear arch supports in their shoes. If having flat feet is causing leg pain, the child should be seen by a doctor.
- **In-toeing**: A rigid, inward-pointing forefoot is usually detectable in infancy and treated by physiotherapy or corrected with a cast. Other forms of in-toeing (e.g., pigeon-toe) rarely require treatment and are usually outgrown.
- **Out-toeing**: Many children walk in a slightly out-toed position. This usually improves with time and doesn't require intervention.
- **Limping**: In a typically developing child, the appearance of a limp is a sign that

something is wrong and requires investigation by a doctor. If a child with a chronic orthopedic condition develops a new limp or weakness, this also needs to be investigated.

What you can do

Be familiar with the stages of physical development and alert parents if you have concerns about their child's progress. Your observations may help their doctor diagnose a problem.

Teething

Teething refers to the emergence of a child's first set of teeth through the gums. On average, babies get their first tooth at around 6 months of age, although that first tooth can emerge as early as 3 months or as late as 1 year of age. The first teeth to emerge are usually the central incisors—the two top front and bottom teeth—followed by the lateral incisors and the canines and molars. (See Figure 4.1, page 54.) For most babies, teething is painless. However, some children experience minimal discomfort, particularly when the canines and molars are coming in.

Signs that a baby is teething include drooling (and possibly a face rash caused by saliva), more gumming of toys or other objects, irritability, waking at night, and some gum redness and swelling.

ALERT

Fever, diarrhea, prolonged crying, a runny nose or coughing are **not** associated with teething, but they are signs of infection and need to be monitored accordingly.

Don't use teething gels that are rubbed on the gums. They can lower a child's gag reflex, may cause an allergic reaction and are not safe to swallow.

What you can do

You can help relieve the discomfort of teething by applying pressure or cold (or both) to the gums. Offer the baby a clean, chilled, wet washcloth or a cold teething ring to chew on. Some babies appreciate having their gums rubbed with a clean finger. Don't offer a baby teething biscuits, as they usually contain sugar. If a child is in pain, a medication like acetaminophen can help. Be sure to obtain specific parental permission before giving it. (See Appendix 7.1 for a sample *Medication consent form and record sheet*.)

Thumb-sucking

Sucking a thumb (or fingers or a fist) is a favourite baby activity and a normal part of healthy development. Infants not only suck for nourishment; they suck for pleasure and to soothe themselves. Many babies continue to suck long after they have been weaned and stop on their own some time during early childhood. The relationship between thumb-sucking and dental problems begins to appear only at 4 to 5 years of age, when permanent teeth begin to come in. Most children do no damage to their teeth unless they are still sucking vigorously after 5 years of age.

What you can do

Don't discourage thumb-sucking, which is a means of self-soothing for babies. If a child is 4 to 5 years old and parents have decided to discourage thumb-sucking, some behavioural strategies may help. A parent might explain how thumb-sucking can damage teeth and choose a low-stress period of time to help their child gradually break the habit. You can reinforce this process by offering the child emotional encouragement, distractions and small rewards for not sucking her thumb.

Rites of passage

All these conditions are common enough that you are sure to encounter them in child care more than once and perhaps many times. Each encounter is likely to be unique, not only because a condition may be more or less serious but because each child is different. Being sensitive to how a child experiences her condition, how she is coping, and whether a condition seems more persistent or problematic than usual can be a challenge. Yet responding personally to each child's needs can be richly rewarding if you and the family work together to help that child feel better or simply get past one of life's early hurdles.

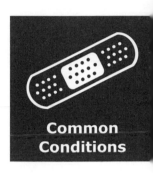

Common Conditions

Selected resources

General

The Canadian Paediatric Society's website for parents and caregivers, Caring for Kids, has information on conditions described in this chapter. Parent notes can be downloaded at www.caringforkids.cps.ca, reproduced and shared with families.

Saunders, Norman and Jeremy Friedman, eds. 2006. *Caring for Kids: The Complete Canadian Guide to Children's Health*. Toronto, Ont.: Key Porter.

Colic

Canadian Paediatric Society. 2008. Colic and crying. Brochure and parent note.

———. 2002. Never Shake a baby. Brochure and parent note.

Centres of Excellence for Children's Well-Being, Early Childhood Development. 2007. *Bulletin* 6(2). This issue is dedicated to crying behaviours.

Constipation

Canadian Paediatric Society. 2008. Healthy bowel habits for children. Brochure and parent note.

———. 2008. Toilet learning. Brochure and parent note.

HealthLink Alberta. 2005. Constipation in Toddlers 1-3 years. www.healthlinkalberta.ca

Diaper rash

Canadian Paediatric Society. 2006. Skin care for your baby. Brochure and parent note.

Diarrhea

Canadian Paediatric Society. 2008. Common infections and your child. Brochure and parent note.

———. 2006. Diarrhea in children: Prevention and treatment. Brochure and parent note.

Drooling

Hospital for Sick Children. 2004. Drooling (excessive). www.aboutkidshealth.ca

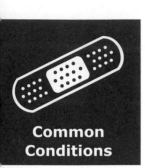

Common Conditions

Eczema

Canadian Dermatology Association. www.dermatology.ca

Canadian Paediatric Society. 2006. Skin care for your baby. Brochure and parent note.

Eczema Society of Canada. www.eczemahelp.ca

Enuresis (bedwetting)

Canadian Paediatric Society. 2008. Bedwetting. Brochure and parent note.

Government of Ontario, Ministry of Health Promotion. Bedwetting. www.healthyontario.com

Hospital for Sick Children. 2004. Bed-wetting (Enuresis). www.aboutkidshealth.ca

Manitoba Health. *Bed-wetting*. www.gov.mb.ca

Gastroesophageal reflux (spitting up)

American Academy of Pediatrics (AAP). www.aap.org

Children's Digestive Health and Nutrition Foundation. www.KidsAcidReflux.org or www.CDHNF.org

Government of Ontario, Ministry of Health Promotion. Gastroesophageal reflux. www.healthyontario.com

North American Society for Pediatric Gastroenterology, Hepatology and Nutrition. www.NASPGHAN.org

Thumb-sucking

Hospital for Sick Children. 2004. Thumbsucking. www.aboutkidshealth.ca

Appendix 7.1: Medication consent form and record sheet

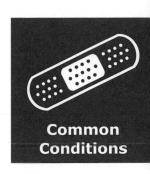

Common Conditions

Program name / logo

Name of child: _____

Date: _____

I: To be completed by child's parent or guardian

I, _____ [parent or guardian's name], give permission

for _____ [child's name] to be given the following

medication by child care staff according to instructions stated below.

Parent/guardian's signature: _____

Name of medication: _____

_____

Amount(s) to be given: _____

Dates(s) to be given [at child care]: _____

_____

Time(s) to be given: _____

_____

Name, address and phone number for child care centre or home setting

Special instructions: _____

_____

Storage: _____

_____

Start date: _____ End date: _____

My child received _____ [number] doses at home.

Are there any possible side effects from the medication? Please specify: _____

_____

_____

_____

Stop medication if the following reaction(s) is observed: _____

_____

II: To be completed by child care practitioner when the medication is given

Date	Time(s)	Amount	Given by (initials)

Comments: _____

_____

Name, address and phone number for child care centre or home setting

Common Conditions

chapter

8

Preventing
Infections

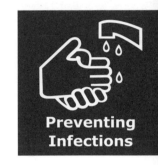

**Preventing
Infections**

Protecting young children against infections is an everyday process with special challenges. Children's immune systems are still developing, which means they are more vulnerable to infection when exposed to new germs. Also, young children are far more likely to transmit an infection in a group setting by doing what comes naturally to them—mouthing toys, sharing utensils, playing closely with other children, holding hands, drooling and sometimes forgetting to wash their hands.

Health promotion is a key part of quality child care. Keeping children healthy involves establishing and following precautionary routines every day to prevent the spread of infection—but to be effective these routines need to be well communicated, understood and enforced. This chapter sets out general protocols and guidelines for preventing infection, while Chapter 9 outlines what to do to reduce the spread of infection when children are ill. Although it's not possible to prevent all infections, reducing their frequency benefits children, caregivers and parents alike—resulting in less physical discomfort, fewer disruptions to programming, and fewer sick days lost by parents and staff.

How infections spread

Children enrolled in child care programs tend to get more infections in early childhood than children cared for at home. Not only are they exposed to more new germs, but the risk of infection is increased by common interactions:

- Large numbers of children from different families spend many hours together in one place most days of the week. Young children who might be infectious (carrying germs that can spread) mix with others who are susceptible (likely to get sick because these germs are new). The more children you have in a group, the more potential contact there is between infectious and susceptible children.
- Children touch each other often when they play. Babies and toddlers who are crawling or walking have more opportunities to transmit infection than infants who are not yet mobile.
- Young children explore by putting things in their mouths, and other children share or touch those objects.
- Young children, especially those under 2 years of age, are just beginning to develop good hygiene. Developmentally, they may or may not be ready for toilet learning, they may drool, they can't always cover their mouth or nose when they cough or sneeze, and they may not be able to wash their own hands or remember to do so.
- Children who are still in diapers can spread certain infections much more readily than children who are toilet trained.
- Young children need a lot of hands-on care by staff, who may inadvertently transmit an infection if they don't wash their hands properly before turning their attention to other children.

Figure 8.1: The chain of infection

Infection spreads through a chain with four main links:

Germs (e.g., viruses or bacteria)

Infectious child or caregiver

Route of transmission (e.g., how germs travel from person to person)

Susceptible child or caregiver

1. Germs

Germs are viruses, bacteria, parasites or fungi that may produce an infection. Visible only under a microscope, some germs (micro-organisms) can survive for hours or even days under the right conditions. For example, the influenza virus can survive 5 minutes on human skin, 12 hours on cloth, and up to 48 hours on a smooth surface such as a countertop or plastic toy.

Not all germs are harmful. "Good bugs," which normally live in our throat, intestines or on the skin, actually help us fight "bad bugs," which cause disease.

REMEMBER

Antibiotics can destroy good germs as well as bad ones, and need to be used carefully—only taken when necessary, as prescribed by a doctor, and only given as directed.

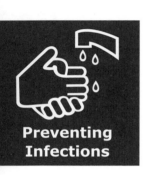

Preventing Infections

2. Infectious child or caregiver

The person with an infection may or may not show signs of illness. In general, people who are ill are more infectious. They carry more germs and—as with the common cold—are likely to cough and sneeze often. However, it's also common for children who don't yet show signs of illness to be infectious before the illness begins (e.g., as with chickenpox) or to remain asymptomatic (never show any sign of illness) even though they are infected (e.g., hepatitis A).

3. Route of transmission

The "route of transmission" means the way germs get from one person to another (e.g., by touching contaminated surfaces or toys, or by floating through the air).

Figure 8.2: Contact transmission of germs

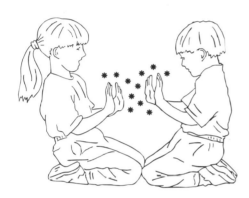 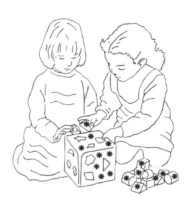

Direct contact   Indirect contact

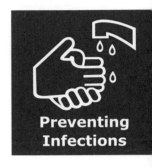

Preventing Infections

In **direct contact transmission**, a person carrying germs in the nose, mouth, eyes, stool or skin lesions usually contaminates her hands, then spreads these germs by touching or being touched by others. In **indirect contact transmission**, an infected person transfers germs by touching or mouthing an object—such as a toy, a doorknob or a used tissue—that is then touched by another person. Once germs are on another's hands, they can cause infection when this person touches her eyes, nose or mouth.

Respiratory viruses (e.g., the common cold) can live on objects for several hours and transfer to the hands of children who touch the objects. Fungal infections, such as ringworm, can also spread this way.

Infections are sometimes spread through **direct or indirect contact with blood**. Blood-borne viruses such as hepatitis B, hepatitis C and human immunodeficiency virus (HIV)

ALERT

Rotavirus, the most common cause of infectious diarrhea in young children, is usually spread through indirect contact. This virus can survive for long periods on hard surfaces, in contaminated water and on hands.

can spread through **direct contact** with blood, specifically when an infected person's blood comes into contact with an open skin lesion or the lining (mucous membrane) in the mouth, nose or eyes of another person. A needlestick injury (e.g., when someone picks up or steps on a discarded needle) can also cause direct contact transmission. **Indirect contact** transmission may occur if a person touches blood while cleaning up a spill, then touches an open skin lesion with a contaminated hand.

Biting may expose children to germs. Both a biting child and a bitten child are at risk. Usually, the bites of young children cause bruising or minor wounds but don't break the skin. However, bites that cause bleeding could transmit infection and should be promptly reported to your local public health unit. (For more about blood-borne infections and responding to bites, see Chapter 9, *Managing Infections*, pages 212–16.)

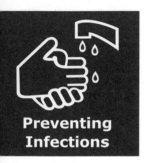

Preventing Infections

Figure 8.3: Droplet and airborne transmission of germs

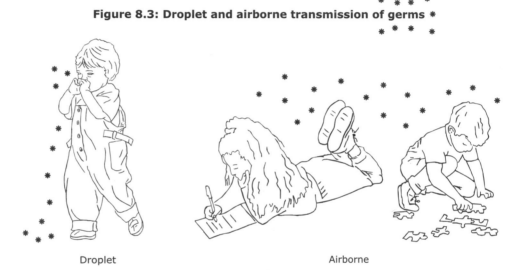

Droplet   Airborne

In **droplet transmission**, germs in the nose or throat of an infected person are expelled as droplets when a cough or sneeze isn't covered. They can transfer to another person up to 1 m (3 ft.) (and sometimes farther) away. While these germs don't stay in the air for long, they're heavy and contain enough water to fall onto surfaces, where they can live quite a long time. Many viral respiratory infections (e.g., colds and influenza) and some serious bacterial infections (e.g., pertussis) spread this way.

Airborne transmission occurs when germs stay in the air as particles carried on air currents—sometimes over a considerable time and distance—to infect people farther than 1 m (3 ft.) away from the infected person, or even in other rooms. Chickenpox and measles viruses spread this way.

Common vehicle transmission refers to the spread of infection by contaminated products, usually food or water, which are distributed to many people. Food may be contaminated at the source by the producer or manufacturer, or by an infected person when preparing or handling it.

Many food sources normally contain low levels of bacteria, which do not cause harm but can grow to dangerous levels if food is not stored and prepared properly. In child care settings, unsafe food-handling practices are the most frequent cause of food contamination.

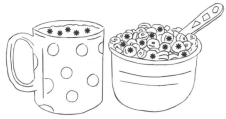

Figure 8.4: Common vehicle transmission of germs

Vector-borne transmission occurs when insects—acting as "vectors" or carriers—transfer infectious germs to humans. Some germs live inside insects. For example, West Nile virus is not transmitted from person to person. Instead, mosquitoes spread West Nile virus by biting an infected bird, growing the virus in their saliva, then injecting it into humans when they bite. Other germs are carried from place to place on the insect (e.g., flies may carry germs from garbage to food).

Figure 8.5: Vector-borne transmission of germs

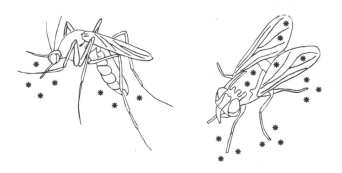

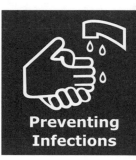

Preventing Infections

4. Susceptible child or caregiver

Germs usually enter the body through the mucous membrane in the nose or eyes, through the mouth, through the lungs, or through a cut or sore. Fortunately, the body's natural defences stop most germs. These defences include the skin, the immune system, and the acids in the human stomach. A person's state of health, age, previous exposure to infection and immunization status will affect the likelihood of infection if exposure occurs. If children have a weakened immune system (e.g., because of a chronic illness), they're at higher risk of both getting an infection and experiencing more serious illness or complications when they do.

Factors influencing the transmission of infection

Important factors that influence the exposure rate and spread of infection in child care settings include group size and the ages of children grouped together, the child-to-adult ratio, and staff orientation and in-service training. Generally, children are healthier when groups are small, when children in groups are close in age, and child-to-adult ratios reflect best practice. Environmental factors that can help or hinder the spread of infection include the physical layout of a centre or home (e.g., the size and placement of rooms, the number and accessibility of sinks and toilets, cot and crib spacing), and whether a facility is clean and properly ventilated.

10 steps for infection prevention and control

Just one exposure to germs can be enough to spread an infection. But children will stay healthier if all staff know and practice appropriate hand-hygiene, diaper-changing and toileting routines. The keys to keeping everybody in your program healthy are consistency and thoroughness in daily routines—especially frequent, thorough handwashing.

1. Practice and promote hand hygiene

Hand hygiene—washing thoroughly with soap and water or cleaning with an alcohol-based hand rub—is the single most effective strategy for both preventing infection in any community setting and stopping its spread once infection is present. In child care facilities or home settings, adults and children must:

- practice proper hand hygiene at all times,
- be reminded about washing or cleaning hands more often whenever infection is present, and
- be monitored for hand-hygiene compliance if an outbreak has occurred.

To wash a baby's hands, or the hands of any child too young to use the sink, use a wet, single-use cloth and soap. Rinse, and dry with a single-use towel (or a towel designated for that baby).

Teach toddlers to wash their hands in a relaxed and fun way, for at least 15 to 30 seconds whether their hands are visibly dirty or not. Singing the alphabet or a handwashing

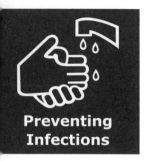

Preventing Infections

The golden rules for preventing and controlling infection

1. Practice and promote hand hygiene
2. Have a written illness policy for children and staff
3. Observe children daily for signs of infection and share concerns and information with parents
4. Require children and staff to be fully immunized, on schedule, and keep up-to-date vaccine records on file.
5. Follow proper diapering and toileting routines
6. Institute routine practices to prevent infection
7. Keep physical environments clean
8. Ensure routine practices are followed when cleaning up and disinfecting blood or body fluid spills
9. Follow food safety standards
10. Limit contact with animals, and control pests

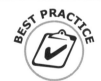

BEST PRACTICE

Hand hygiene is the single most effective way to prevent infection and stop its spread once it is present. An adult should always help children wash their hands until they've mastered this skill for themselves.

Handwashing songs

Twinkle, twinkle little star,
Look how clean my two hands are.
Soap and water, wash and scrub.
Get those germs off rub-a-dub dub.
Twinkle, twinkle little star,
Look how clean my two hands are.

Wash, wash, wash your hands
After work and play
Scrub, rinse, shake and dry
Keep the germs away.

song can be a motivator for both of you, and is easy to incorporate into hand-hygiene routines. Children should wash until they finish singing both songs, especially if their hands are visibly dirty.

The following guidelines for the "how" and "when" of proper hand hygiene apply to both children and staff.

How to wash hands with soap and water

1. Turn on taps and wet hands from wrists to fingertips. Leave the water running. It isn't necessary for the water to be hot because water temperature doesn't matter as much as rubbing (friction) for cleaning hands. Apply liquid soap and lather well.

2. Wash hands thoroughly, including the backs and between the fingers, for 10 to 15 seconds. Rubbing removes germs. Don't use or share a nailbrush, which can spread germs. Ask parents to keep children's nails trimmed.

3. Rinse hands under running water for 5 to 10 seconds.

4. If you don't have elbow faucets, turn off taps with a disposable paper towel.

5. Dry hands on a second paper towel or personal cloth towel.

6. Dispose of paper towels in a foot-activated, plastic-lined and covered garbage container **or** hang a personal cloth towel back on its own hook to dry.

7. Ensure that staff use hand lotion after washing. Skin cracks trap germs that can be passed along to others.

Using personal cloth towels in child care is feasible **only** if they're:

- clearly labelled with a person's name,

- hung separately (without touching),

- not shared,

- changed daily, and

- laundered, preferably every day (to prevent mould) in hot soapy water.

Having towels designated for individual children and staff may be more workable and enforceable in a home setting. Even then, you may need to switch to using disposable paper towels exclusively when there's an outbreak of infection.

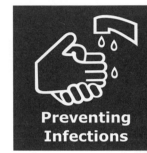

Preventing Infections

Soap: A mild, liquid soap in a dispenser works best. **Germicidal or antimicrobial hand soaps are not necessary.** Although these products are used in hospitals, they kill both helpful and harmful bacteria and are **not** recommended for any child care setting. Bar soap is shared by too many hands and may spread germs. Germs can also grow on the bar and in the soap dish. Bar soap is **not** recommended in child care.

 Either discard and replace your soap dispenser when it is empty or clean and refill it. **Don't top it up** with fresh soap—this practice has been shown to spread germs. For the same reason, make hand lotion available in pump containers that can be discarded and replaced or washed and dried before refilling.

Alcohol-based hand rubs: Waterless hand rubs are the preferred cleaning agent in health care settings but are not recommended for routine use in child care. However, hand rubs are useful when a sink or running water isn't available. For outings or picnics, they can be carried in a pocket and used anywhere at any time. Be sure to choose a product that is alcohol-based. Some waterless hand cleaners don't contain alcohol and won't destroy germs. Because they contain 60 to 90 per cent alcohol, hand rubs are a fire hazard and can be harmful to children if swallowed. Keep them safely out of reach, avoid contact with eyes and, because hand rubs are flammable, make sure hands are dry before moving on to the next activity.

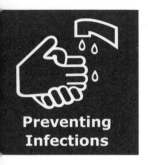

Preventing Infections

How to wash hands with an alcohol-based hand rub

1. Put about 2.5 mL (½ tsp.) onto your palm. Rub your hands together over all surfaces —paying special attention to backs of hands, between fingers, fingernails, thumbs and wrists—until hands are dry, usually 10 to 15 seconds.

2. For young children, dispense the rub into your own hands, then rub the surfaces of a child's hands between yours.

3. For visibly dirty hands, use paper towels or disposable moist towelettes to remove as much dirt as possible, apply the hand rub, then use a fresh hand wipe or paper towel to remove residue. Alcohol-based hand rubs are less effective than soap and water for cleaning hands that are visibly dirty, but they still kill micro-organisms, which makes them a good second choice if you don't have access to a sink.

4. Wash hands with soap and water as soon as possible to remove any remaining dirt.

Disposable moist towelettes can be as effective as soap and water. They're a good third choice when a sink or alcohol-based hand rub is not available or practical to use.

Knowing **when** to clean hands is just as important as proper technique. Post these checklists for staff as a reminder beside all sinks, at building entrances, and in the kitchen and diapering areas.

WHEN TO WASH HANDS

Staff must wash their hands:

- ☐ Whenever they're visibly dirty
- ☐ After arriving for work
- ☐ After using the toilet, changing a diaper or helping a child to use the toilet
- ☐ Before and after preparing food, before feeding a child and before eating
- ☐ After sneezing, coughing or blowing their nose and after wiping a child's nose
- ☐ After caring for a child with an infection
- ☐ Before and after giving medication or applying an ointment, cream or sunscreen
- ☐ Before and after applying a bandage or performing other first aid
- ☐ After cleaning up any body fluid (blood, mucus, vomit, feces, urine, drool)
- ☐ After household (environmental) cleaning and disinfection
- ☐ After handling contaminated or soiled clothing or bed linens
- ☐ After removing disposable (e.g., plastic or vinyl) or household rubber gloves
- ☐ After handling or caring for pets

Help children wash their hands:

- ☐ Whenever they're visibly dirty
- ☐ When they arrive
- ☐ After a diaper change or after using the toilet or potty
- ☐ Before eating or drinking
- ☐ Before and after water play
- ☐ After playing with sand or clay
- ☐ After sneezing, coughing, or wiping their nose with a hand or tissue
- ☐ After handling pets or other animals

Sinks: The number, location and function of handwashing basins or sinks will depend on your child care setting (centre or home-based), provincial/territorial public health regulations and the number of children in your program. In centres, a separate sink for washing hands must be available at each diaper change station/toileting area, in the food preparation area and near play areas. These sinks should **not** be used for rinsing contaminated clothing or for cleaning potties. Always keep them supplied with hot and cold running water, liquid soap in dispensers and disposable paper or (where practical) personal cloth towels. You must provide separate utility sinks for cleaning contaminated objects (in the bathroom) and for doing dishes or washing toys (in the kitchen).

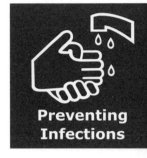

Preventing Infections

In home settings, the number and location of sinks are usually limited. The kitchen sink is used for hand hygiene before and after food preparation, and the bathroom sink is used for hand hygiene after toileting and diaper changing. However, there should be at least one utility sink available for cleaning potties or objects contaminated with urine or stool. If you don't have a utility sink, use one bucket just for cleaning these items and empty waste water into the toilet. Keep this utility bucket tightly sealed at all times.

Use each sink only for its prescribed purpose to avoid cross-contamination. Wash, rinse and disinfect all sinks regularly. (For a cleaning and sanitizing schedule, see Appendix 8.1.)

Towels: Whether you have the option of using cloth towels will depend on your child care setting (centre or home-based), provincial/territorial public health regulations and the number of children in your program. In a home setting, having accessible storage space, good laundry facilities and enough room to dry personal cloth towels on separate hooks without their touching are essential for cloth towels to be a practical option. Even then, you may need to switch to using disposable paper towels when there's an outbreak of infection. Don't use cloth towels to turn off taps, which likely carry germs. Each child care practitioner should have two cloth towels—one to use after food preparation and another after diapering or toileting. It helps to use towels of different colours and sizes for one designated purpose—to dry children's hands, or your own after food preparation or toileting.

Using disposable paper towels and/or single-use cloths at all times will be the only option for many programs. Use disposable paper towels to turn off taps if you don't have elbow faucets. Dispose of paper towels in a foot-activated, plastic-lined and covered garbage container.

2. Have a written illness policy for children and staff

Review the illness policy for your child care centre or home setting once a year and update it regularly. This policy is part of the orientation information you give to families at the time of enrolment, and should cover:

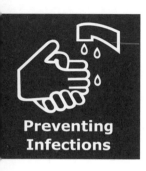

Preventing Infections

- The rules for hand hygiene, diaper changing and toileting, cleaning and disinfection, and food safety, and where these are posted for staff to review.
- The need for up-to-date immunization records for all children and staff.
- The need for an ongoing health record for each child in the program.
- The circumstances in which a parent will be contacted for early pick-up (e.g., which signs of illness will prompt a call).
- The need for current contact information for parents and one alternate caregiver (specify this person's relationship to the child), if a parent cannot be reached.
- A general description of when a sick child or staff member should stay at home (be excluded).
- Consents, permissions and special instructions for giving medication, as well as the use of a medical device if needed.
- The circumstances in which the local public health unit needs to be notified about health concerns. Requirements vary between regions.

(For more information about public health notification, exclusion and giving medication, see Chapter 9, *Managing Infections*.)

3. Observe children daily for signs of infection and share concerns and information with parents

Every day, as children arrive, make it part of your routine to check each child for a change in behaviour or appearance, or for some sign that may indicate illness—a flushed face, lethargy, a cough or a runny nose. Take a minute to ask about the child's well-being at drop-off time. Invite parents to share information about a restless night or lack of appetite. Throughout the day, watch for any sign of illness, especially monitoring children that you know are feeling under the weather.

When enrolling a child in your program, let parents know they need to tell you about illnesses at home or any early sign of infection their child might exhibit, including a low-grade fever, a cough, a loose bowel movement, a new rash or vomiting. They must tell you if their susceptible child has come into contact with someone who has a contagious infection (e.g., chickenpox), so that you can watch for signs of illness.

Let families know when a child is to be kept at home (excluded). They should also be aware that, for some illnesses, their child may need to be excluded until they provide a doctor's note stating that she is not contagious and/or can take part in program activities. Reassure parents that infections are common in child care and that very few require exclusion.

4. Require children and staff to be fully immunized, on schedule, and keep up-to-date vaccine records on file.

Although immunization is the most effective way to prevent serious childhood illnesses, a significant percentage of children in Canada are not fully immunized. It's usually because parents have missed an appointment or are unaware of recent changes to the routine schedule for childhood immunization, but sometimes it's because they oppose a given vaccine or immunization in general. In some jurisdictions (e.g., Ontario), immunization is a legal requirement for all children attending child care, as well as for employees. Where you know a parent or staff member has refused vaccines, advise them of the risk of infection—both to themselves and to their community. Inform them that public health authorities may need to treat them differently or exclude them for longer if there's an outbreak of infection in your facility or community.

Each child's immunization record must include the dates that routine vaccines were given and be consistent with the provincial/territorial schedule. This record needs to be checked for currency every 6 months, until a child is 2 years of age. After that, if a child has received all required vaccines for her age, an annual review at re-enrolment is sufficient. Keep this immunization record with the child's health record so it can be produced on demand (e.g., for your local public health unit in case of an outbreak of infection). The immunization records of child care practitioners should also be kept up-to-date.

Immunization schedules vary somewhat across Canada. Visit the website of the National Advisory Committee on Immunization at the Public Health Agency of Canada (www.phac-aspc.gc.ca) for current immunization schedules for your jurisdiction. These change, so check this website periodically. If the immunization record of a child in your care differs from the posted schedule for your province or territory, ask his parents to consult their doctor. You can also contact your public health unit for advice and direction.

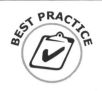

BEST PRACTICE

Raise awareness about immunization and help to ensure that families in your program are fully immunized by:

- being familiar with the routine schedule for your province or territory, and

- sharing this schedule and credible information about vaccines with families of children in your care. Many excellent resources are available at no charge.

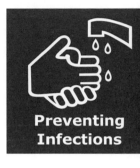

Preventing Infections

5. Follow proper diapering and toileting routines

Following appropriate diapering and toileting routines is critical to prevent and control infections in child care settings. The following precautions are particularly important:

- Diapering and/or toileting areas must be separate from the area where food is prepared. To prevent contamination, the diapering area should not be used for any other purpose.

- Children should be diapered only on a dedicated diaper-changing surface. Diapering a child "on the run" increases your risk of contaminating other surfaces.
- You should assemble all supplies necessary for a diaper change beforehand. This ensures the child's safety and makes the change more efficient.
- You don't need gloves for diapering or toileting if you can do it without direct hand contact with stool or urine, but you must wash your hands (and the child's hands) after every change.
- Children should wear clothing over their diapers throughout the day, and reusable or disposable swim diapers during water play.
- Ideally, no child care practitioner who is responsible for diapering/toileting should prepare food on the same day. However, in home settings, where this is impractical, you need to practice meticulous hand hygiene after diaper changing and before meal preparation.

Post the 10 steps for diaper changing and for toileting toddlers prominently in all diapering and toileting areas:

Preventing Infections

10 steps for diaper changing

1. Remove the diaper. Fold it closed and put it out of the child's reach.

2. With warm water, clean the child's diaper area with a disposable paper towel, baby wipe or single-use cloth. Dry well, patting rather than rubbing. Use soap only if it's needed to remove stool. Use diaper cream only if there's redness or a rash. Remove cream from a container with a tissue or tongue depressor to avoid contamination and apply it with your fingers.

3. Diaper the child, keeping one hand on him at all times to prevent a fall.

4. Wash your hands well. Wash the child's hands too.

5. Move him to a safe place, such as a crib.

6. Avoid handling the diaper if you don't need to—this increases the risk of hand contamination. Don't rinse reusable (cloth-lined) diapers, because this will spread germs to the toilet, floor or other surfaces.

7. Dispose of the dirty diaper. Wrap disposables before putting them into a secure, foot-activated, plastic-lined and covered garbage container. Bag soiled **reusable** diapers without disturbing the contents and send them home for laundering at the end of each day.

8. If you use a disposable paper liner on the diaper-changing surface, discard it into the garbage container after each change. If the diaper-changing surface is wet or soiled, you must clean and disinfect it and allow it to air dry (see step 9, below) before covering it again. Keep diaper pails and garbage containers tightly sealed and out of children's reach, preferably in a closed cupboard.

9. If you don't use a paper liner, disinfect the diaper-changing surface with a mild (1:100) bleach solution (see Table 8.1), for a contact time of at least 2 minutes, and allow it to air dry.

10. Wash your hands.

Child-sized toilets or an adult toilet modified for children's use with steps or a special seat are easier to clean properly than potty chairs, which are increasingly discouraged in child care settings.

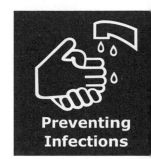

---

10 steps for toileting toddlers

1. Remove the child's diaper or pull-up and place her on the toilet or potty chair.

2. Wipe the child from front to back. Teach children to do the same.

3. Flush the toilet.

4. Diaper the child, as above, and help her to dress.

5. Wash your hands and help the toddler wash her hands too. Another staff member may also help the child while you continue cleaning.

6. Return the child to a safe place.

7. Empty the contents of the potty into the toilet carefully, to avoid splashing. Rinse the potty in a utility sink and flush this water down the toilet. Wear reusable household rubber gloves if hand contact with stool is possible. Wipe away any remaining stool with toilet paper and flush this at the same time.

8. Disinfect the potty and utility sink with a mild (1:100) bleach solution (see Table 8.1), for a contact time of at least 2 minutes, and allow them to air dry.

9. Remove gloves and wash them in soap and water. Then disinfect by soaking them in a mild (1:100) bleach solution for at least 2 minutes. Hang them to air dry.

10. Wash your hands.

---

6. Institute routine practices to prevent infection

Routine practices in health care are universally recognized strategies to prevent and control infection. Developed for use in hospitals, these strategies apply in any community setting and are now considered a key component of quality child care. Routine practices are based on the principle that any person may be carrying an infection and that their bodily excretions (e.g., blood and body fluids) potentially contain illness-causing micro-organisms. Consequently, specific preventive actions must be taken whenever there is risk of contact with, or exposure to, any person's bodily excretions. Practicing proper hand hygiene, covering a cough or sneeze, using protective barriers (e.g., gloves), and cleaning and disinfecting environmental surfaces are all basic routine practices.

Take these essential precautions to prevent infection in child care settings:

- Keep any cut or sore (yours or a child's) covered with a dry, clean bandage.
- Wipe or blow runny noses promptly.
- Immediately dispose of used tissues in a foot-activated, plastic-lined and covered garbage container. Wash your hands **and** a child's hands if you suspect he's wiped his nose.

- Cover your mouth and nose with a tissue whenever you cough or sneeze. If a tissue isn't within reach, cough or sneeze into your sleeve—on your upper arm—not into your hands.
- Use disposable non-latex gloves:
  - ➤ if touching a child's open skin lesion (e.g., a blister, cut or open sore),
  - ➤ for direct contact with children if you have an open sore or wound on your hands.

Teach children not to share combs, hairbrushes, toothbrushes, clothing or bedding. Require all personal items (e.g., toothbrushes and toothpaste) to be labelled with their owner's name to avoid mix-ups.

7. Keep physical environments clean

In any child care setting, keeping work and play surfaces and objects as clean and free of germs as possible is an ongoing challenge. Proper cleaning requires regular, rigorous and enforceable routines, specifically:

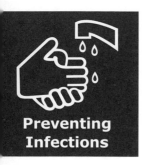

Preventing Infections

- **Cleaning**, which means removing all visible dirt or contamination with household soap or detergent. Most germs are removed through the friction of cleaning. Wiping or scrubbing removes surface dirt or contamination, allowing a disinfectant to reach germs underneath. **Always clean before disinfecting.**
- **Low-level disinfection**, also called sanitizing, which means destroying most germs by applying a disinfectant such as a mild (1:100) bleach solution (see Table 8.1) and leaving it on a surface for 2 minutes. Bleach can be diluted in advance and applied with a cloth rinsed in the solution. This solution can also be squirted onto a cloth, rather than sprayed on a surface. Wiping is always preferable to spraying, but if you do spray, be sure to cover the surface to be disinfected completely before wiping it down. Small items, such as plastic toys, can be dipped in fresh mild bleach solution to remove germs and allowed to air dry. Cleaning with a commercial detergent and/or disinfecting with a mild (1:100) bleach solution is sufficient for most housekeeping tasks.

TABLE 8.1

Solutions for disinfection (conversions)

Solution	Bleach:water ratio	Metric bleach:water ratio	Household measures
Very mild bleach solution (for sanitizing dishes only)	1:400	10 mL of bleach to 4 L of warm water	2 tsp. of bleach to 1 gallon of warm water
Mild bleach solution (for low-level disinfection or sanitizing)	1:100	5 mL of bleach to 500 mL of water	1 tsp. of bleach to 2 cups of water
Strong bleach solution (for disinfecting large blood and body fluid spills)	1:10	50 mL of bleach to 500 mL of water	¼ cup of bleach to 2 cups of water

Cleaning agents: Use store-bought household detergents or disinfectant detergents in child care settings. Homemade preparations—other than bleach solutions—are less suitable for cleaning because they aren't always powerful enough to kill germs, may release harmful fumes, and can be more difficult to prepare correctly. Follow product directions for any household cleaner. Store all cleaning products in a locked cupboard, out of children's reach.

Bleach: Household chlorine bleach is the most common chemical used to disinfect objects and surfaces in child care settings. Pre-mix a fresh batch of mild (1:100) bleach daily or as needed. For maximum effectiveness, don't store this solution for more than 1 week. Bleach solutions are perishable but last longer if they're stored in a tightly sealed container out of direct light. Handle bleach solutions with care—even diluted bleach is corrosive to some metals. It will discolour fabric and irritate skin.

Gloves: Wear protective household rubber gloves to clean or disinfect. Use a separate pair of clearly labelled household rubber gloves for each of the following tasks:

- dishwashing by hand,
- cleaning toys and general environmental cleaning, and
- cleaning bathrooms, potties, and blood and body fluid spills.

Before pulling gloves on, roll up your sleeves and remove any jewellery that might tear them. **Always wash your hands after removing gloves.** Rinse household rubber gloves as necessary in a mild (1:100) bleach solution for 2 minutes, then hang them to air dry.

Mops: Rinse a wet mop in fresh detergent or disinfecting solution and hang it head-side up to air dry. Shake a dry mop outside after each use and launder when visibly dirty.

Cloths and towels: Clearly identify single-use cleaning cloths and towels and store them separately from other linen.

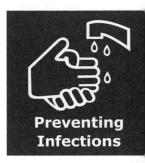

Preventing Infections

Dishwashing

Consult your local public health unit to make sure your dishwasher meets local specifications. Commercial dishwashers have shorter, more efficient cycles, and are mandatory in licenced child care centres. Domestic or residential dishwashers are common in home settings. These models must meet Canadian Standards Association (CSA) specifications and be properly maintained. The water temperature needed to clean dishes properly in a residential dishwasher is 60°C to 65°C (140°F to 150°F). This is considerably hotter than water from faucets which, to prevent scalding, should not be above 49°C (120°F). Water draining from a portable dishwasher into the sink is a scalding hazard, and children should not be in the kitchen while a portable dishwasher is operating. Always use the full wash/rinse/dry cycle rather than an "energy-saver" (or air-dry) cycle. Residential dishwashers clean dishes properly only if the full heat-dry cycle is used. Wash any dishes left out of the dishwasher by hand, promptly.

Legislation in most jurisdictions requires child care centres to have a three-compartment sink in the food preparation area for dishwashing by hand. Using a two-compartment sink is considered acceptable only for cleaning pots, pans and utensils. In home settings, kitchen sinks usually have only one or two compartments. It's still important to use a "four-step" method (wash, rinse, sanitize, dry) when dishwashing by hand in either setting.

When washing dishes by hand in a three-compartment sink:

1. Scrape or rinse off sticky or baked-on food.
2. Wash dishes in the first sink, using dish detergent. Germs are removed by friction (scrubbing) rather than by water temperature, which should be about 43°C (110°F). Change the water when it's visibly dirty.
3. Rinse dishes in hot water in the second sink. Rinsing is important for removing organic residue.
4. Sanitize dishes in the third sink for 45 seconds using a very mild (1:400) bleach solution (see Table 8.1). You can buy test strips for checking the concentrations of chemical sanitizing solutions. Make up a fresh sanitizing solution between batches of dishes.
5. Air dry dishes on a clean non-absorbent surface or rack, protected from splashing.
6. Clean and sanitize the sinks after doing dishes by hand. Wash your hands if you've used household rubber gloves.
7. Avoid reusing cloths to wipe food surfaces—they can spread bacteria. Instead, use disposable cloths **or** rinse and disinfect reusable cloths in a mild (1:100) bleach solution. Allow them to air dry between uses. Sponges break down quickly in any bleach solution and shouldn't be used.
8. Store dishes in a clean dry place where children can't reach or touch them.
9. Make sure the dish drainer or countertop space set aside for clean dishes and utensils is on the opposite side of the sink from dirty dishes.

Follow all the same steps when washing dishes by hand in a two-compartment sink, but use the first sink for both washing and rinsing dishes under the faucet.

Keeping toys, play areas and sleep areas clean

- For babies and children in diapers, choose toys that can be easily washed or laundered. If toys can't withstand multiple washings in hot, soapy water, discard them. You can clean plastic toys in the dishwasher, but not at the same time as dishes or cutlery. Minimize the sharing of mouthed objects (e.g., soothers) and, whenever possible, clean any toy that has been mouthed before another child plays with it.
- For babies and toddlers, clean and sanitize larger toys, play mats and activity centres **daily** and when soiled with a mild (1:100) bleach solution (see Table 8.1).
- For preschoolers, clean toys, mats and play surfaces **weekly** and when soiled. Disinfection isn't necessary unless babies share these play areas and/or toys become soiled with body fluids. Don't provide mouth toys (e.g., harmonicas), which are sure to be shared.
- Launder all dress-up clothes and soft washable toys **weekly** and when soiled.

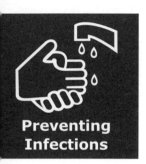

Preventing Infections

REMEMBER

What you clean and disinfect—and how frequently—often depends on the age and developmental stage of children in your care (e.g., whether a toy is mouthed or pushed along the floor). Generally, any object or area that is touched or used a lot needs to be cleaned every day.

Cover your sandbox with screening or mesh when it's not in use to:

- keep animals out,
- allow air circulation, and
- let in enough sunlight to kill bacteria.

Rake the sand and the area around the sandbox before play to aerate it. If you find animal or human feces, empty the sandbox, discard the contaminated sand, clean and disinfect the sandbox, and allow it to air dry before refilling it with clean sand. If only urine is present, rake the sand to aerate it, leave the sandbox open to sunlight and don't allow children to use it for 24 to 48 hours. Keep sandbox toys indoors between uses and clean and disinfect them weekly.

Cover your sand table when it's not in use. Sweep up any sand that falls on the floor and discard it. If the sand becomes contaminated with body fluids, replace it and follow the cleaning and sanitizing instructions for a water table (see below).

Individual containers for water play—rather than a shared water table—are recommended for children still wearing diapers. Individual containers are easier to clean and sanitize between uses. They can be grouped together on the floor or a table so that children interact during play. Individual water play is also recommended for any child with an infection.

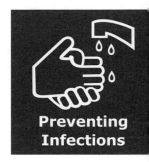

Preventing Infections

For preschoolers, be sure to empty and disinfect a shared water table daily and whenever you suspect contamination. If the water looks cloudy, it needs to be changed. Fill the water table with clean tap water just before use. **Do not add bleach, disinfectant or vinegar to the play water.**

Because shared water play can spread infection, it's important to choose a water table that is easy to move, clean and disinfect. It should be small and light enough to handle easily, have a smooth, non-porous and non-corrosive surface, and have rounded corners and edges for easy cleaning. Remove any water toy that comes into contact with a child's mouth during shared water play, and clean, sanitize and air dry all water toys between sessions.

Fill a portable wading pool with fresh water before each use. Empty, clean and disinfect pools after each use with a mild (1:100) bleach solution.

---

5 steps for cleaning a water table

1. Empty the water and wash out the table with detergent.

2. Rinse off the detergent with clean water.

3. Apply a sanitizing solution following the manufacturer's directions **or** use a mild (1:100) bleach solution.

4. Sanitize for at least 10 minutes or for whatever time the manufacturer recommends.

5. Allow the water table to air dry.

In sleeping areas, use moisture-resistant or easily washable covers for mats, resting pads and crib mattresses. Designate bedding (sheets and blankets) for each child in your care and launder it weekly and when soiled. Clean and disinfect crib mattresses, cots and mats if soiled and before assigning them to another child. Sleeping mats should be stored upright, separated by partitions, so their surfaces don't touch. Try to place cots or cribs at least 1 m (3 ft.) apart.

Laundry

Sort laundry into two groups, keeping all items used during cleaning, disinfecting, diapering and toileting routines separate from other laundry. **Wash everything in hot, soapy water.**

Group 1 includes:

- kitchen linens,
- cloth towels for hands and faces,
- cloth and plastic bibs (plastic bibs may last longer if cleaned and sanitized by hand),
- bed linens, and
- dress-up clothes and washable toys.

Group 2 includes:

- cloths used for cleaning and disinfecting,
- washcloths used during diapering, and
- mops.

Garbage disposal

Indoors: Use plastic-lined, waterproof garbage containers with tight-fitting lids, preferably operated by a foot pedal, in the diapering area, washrooms, kitchen, eating and play areas. Keep replacement liners out of reach of children. Empty each container and change the liner daily. Clean and disinfect containers weekly and when soiled.

Outdoors: Keep outdoor garbage containers in a secure, closed structure to discourage pests. Rinse outdoor garbage containers with water when soiled and air dry.

General housekeeping tips

- Store children's personal belongings, including one extra change of clean clothes, in individual cubbies or lockers.
- Place a child's soiled clothes or reusable diapers in a sealed plastic bag, safely out of children's reach. Return them to parents daily, or as necessary, to be laundered at home.
- Choose equipment with surfacing that is non-porous and easy to clean (e.g., a diaper-changing table with heavy vinyl covering).
- Don't use carpeting in the kitchen, eating area, bathrooms or infant/baby areas. Carpeting is much harder to keep clean than solid flooring. Use throw rugs in other

Preventing Infections

areas, taking care when cleaning to choose a product or process that leaves no chemical residue that may harm children.

- Minimize dirt by removing outdoor shoes and boots (both yours and the children's) just inside the facility's entrance. Set aside a specific area for this.
- Sweep or vacuum all uncarpeted floors and damp mop them with detergent every day.
- Clean and disinfect bathroom sinks, countertops and toilets at least once a day and when soiled.
- Vacuum throw rugs daily. Don't change vacuum bags or empty the vacuum when children are in the room. Clean rugs in infant areas once a month and in preschooler areas once every 3 months.
- Clean all other surfaces, furniture and equipment as needed to maintain a clean and dust-free environment.

Composting

If you're composting on site, outdoor bins should be covered and well maintained to prevent them attracting rodents or vermin. For indoor composting, collect food scraps in a plastic container with a tight lid and keep it out of children's reach. Empty the contents and wash this container at least once a day. An indoor composter should be inaccessible to children—preferably inside a locked kitchen cupboard. Materials that should not be added to a backyard composter include:

- pet wastes, which contain harmful bacteria, and
- meat, fish, fats and dairy products, which will attract vermin as they decompose.

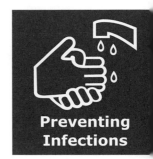

Preventing Infections

If your municipality is composting, then meat, fish, fats and dairy scraps are picked up regularly and can be collected and kept in your compost bin. Recycling and composting reduce the amount of garbage your facility produces day to day—and help children learn to protect their environment.

8. Ensure routine practices are followed when cleaning up and disinfecting blood or body fluid spills

Because bodily excretions, blood and body fluids from any person may contain micro-organisms that cause illness, take extra care to prevent contact whenever you need to clean up these substances. Routine practices include the use of protective barriers (e.g., gloves), careful disinfection and proper hand hygiene.

When there is a spill, a two-step process is required: clean first, then disinfect. Usually, wearing disposable gloves, cleaning up the spill with paper towels or a cloth soaked in detergent and water, and disinfecting with a mild (1:100) bleach solution (see Table 8.1) for 30 seconds are adequate precautions.

Extra precautions are needed when:

- the size of the spill exceeds the volume of the disinfectant used, and
- broken glass or other sharp objects may be present in the spill.

BEST PRACTICE

- Wear gloves to clean up larger spills of blood, stool, urine or vomit, where direct hand contact with the material may occur. You don't need to wear gloves to clean up small amounts of these substances, **if you can do it without direct hand contact with the material**.

- Wear gloves for cleaning if you have an open scratch or sore on your hands.

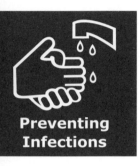

Preventing Infections

10 steps for cleaning up a large blood or body fluid spill

1. Protect mucous membranes (your eyes, nose and mouth) from splashes of blood or body fluid when cleaning up spills (i.e., turn your face away).

2. If broken glass or other sharp objects may be present in the spill, put on a pair of heavy-duty household rubber gloves. Otherwise, use disposable gloves.

3. Clean up the bulk of the spill using paper towels, then wash the area with detergent and water.

4. Safely discard contaminated materials in a foot-activated, plastic-lined and tightly covered garbage container.

5. Disinfect the area with a strong (1:10) bleach solution (see Table 8.1) for a contact time of at least 30 seconds. This will kill any germs left on the surface.

6. Discard single-use bleach-soaked cloths in the garbage container (see step 4, above) or a closed laundry container if the cloths are reusable.

7. To prevent cuts, keep your gloves on to sweep up broken glass or other sharp objects. **Never handle sharp objects with your hands or fingers**: use a broom or dust pan or two pieces of cardboard instead. Put sharp objects into a sealed box or puncture-resistant container.

8. Remove gloves by grasping the cuffs on the inside of your wrist and pulling the gloves off inside-out. Discard disposable gloves in the garbage container.

9. Wash reusable household rubber gloves in soap and water and disinfect by soaking them in a mild (1:100) bleach solution for at least 2 minutes. Hang them to air dry.

10. Wash your hands.

9. Follow food safety standards

For safe food practices, see Chapter 3, *Nutrition*, pages 46–49.

10. Limit contact with animals, and control pests

Animals

Pets can be brought into child care facilities for closely supervised visits but shouldn't live there permanently. Many animals can carry bacteria, parasites or zoonoses—diseases that people can get from animals. Pets can also cause difficulties for:

- children and staff who are allergic to animal fur, hair, saliva or dander,
- children and staff with weakened immune systems, and
- caregivers who are pregnant.

In home settings where pets may already be living, you should:

- **Always wash your hands after handling pets, and ensure that children do too.**
- Keep pets away from areas where food is prepared, served or stored.
- Supervise closely whenever children and pets are together.
- Make sure pets are healthy, free of fleas, ticks and worms, and properly immunized. Tick and flea collars containing organophosphates are toxic, and shouldn't be used in homes with young children.
- Clean up carefully after pets:
  - ➤ Change litter boxes often and make sure young children cannot access them.
  - ➤ Wipe up "accidents" promptly and disinfect the area with a mild (1:100) bleach solution (see Table 8.1).
  - ➤ Keep sandboxes covered and wash animal bedding regularly to prevent contamination.
- Keep pet food off the floor between feedings, and store bags of kibble in a latched cupboard.
- Discourage pets from licking faces.

ALERT

Clean animal scratches immediately with soap and water and watch for any sign of infection.

All bites that are serious enough to require medical attention (e.g., if the skin is broken and/ or if rabies is a concern) are reportable to your public health unit.

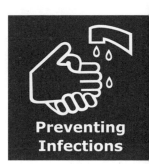

Preventing Infections

Cleaning animal cages

Animal cages should have removable bottoms, and cage liners should be changed often.

1. Wear household rubber gloves.
2. Remove loose dirt.
3. Scrub surfaces with soap and a detergent solution.
4. Rinse with water and allow to air dry.
5. Sanitize using a mild (1:100) bleach solution (see Table 8.1).
6. Remove used animal litter from the children's area immediately and discard in a closed garbage container or bin.
7. Remove gloves and wash hands.

Source: Region of Peel (Ont.) Public Health, *Keep on Track: A Health and Resource Guide for Child Care Providers in Peel*. Adapted with permission.

Certain animals present a much higher risk of causing infection and should never be allowed to live in a child care setting. These are:

- reptiles (e.g., turtles, lizards and snakes) or amphibious or aquarium animals (e.g., newts, toads or frogs), which can carry harmful bacteria on their skin,
- exotic animals, such as hedgehogs, parrots or monkeys, which are known to carry germs that are dangerous to humans, may bite, and need special care that young children can't provide, and

- wild animals, such as squirrels and raccoons, which are more likely to bite or scratch and can carry rabies.

Keep insects or spiders in a covered aquarium or other see-through container to prevent children from touching them and potentially being bitten. If you're uncertain about whether bringing an animal or pet into your facility is appropriate, consult your local public health unit. (For more on children and animals, see Chapter 5, *Keeping Children Safe*.)

Pests

Pests such as cockroaches, flies, mice and rats carry germs and contaminate food. You can prevent infestations of insects or rodents through regular cleaning, basic building maintenance and food safety.

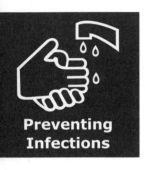

Preventing Infections

- Check food supplies entering your facility in boxes. Insects can travel from store to facility this way.
- Clean food, drink or grease spills promptly, even under equipment.
- Repair leaky water pipes and faucets—water attracts pests. Cover your drains.
- Keep garbage containers tightly covered, and store them well away from the facility in leak-proof, waterproof, rodent-proof storage bins.
- To prevent mosquito propagation, clean eavestroughs, gutters and run-off channels, and minimize standing water.
- Have screens on your windows and keep them in good repair.
- To prevent access by insects and rodents, repair any holes in walls or window frames, and caulk cracks and crevices.
- Install thresholds at the bottom of doors and vapour barriers under buildings.
- Keep doors closed.

If an infestation does occur on your premises, consult your local public health unit about appropriate extermination measures. Remember that **all** pesticides are toxic and should never be used inside while children are present or while food is being prepared or served.

- Use mousetraps only in areas that are inaccessible to children.
- Make sure the exterminator crew applies pesticide only in appropriate areas.

Adhere to all instructions for ventilation and for cleaning up chemical residues, and follow recommended times before staff and children can return to the premises.

Preventive routines

Keeping children healthy in child care is an ongoing challenge. A healthy program is one where your routines to prevent infection—from proper hand hygiene to cleaning mouthed toys, from reinforcing protocols to communicating with families about early signs of illness—are in action every day.

Selected resources

Immunization

Canadian Coalition for Immunization Awareness and Promotion. www.immunize.cpha.ca

The Canadian Paediatric Society's website for parents and caregivers, Caring for Kids, has information on immunization that can be downloaded at www.caringforkids.cps.ca, reproduced, and shared with families. Brochures on the following topics are also available:

———. 2008. Common infections and your child.

———. 2008. Vaccination and your child.

———. 2008. Getting your shots: 5-in-1.

———. 2005. Getting your shots: Chickenpox.

———. 2005. Getting your shots: Diphtheria-tetanus-acellular pertussis.

———. 2004. Getting your shots: Hepatitis B.

———. 2003. Getting your shots: Measles, mumps, rubella.

———. 2003. Getting your shots: Meningococcal vaccine.

———. 2002. Getting your shots: Pneumococcal vaccine.

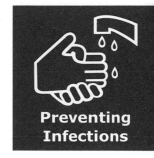

Preventing Infections

———. 3rd ed., 2006. *Your Child's Best Shot: A Parent's Guide to Vaccination*. Ottawa, Ont.: Canadian Paediatric Society. This book is the definitive guide to childhood vaccines in Canada.

Fisher, Margaret C. 2006. *Immunizations and Infectious Diseases: An Informed Parent's Guide*. Elk Grove, IL: American Academy of Pediatrics. www.aap.org

National Advisory Committee on Immunization. 7th ed., 2006. *Canadian Immunization Guide*. Ottawa, Ont.: Public Health Agency of Canada. www.phac-aspc.gc.ca

Public Health Agency of Canada. National Advisory Committee on Immunization. www.phac-aspc.gc.ca

Hand hygiene

Canadian Patient Safety Institute. Stop! Clean your hands: Canada's hand hygiene campaign. www.handhygiene.ca

Community and Hospital Infection Control Association, Hand hygiene. Includes numerous standards, fact sheets and links on hand hygiene. www.chica.org

General

American Academy of Pediatrics, American Public Health Association, National Resource Center for Health and Safety in Child Care. 2nd ed., 2002. *Caring for Our Children: National Health and Safety Performance Standards; Guidelines for Out-of-home Child Care Programs*. Elk Grove, IL: American Academy of Pediatrics. www.aap.org

Aronson, Susan S. and Timothy R. Shope, Eds. 2004. *Managing Infectious Diseases in Child Care and Schools: A Quick Reference Guide*. Elk Grove, IL: American Academy of Pediatrics. www.aap.org

Association of Professionals in Infection Control and Epidemiology (APIC). www.apic.org

Canadian Paediatric Society. 2000. Healthy pets, healthy people: How to avoid the diseases that pets can spread to people. Parent note. www.caringforkids.cps.ca

Centers for Disease Control and Prevention (CDC, U.S.). www.cdc.gov

————. 10th ed., 2008. *Epidemiology and Prevention of Vaccine-preventable Diseases*. Washington, DC: Public Health Foundation.

Community and Hospital Infection Control Association Canada. www.chica.org Provincial/territorial infection control resources can be found at this website.

Department of Health and Human Services (Newfoundland and Labrador). 2005. *Standards and guidelines for health in child care settings*. www.health.gov.nl.ca

Government of British Columbia, B.C. Community Care Facilities. 2003. *Preventing illness in child care settings*. www.health.gov.bc.ca

Heyman, David L. 18th ed., 2004. *Control of Communicable Diseases Manual*. Washington, DC: American Public Health Association.

Region of Peel (Ont.) Public Health. 2004. *Keep on track: A health and resource guide for child care providers in Peel*. Section 3. Keeping your facility clean, and resources. www. region.peel.on.ca/health/keep-on-track/pdfs/entiremanual.pdf. See also free educational resources on respiratory infection control and hand hygiene at www.peelregion.ca.

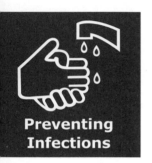

Preventing Infections

Appendix 8.1: Cleaning and sanitizing schedule

How often	Cleaned *and* sanitized	Other cleaning methods and notes
Before *and* after each use		
Kitchen		
Food preparation surfaces	X	
After each use		
Bathroom		
Potty chairs	X	
Change tables—without paper liner	X	
Utility sinks	X	
Kitchen		
High chair trays	X	
Tabletops	X	
Plastic bibs	X	
Blenders and food processors	X	
Toys		
Babies' plastic mouthed toys	X	Or run them through a full wash/rinse/dry dishwasher cycle (not at the same time as dishes or cutlery).
Other items		
Soothers	X	Reserve for use by one child.
Daily *and* when soiled		
Bathroom		
Change tables—with paper liner	X	Discard paper after each change. Clean and sanitize if surface becomes soiled.
Handwashing sinks	X	
Toilets	X	
Floors		Mop using household cleaner.
Diaper pails	X	
Countertops and fixtures	X	
Kitchen		
Floors		Mop using household cleaner.
Stovetops and tabletops	X	
High chair trays	X	
Can openers	X	
Countertops and sinks	X	
All areas		
Doorknobs, door handles, light switches	X	
Throw rugs and carpets		Vacuum daily, clean as needed and shampoo every 3 months. Avoid using carpet in infant/baby areas.
Floors		Sweep or vacuum.
Toys		
Activity centres, play mats	X	
Shared plastic toddler toys	X	Or run them through a full wash/rinse/dry dishwasher cycle (not at the same time as dishes or cutlery).
Water tables	X	
Shared puzzles, board books	X	Only clean before sanitizing if visibly soiled.
Cleaning items		
Dusting/cleaning cloths		Launder.

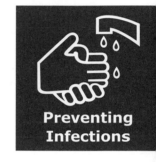

Preventing Infections

How often	Cleaned *and* sanitized	Other cleaning methods and notes
Weekly *and* when soiled		
Kitchen		
Microwaves	X	
Sleeping areas		
Bedding		Launder. Where possible, reserve for use by one child.
Cribs/cots/mats	X	Where possible, reserve for use by one child.
All areas		
Floor mats	X	
Garbage containers (inside)	X	Clean whenever garbage has leaked.
Tabletops not used for food preparation and eating		Clean.
Sofas, chairs		Vacuum.
Pillows and cushion covers used in activity areas		Launder.
Toys		
Soft washable toys		Launder. Where possible, reserve for use by one child.
Dress-up clothes		Launder.
Sandbox toys	X	
Sand table toys	X	
Cleaning items		
Sponge mops	X	Hang head-side up to air dry.
Monthly *and* when soiled		
Kitchen		
Refrigerators		Clean. Clean out the freezer every 6 months.
Ovens		Clean.
All areas		
Woodwork and cubbies		Damp-wipe.
Garbage containers (outside)	X	Clean whenever garbage has leaked.
Drapes and curtains		Vacuum. Launder or dry clean yearly.
Air vents		Vacuum.
Door ledges and shelving		Damp-wipe.
Windows		Wash inside and out at least twice a year.
Toys		
Sand tables	X	
Preschoolers' toys	X	

Source: Department of Health and Human Services (Newfoundland and Labrador). 2005. *Standards and Guidelines for Health in Child Care Settings*. Adapted with permission.

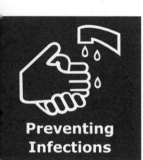

Preventing Infections

c h a p t e r

9

Managing
Infections

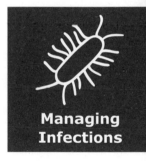

**Managing
Infections**

Keeping children healthy is the goal of every child care practitioner. However, despite best efforts, you can expect certain childhood infections to occur in your child care centre or home setting. As with prevention, the first line of defense in managing infections involves working together with parents. Sometimes your combined protection isn't enough. If the infection is serious or there's a disease outbreak, proper management will involve following a doctor's directions for treatment or, possibly, a public health intervention.

Chapter 8, *Preventing Infections*, describes how any child care program needs an illness policy to share with families so that both parents and child care practitioners know what is expected of them when a child shows the first sign of infection. Promptly identifying a possible symptom, having correct contact information in case an early pick-up is required, and recognizing when a sick child or staff member should stay at home are all things to be done before consulting a doctor. If a doctor's visit is in order, parents usually notify you afterward of the diagnosis and the doctor's recommendation that their child stay at home (be excluded). Once their child returns, they should provide you with written directions from the doctor about any continuing treatment that will affect the child's routine care in your program. (See, for example, Appendix 9.1, *Administering Medication*.)

This chapter describes the effects of illness in child care: where infections come from, how they spread, what can be done to control them, and what to do if you suspect an outbreak. With infections like the common cold, taking precautions, proper care, and riding out the symptoms are about the only things to do. For other infections, or if you suspect an outbreak of a communicable illness, additional steps are necessary.

If you've advised parents to take their child to a doctor, remind them to mention that she is attending a child care program.

The definition of an outbreak depends on the type of infection, normal seasonal variations, as well as provincial/territorial public health guidelines. Whether an outbreak is occurring is determined by public health authorities. If you suspect an outbreak, determine how many people in your facility have similar symptoms before contacting your public health unit. Include children and staff who are absent from the program in your count if they may be ill at home. Managing certain infections in child care may also mean reporting a confirmed diagnosis to public health authorities—if a treating physician or testing laboratory hasn't already done so—notifying the parents of all other children in your program about the presence of infection, or distributing information or a public health letter.

Public health's role in managing an infection in child care is often consultative: guiding or advising on community health issues. A public health intervention usually involves specific medical referrals, prophylaxis (preventive treatment) for peers, families and for close contacts who may have been exposed to a sick child. If a child is diagnosed with a serious or very contagious infection (e.g., measles, mumps, rubella or chickenpox), you'll need to consult your local public health unit **before** distributing information to parents of other children in your program.

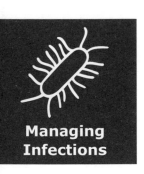

Managing Infections

Physicians are required to report occurrences of certain diseases to public health authorities. Reportable diseases are tracked because they're potentially dangerous to human health, have the potential to spread and require some level of intervention by health care personnel. The list of reportable diseases varies somewhat among provinces and territories in Canada. **Contact your local public health unit for a list of reportable illnesses in your area.** Be sure to notify public health authorities (if a physician or local laboratory hasn't already done so) whenever a child in your care is diagnosed as having a reportable illness. At a minimum, public health authorities will advise you about taking steps to protect the health of other children and staff.

Signs and symptoms of infection

Adhering to daily routine practices to prevent the spread of germs is a cornerstone of health in child care. The next best way to manage infection is to be alert for telltale signs of illness. Every day, for every child, ask yourself: "Is there anything different about this child today?" If you observe just one sign or symptom of infection, it may mean that you have a sick child on your hands. It should also prompt early and effective steps to manage the infection.

Each occurrence of illness in your program should trigger a review of procedures to ensure that all the proper steps are being taken to prevent spread. For example, a case of diarrhea should activate a full review of diapering procedures; a case of impetigo, a careful look at hand towel use.

1. Unusual behaviour

Behaviour is an important signal of how serious an infection may be. A child who can play, be active, laugh or smile likely doesn't have a serious infection. But a child who shows a definite change in normal patterns of behaviour (e.g., unusual lethargy or lack of interest, loss of appetite, irritability or persistent crying, or excessive sleepiness) may have a serious infection and should see a doctor as soon as possible. This child should be excluded from your program until a doctor approves his return.

2. Runny nose, cough, difficulty breathing

The most common cause of a runny nose in young children is a viral infection, such as the common cold. Nasal discharge usually begins as clear colourless mucus and becomes thick yellow or green within a day or two. The colour change is **not** a signal of a more serious infection and is no reason to exclude or isolate a child. However, if nasal discharge persists for 10 to 14 days, the child should be checked for the possibility of a secondary bacterial infection.

Coughing can be triggered by irritation anywhere in the respiratory tract, from the nose to the lungs. There are many causes of coughing, from allergies to chemical irritation (e.g., cigarette smoke), but the most frequent cause is the common cold. Of all the symptoms of a viral infection in the respiratory tract, coughing lasts the longest.

Difficulty breathing may be caused by a stuffy nose during a mild viral infection, or it may be a sign of a more serious infection such as croup, bronchiolitis or pneumonia.

Wheezing refers to noise (often "musical" sounds) made when breathing, mainly while exhaling (breathing out). Wheezing is caused by a combination of narrowing of and excess mucus in the smaller airways of the lungs. The most common cause of wheezing in young children is a viral infection, but it may also be caused by asthma.

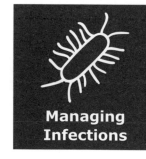

Managing Infections

ALERT

Difficulty breathing, how fast a child breathes, and the extra effort required to breathe can indicate a serious problem. You may see that the muscles located between the ribs at the bottom of the rib cage, just above the chest bone (sternum), are "tugging" (sucking inward).

Inflammation of the windpipe (airway) and vocal cords may cause a child's voice to get hoarse and his breathing to get very laboured, noisy or "croupy" (like a bark). In severe cases, the windpipe may become obstructed. This is a true emergency. Seek immediate medical attention. The harder a child is working to breathe or inhale when at rest, the more serious the airway obstruction.

3. Vomiting

Children vomit much more easily than adults and often with less apparent discomfort. Vomiting may be due to the general effects of an infection rather than specific irritation of the stomach. Vomiting itself is not usually dangerous unless:

- the child chokes and inhales vomit,
- the child vomits so frequently that dehydration occurs, or
- vomiting is combined with lethargy.

In young infants, it's important to distinguish vomiting from spitting up after feeding, which is very common. (See Chapter 7, *Common Conditions*.)

4. Diarrhea

Diarrhea means a change in the normal pattern of bowel movements, resulting in a substantial increase in the number of stools **and** a change in the consistency of the stools to watery or unformed.

Diarrhea occurs when the bowel is stimulated or irritated by infection, a change in diet or other causes. It can be dangerous if **dehydration** occurs. Dehydration means that the amount of water lost through the stool is greater than the amount a child drinks. Dehydration impairs blood circulation and occurs far more rapidly in babies and toddlers with diarrhea than in older children. The risk of dehydration is even greater if a child is also vomiting. Abdominal cramps or stomach ache often accompany vomiting or diarrhea.

5. Any change in skin colour

A sudden loss of colour in the face that seems to persist may be a sign of decreased blood circulation because of an infection. It may also be a sign of bleeding. Yellowing of the skin or the whites of the eyes (jaundice) can be a sign of infection, but there are many other causes. In either case, the child should see a doctor.

6. Rash

Rashes take many forms, have many different causes, and often require a doctor's examination before a cause can be determined. Children who have a rash without a fever or change in behaviour can attend child care, but should still

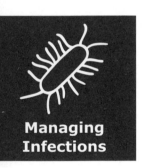

Managing Infections

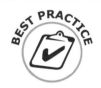

BEST PRACTICE

A fever is one of the body's best defence mechanisms against infection and a valuable warning sign. Although a fever doesn't hurt a child and usually goes away within 72 hours, babies younger than 3 months old should be taken to a doctor whenever they have a fever. Toddlers and preschoolers should see a doctor if their fever is above 39°C (102°F) and lasts longer than 48 hours.

be seen by a doctor, especially if the rash is extensive or persistent. Rashes are a valuable early warning sign for child care practitioners who are on the alert for further cases of a communicable disease in their facility.

7. Fever

Having a fever means having a body temperature that's higher than normal. It's defined as a reading above 38°C (100.4°F) when measured rectally or by ear, above 37.3°C (99.1°F) when measured in the armpit, and above 37.5°C (99.5°F) when measured by mouth.

The degree (height) of a fever doesn't necessarily tell you how serious a child's illness is. How the child is acting is usually a much better indicator. A child with a mild viral infection may have a fever as high as 40°C (104°F), while a child who is severely ill with meningitis may have a fever of only 38.5°C (101.3°F). Infants under 3 months of age with a serious infection can also run a temperature that's **below** normal.

When to take a temperature

Confirm that a child is running a fever once you've noticed possible signs: a flushed face or glassy-eyed look.

REMEMBER

- A child's face or forehead feeling warm or cool doesn't necessarily reflect body temperature or whether fever is present.
- A child's normal body temperature range varies somewhat throughout the day.
- A fever sometimes occurs after vaccination (usually within 24 hours of receiving most vaccines).
- Teething doesn't cause fever.
- The accuracy of your temperature reading depends on which method you use.

Temperature-taking tips

- You should never use a mercury thermometer. If it breaks, you and the children in your care may be exposed to this toxic substance.

- A digital thermometer made of unbreakable plastic is easy to read and measures temperature quickly. If it is reusable, meticulous cleaning and disinfection are important to prevent the transmission of infections.

- **Taking a child's temperature orally (by mouth) is not recommended for children under 5 years of age.** It's hard for them to hold the thermometer under the tongue for long enough.

- Ear thermometers are simple to use for detecting fever in young children, but they can be expensive and tend to give low readings, even when the manufacturer's instructions are followed.

- Fever strips are not recommended because they're very inaccurate.

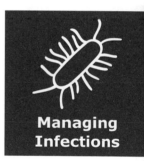

Managing Infections

How to take a temperature

Follow your facility's policy and comply with parents' wishes when taking a temperature. A rectal reading is the most accurate but may not be appropriate in child care facilities. Many child care facilities prohibit this method, parents may not permit it, most children don't like it, and reusable rectal thermometers are harder to disinfect properly. Although taking a temperature in the armpit or by ear isn't as precise, both methods show whether a child has a fever and can be used as screening tools.

Axillary method (in the armpit)

- Clean a digital thermometer with cool, soapy water, and rinse.
- Place the tip of the thermometer in the centre of the armpit.
- Make sure the child's arm is tucked snugly against her body.
- Listen for the beep, which may take up to a minute.
- Remove the thermometer and read the temperature.
- Clean the thermometer with cool, soapy water, rinse, and disinfect with a mild (1:100) solution of bleach (see Table 8.1, page 154).

Tympanic method (by ear)

- **Use a clean disposable plastic sleeve each time**, and follow the manufacturer's instructions carefully.
- Gently tug on the ear, pulling it back. This helps to straighten the ear canal and make a clear path inside the ear to the eardrum.
- Gently insert the thermometer until the ear canal is fully sealed off.
- Squeeze and hold down the button for 1 second.
- Remove the thermometer and read the temperature.
- Discard the disposable sleeve.
- Clean all other parts of the thermometer, including the box housing the electronic components, with cool, soapy water, rinse, and disinfect using a mild (1:100) bleach solution.

Oral method (by mouth, only if a child is older than 5 years)

- Clean a digital thermometer with cool, soapy water, and rinse.
- Carefully place the tip of the thermometer under the child's tongue and have the child close her mouth.
- Listen for the beep, which may take up to a minute.
- Remove the thermometer and read the temperature.
- Clean the thermometer in cool, soapy water, rinse, and disinfect using a mild (1:100) bleach solution.

What to do when a child has a fever

1. Notify the parents.
2. Offer plenty of fluids.
3. Keep the child comfortable. Make sure she is neither shivering nor sweating (overdressed).

BEST PRACTICE

Thermometers can be an infection risk. Whenever possible, use electronic thermometers with a permanent base and disposable sleeve.

The non-disposable parts are easily contaminated with germs from handling when taking a temperature, and they must be carefully washed and disinfected after each use.

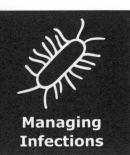

Managing Infections

4. Don't sponge the child with lukewarm water, alcohol baths and/or rubs, as they can cause discomfort. They are not effective for lowering body temperature, and are not recommended.
5. Fever alone doesn't need to be treated with medication. Giving medication may ease aches and pains and make the child feel more comfortable.

Fever medication

Be sure to follow your facility's policy when administering a fever medication. **Remember that provincial/territorial child care regulations for administering medication to children (i.e., safe procedures and consents) apply to fever reducers.** Acetaminophen (e.g., Tylenol, Tempra, Panadol and others) is the best medication for lowering fever. Provided you have obtained physician and parental consents, the recommended dose of acetaminophen can be given every 4 to 6 hours. Ibuprofen (e.g., Advil and Motrin) may be used for children over 6 months old and given every 6 to 8 hours, as long as the child is drinking fluids well.

When treating a child for fever

- **Don't give "over-the-counter" (OTC) cough and cold medicines to children in your care. There is no proof that they work, some side effects can make a child feel worse, and they are not recommended for children under 6 years of age.**

- **Don't** give acetaminophen and ibuprofen at the same time, and **don't** give acetaminophen to a child who is already taking an OTC at home. Many OTCs already contain acetaminophen.

- **Always** recheck the child's temperature before giving a second dose of medication.

- **Never** exceed the recommended dose and schedule.

- **Never give aspirin (acetylsalicylic acid or ASA), unless it is prescribed by the child's doctor.** For certain infections, taking aspirin can increase the risk of Reye's syndrome, a very serious condition that can damage the liver and brain.

Be sure to record giving fever medication on the *Medication consent form and record sheet* (see Appendix 7.1, pages 139–40) and note the following information in the child's file:

- the date and time(s) the child's temperature was taken,
- the method used and the child's temperature reading,
- how the child was feeling (i.e., why the temperature was taken), and
- if/when a parent was informed before the medication was given.

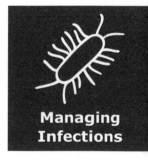

Managing Infections

Febrile seizures

Febrile seizures are convulsions caused by fever and are fairly common. Often, the seizure is the first signal of a child's fever and is characterized by stiffening of the body, upward rolling of the eyes, and jerking movements of the head and limbs. Most febrile seizures last from 30 seconds to 2 minutes and are harmless despite their frightening appearance. They occur in 2 to 5 per cent of children between 6 months and 5 years of age, are particularly common in babies and toddlers, and tend to run in families. In rare instances, seizures may be triggered by a serious infection, such as meningitis. Any child who has a seizure while in child care should see a doctor promptly. (For more about seizures, see Chapter 11, *Emergencies*.)

Isolation and exclusion strategies for a sick child

Many childhood infections are communicable—that is, passed from one person to another. Effectively managing infection means taking steps to prevent it from spreading. One strategy is to contain infection by separating one or more sick children from the rest of the group. This step is usually taken to control the spread of serious illnesses, but it may also be useful for containing milder contagious infections, such as conjunctivitis (pinkeye).

Isolation involves physically separating one child from the group when he has—or is suspected of having—an infectious illness. In child care centres, space should be available for temporarily isolating a child who becomes ill. Also, there should be sufficient staff for at least one adult to stay with the sick child. Many facilities use a cot in the director's office for this purpose. Larger facilities may have a separate room or cubicle for isolation. However, isolation is difficult and may be impossible for most home settings. Instead, you'll need to call a parent or other designated caregiver for an early pick-up.

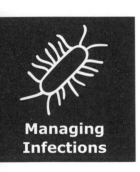

Managing Infections

Cohorting is the term used for isolating several children together who are known to have the same infection. While cohorting is beyond the limited space and budget constraints of most facilities, local cohorting of entire facilities (using selected facilities for infected and immune children and others for susceptible children) may become necessary in unusual emergency circumstances (e.g., pandemic influenza). This strategy would be coordinated by local public health authorities. Ideally, staff caring for infected children would also be cohorted and would have no direct contact with uninfected children or caregivers. Toys, equipment and other materials would not be shared among groups.

Excluding children from your program for as long as they're considered infectious may be necessary for certain illnesses. Exclusion isn't recommended for infections that are mild and/or common in the community (e.g., the common cold or parvovirus B19), or where this strategy isn't considered effective in preventing spread (e.g., head lice, chickenpox). However, a sick child should be excluded from the regular child care program if one or more of the following conditions exists:

1. The illness prevents the child from participating comfortably in all program activities, including going outside.

2. The illness results in a greater need for care than the staff can provide without compromising the health, safety and care of other children.
3. The illness poses a serious health risk if it spreads to other children or staff, and/or local public health authorities require exclusion. (Consult your local public health unit for a list of these infections, and see Appendix 9.2, pages 225-34.)

A public health intervention can often prevent an outbreak of certain serious infections, such as measles, by immunizing children or staff who have been in contact with a sick child and exposed to his germs. Other infections, such as pertussis, involve a public health mandate to treat people at risk with preventive antibiotics.

Respiratory infections

Influenza

There are many viruses that cause respiratory infections, including the cold viruses, respiratory syncytial virus, influenza and others. In young children, any of these viruses can cause a cold, croup, bronchiolitis or pneumonia. In school-aged children and adults, the influenza virus tends to cause a more severe illness than other respiratory viruses, with high fever, cough and body aches, and strikes more quickly than a cold. However, in younger children, infection with influenza is often not different from that with other respiratory viruses, although some infants may have a high fever only, and febrile seizures are more common.

A vaccine is available for the influenza virus but not for the other viruses that cause respiratory infections. Influenza vaccine is routinely given each fall to all children between 6 months and 2 years of age, to all their family members and to those who provide child care for children under 2 years of age. It is also routinely given to older children with certain chronic illnesses. Influenza vaccine should be considered for all children, because it reduces the chance of developing serious illness.

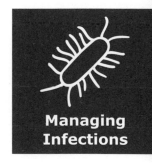

Managing Infections

From time to time, there is a major change in the influenza virus such that no one is immune and large numbers of people around the world develop influenza within a few months. This is called pandemic influenza. In a pandemic, decisions as to whether child care centres remain open and about exclusion policies for children with known or suspected pandemic influenza would be directed by public health authorities.

Common cold

Young children get lots of colds, some as many as 8 to 10 a year before turning 2 years of age. Children attending child care or living with older siblings catch many colds because they're exposed frequently to the more than 100 different cold viruses to which they haven't yet built up immunity (defences). But by the time they start school, children who have attended child care will usually have fewer colds than children who have stayed at home.

Children with a cold usually have a runny nose, cough, sneezing and fever. They may also have a headache and sore throat, and lack energy or appetite. Colds usually aren't serious, but complications such as ear and lung infections can occur. Most colds last for 7 to 10 days, and children usually have enough energy to play and keep up their daily routines.

Some respiratory viruses that cause colds can also cause serious illnesses when they infect infants and toddlers, such as croup and bronchiolitis, or produce symptoms, such as sore eyes, sore throat and swelling of the neck-glands, that are less likely to appear as children get older.

Transmission

Cold viruses are found in the nose and throat. These germs spread easily because young children often touch their nose, eyes and mouth, put objects in their mouth, and have more frequent contact with furniture surfaces and toys without washing their hands. Children also transfer viruses while they play. Cold viruses can live on toys and other objects for several hours and can be picked up by other children as well as their caregivers. The spread of viruses also occurs through the many contacts between child care practitioners and children: holding hands, blowing noses, picking up toys, feeding, changing diapers and so on. Some cold viruses may be spread when a child with a cold coughs or sneezes. Droplets from the cough or sneeze may reach other children's noses or mouths if they are less than 1 m (3 ft.) away.

What to do

There's no cure for the common cold. Colds usually go away on their own. Because colds are viral infections, antibiotics don't help. Antibiotics are used only when children develop complications from bacteria, such as an ear infection or pneumonia. In the meantime:

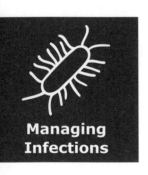

Managing Infections

1. Keep the child as comfortable as possible. If he doesn't want to eat, offer plenty of fluids and small, nutritious meals.
2. Don't use decongestants and antihistamines. They have no effect on cold symptoms and are not recommended.
3. If a baby is having trouble feeding because his nose is stuffed with mucus, use a rubber suction bulb to clear his nostrils. Saline nose drops or saline nose spray may be used if the mucus is very thick. The spray goes well into the nasal passages and may be more effective than drops.
4. Teach children who are old enough to understand to "cover their cough" with a tissue or to cough into their sleeve or elbow if they don't have a tissue handy.
5. Use disposable tissues to blow or wipe a child's nose and throw them out right away.
6. Wash your own hands and a child's hands after contact with nose secretions (or contact with eyes, nose or mouth) and after using a tissue.
7. A cold can sometimes progress to a more serious problem. Advise parents to have their child seen by a doctor as soon as possible if the child also develops an earache, high fever, rash, vomiting or excessive crankiness.
8. **Call 911 first** (or emergency services where 911 service is unavailable), **then notify the parents**, if the child:

- is breathing rapidly or has significant difficulty breathing,
- has bluish or greyish skin or lips, or
- is coughing so hard that it causes choking.
9. A fact sheet is available at www.caringforkids.cps.ca and can be downloaded and given to the parents of children who have a common cold.

Exclusion and reporting

- Children with a cold can continue to attend child care as long as they are well enough to participate comfortably in all program activities, including going outside. If they have a fever or complications, they may need a few days of rest at home.

Croup

This illness, which often begins like a cold, is a viral infection of the throat and larynx (voice box). Croup can be caused by several different viruses. Swelling in the larynx causes the airway to narrow. The child's voice gets hoarse and she develops a cough that sounds like barking. Breathing may become rapid, laboured, very noisy or "croupy."

Any activity that increases the rate of breathing (even crying or excitement) will make the child sound worse. Often when the child is quiet or asleep, the noise is hardly audible. Croup usually sounds worse than it really is, and the best time to assess its severity is when the child is relaxed.

In severe cases, the windpipe may become obstructed and the child will have trouble swallowing and breathing. This is a true emergency: seek immediate medical attention. Some children become so ill with croup that they require treatment in hospital, but most get better without specific treatment. Because croup is a viral infection, antibiotics don't help. Occasionally, a child's doctor will prescribe an anti-inflammatory medication.

Transmission

Same as for the common cold, above.

What to do

1. Advise the parents to have their child seen by a doctor as soon as possible.
2. Encourage the child to drink extra fluids.
3. **Call 911 first** (or emergency services where 911 service is unavailable), **then notify parents**, if a child with croup has:
   - rapid or difficult breathing,
   - trouble swallowing or distress when lying down,
   - inability to swallow saliva, and/or
   - bluish lips or mouth.

BEST PRACTICE

- Cool mist humidifiers are not recommended because of the risk of contamination from bacteria and mould. If used, they must be cleaned and disinfected daily.
- Hot water vaporizers are not recommended because they haven't proved effective for relieving congestion. They also pose a burn risk.

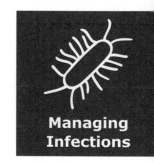

Managing Infections

4. A fact sheet is available at www.caringforkids.cps.ca and can be downloaded and given to the parents of a child who has croup.

Exclusion and reporting

• Children with croup should be excluded from child care until they are well enough to participate comfortably in all program activities, including going outside.

Bronchiolitis and pneumonia

Bronchiolitis and pneumonia are infections of the airways and air spaces of the lungs that are much more severe than colds.

Bronchiolitis involves swelling of the lining of the smaller airways and occurs most commonly in the first 2 years of life. The child experiences difficulty moving air in and out of the lungs. Certain viruses that cause colds (e.g., the respiratory syncytial virus) can also cause bronchiolitis. **Pneumonia** is an infection in the lung tissue that prevents oxygen from moving from the air spaces to the bloodstream. It may be caused by viruses or bacteria.

Signs of infection in the lower respiratory tract are cough and rapid, laboured breathing. Fever may also be present. When a child has difficulty breathing, muscles located between the ribs at the bottom of the rib cage "tug" (suck inward). You may also notice noisy breathing, wheezing or grunting, and poor skin colour.

Transmission

Same as for the common cold, above.

What to do

1. Advise the parents to have their child seen by a doctor as soon as possible.
2. Encourage the child to drink extra fluids.
3. Familiarize yourself with emergency procedures in case the child has respiratory distress (difficulty breathing). (See Chapter 11, *Emergencies*.)
4. Watch for the following signs and, if either appear, **call 911 first** (or emergency services where 911 service is unavailable), ***then* notify the child's parents**:
    • rapid or difficult breathing, and/or
    • bluish lips or mouth.

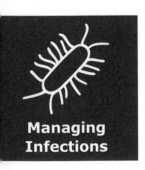

Managing Infections

Exclusion and reporting

• Children with bronchiolitis or pneumonia should be excluded from child care until they are well enough to participate comfortably in all program activities, including going outside.
• Bronchiolitis and pneumonia don't need to be reported to your local public health unit.

Otitis media (middle ear infections)

Ear infections are very common and are usually not serious. Most children will have one or more before they are 3 years old, and these infections can occur with such frequency in child care settings that they seem to be contagious (even though they aren't). Middle ear infections are caused by viruses or bacteria and usually occur with a common cold. These germs travel from the back of the nose through the Eustachian tube, which connects the back of the throat to the middle ear. Also, when babies swallow milk while lying down, the milk can enter the Eustachian tube and increase their susceptibility to ear infections. Children attending child care have more ear infections than those who don't, probably because they have more colds. Having allergies and being exposed to cigarette smoke also increase the risk of ear infections.

Older children will complain of an earache. Younger ones might not say they have an earache, but will become irritable and fussy, have trouble sleeping, tug at their ears or be less responsive to quiet sounds. They may have fluid draining from their ears. Discharge from the ear is considered a body fluid that potentially contains blood-borne viruses. Routine practices apply. Use proper hand hygiene, and clean and disinfect any object or surface that's come into contact with fluid from the ear.

Signs of an ear infection include high fever, lack of energy and loss of appetite. Ear infections can be diagnosed only by examining the child's eardrum (tympanic membrane). Children younger than 2 years of age are usually treated with antibiotics because this infection can lead to other, more serious complications. For older children who don't experience too much discomfort from an ear infection, the doctor may suggest a painkiller, such as acetaminophen, and then re-examine the child 2 or 3 days later to see if antibiotics are needed. Most children are feeling better by then.

Use antibiotics only as directed and only for as long as they are prescribed. A course of antibiotics should not be stopped just because a child feels better. Consider advising the parents to make a second doctor's visit to make sure the ear infection has cleared up.

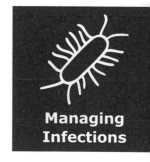

Managing Infections

Children with frequent ear infections and persistent fluid in the middle ear, with hearing loss, may need plastic ventilation tubes. Inserted into the middle ear through the eardrum, ventilation tubes allow air pressure to remain normal on both sides of the eardrum and fluid to drain. Ask the parents of a child with ventilation tubes if the doctor placed limits on bathing or swimming. Advise parents to see a doctor promptly if you see drainage from these tubes that might be fluid from the ear canal. Otherwise, a child with ventilation tubes usually requires no special care.

Transmission

An ear infection is usually a complication of a cold and doesn't spread from child to child.

What to do

1. Advise the parents to have their child seen by a doctor as soon as possible.
2. Watch for complications. Ask the parents to notify a doctor if their child shows any of the following signs:
   * earache that gets worse in spite of treatment,
   * a high fever (over 39°C [102°F]) that doesn't respond to medication, or a fever lasting longer than 3 days,

- tenderness or swelling behind the ear,
- excessive sleepiness,
- excessive crankiness or fussiness,
- skin rash, or
- hearing loss.

3. A fact sheet is available online at www.caringforkids.cps.ca and can be downloaded and given to the parents of a child who has an ear infection.

Exclusion and reporting

- Children with an ear infection can continue to attend child care as long as they are well enough to participate comfortably in all program activities, including going outside.
- Ear infections don't need to be reported to your local public health unit.

Conjunctivitis (pinkeye)

Conjunctivitis, also called pinkeye, is an infection of the covering of the eyeball and the inside of the eyelid. It is usually caused by a virus, but may also be caused by bacteria. Occasionally, pinkeye can also be caused by allergies, exposure to chemicals, smoke and other irritants, injury or excessive rubbing.

A child with pinkeye will experience a scratchy feeling or pain in his eyes, often with lots of tearing. The whites of the eyes are pink or red. Pus or a discharge from the eyes makes eyelids sticky during sleep.

Different kinds of conjunctivitis are treated and managed differently, so it's important to find out as soon as possible from a child's doctor what kind you're dealing with. **Purulent pinkeye**, with a pink or red eyeball, white or yellow discharge, matted or red eyelids and eye pain, is usually caused by a bacterial infection and can be treated with antibiotics. **Non-purulent pinkeye**, in which the eyeball is pink or red, discharge is clear and watery and there is mild or no pain, may be caused by a virus or a non-infectious condition. Antibiotics are not effective.

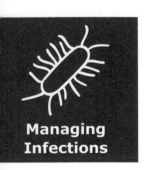

Managing Infections

Transmission

Both kinds of conjunctivitis spread easily through direct and indirect contact. Direct contact occurs when tears or discharge from an infected person's eyes are touched and transferred by the fingers to the eyes of another person. Indirect contact occurs when an object contaminated with eye fluid (e.g., a used tissue) is touched, or touches another person's eyes. When conjunctivitis is associated with a common cold, it is also spread by droplets in a sneeze or cough.

What to do

1. Advise the parents to have their child seen by a doctor as soon as possible.
2. When wiping tears or discharge from the child's eyes, wipe from the inside out, in one direction only. Use a clean part of the cloth each time, and do not reuse the cloth.
3. Good hand hygiene is essential. Wash your hands before and after contact with the child's eyes or contaminated cloths.

4. Avoid touching others unless your hands are washed.
5. Wash the child's hands or have the child wash his hands carefully after touching his eyes.
6. Review the use of cloths, hand towels and tissues to make extra sure they're not shared between children.
7. If possible, move a child with pinkeye to a separate area to prevent exposure to other children while you're waiting for the parent to take the child home. Don't let other children use toys handled by the infected child until they've been cleaned and disinfected.
8. Watch other children for signs of infection.
9. If you suspect an outbreak of conjunctivitis at your facility, notify public health authorities. They can advise you about next steps, and exclusion may be mandated.
10. A fact sheet is available at www.caringforkids.cps.ca and can be downloaded and given to the parents of a child who has pinkeye or distributed to the **parents of all children** in your program if an outbreak occurs.

Exclusion and reporting

- A child with pinkeye should be excluded until he has been seen by a doctor. If the pinkeye is caused by bacteria, the child can return to child care after an antibiotic has been prescribed and given for 24 hours.
- If the pinkeye is caused by a virus, the child can return to the program with a doctor's (or public health) approval. Children with non-purulent pinkeye don't need to be excluded unless there's an outbreak at your facility.
- A case of pinkeye diagnosed as a *Chlamydia* infection is reportable to local public health authorities by the treating physician and testing laboratory.

Streptococcal pharyngitis (strep throat)

Streptococcal pharyngitis (strep throat) is caused by bacteria called Group A *Streptococcus*. This infection is more common in children than in adults. Children with strep throat usually have a very sore throat, fever, and swollen, tender neck glands. They may also complain of headache, nausea or stomach ache. The same bacteria can cause a variety of infections: one type is called scarlet fever. Scarlet fever presents as a red rash all over the body—it looks like a sunburn and feels like sandpaper.

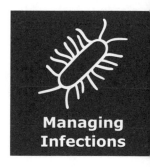

Managing Infections

The two major complications of a strep infection are acute rheumatic fever, which is a disease of the heart and joints, and acute glomerulonephritis, a disease of the kidney. Group A *Streptococcus* can also cause skin infections, bloodstream infections, ear infections and pneumonia.

Some strains of Group A *Streptococcus* may cause severe invasive disease with shock or soft tissue necrosis (flesh-eating disease). (See also Group A *Streptococcus* invasive diseases, page 211.)

It's difficult to identify strep throat visually, and health care providers need to take a throat culture (swab) to make the diagnosis. Strep throat is treated with an antibiotic (usually penicillin or amoxicillin). Although the infection often gets better without treatment, some children can get serious complications if they are not treated. Recovery is faster with an antibiotic.

Transmission

Strep throat is spread by direct contact with secretions of the mouth or nose or direct contact with a skin lesion. It may also be spread through large respiratory droplets.

What to do

1. Advise the parents to have their child seen by a doctor as soon as possible.
2. Watch for signs of fever or sore throat in other children.
3. A fact sheet is available at www.caringforkids.cps.ca and can be downloaded and given to the parents of a child who has strep throat or distributed to the **parents of all children** in your program if an outbreak occurs.

Exclusion and reporting

- Children with strep throat or scarlet fever should return to child care only when they have received **at least** one full day (24 hours) of antibiotic treatment and are well enough to participate comfortably in all program activities, including going outside.
- You should report strep throat to your local public health unit if you suspect an outbreak—defined as more than 2 cases in a month.
- Scarlet fever is reportable in some jurisdictions.

Pertussis (whooping cough)

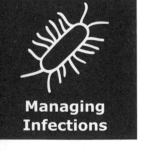

Pertussis (whooping cough) is caused by a bacteria called *Bordetella pertussis*, and is a particularly severe infection for babies. Illness usually begins with a runny nose and cough, with attacks of coughing that become increasingly frequent and severe. Pertussis is called whooping cough because of the characteristic gasping breath at the end of a coughing spell, though in some babies and older children this "whoop" may be absent. During coughing attacks, children with pertussis have difficulty drawing breath, may get blue in the face and will often vomit afterward. Coughing can be triggered by eating, drinking, crying or laughing.

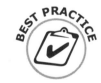

BEST PRACTICE

Young adults should receive a booster shot of acellular pertussis vaccine, especially if they plan to work with children. Outbreaks of pertussis have occurred in child care centres where immunization of children or staff has not been adequate.

Children with pertussis will cough for a long time, usually 6 to 10 weeks. The disease is most severe in babies under 1 year of age: many become so ill that they have to be cared for in hospital. Minor complications include nosebleeds, small hemorrhages in the whites of the eyes because of forceful coughing, swelling of the face and ear infections. Major complications can include weight loss, pneumonia, spells where a child stops breathing, seizures, brain damage and even death. Older children and adults may have rib fractures or hernias from prolonged, forceful coughing.

If given early enough, an antibiotic may improve the symptoms of pertussis and speed a child's recovery. To prevent the spread of infection, antibiotics may be prescribed for contacts in the same household or in home-based child care, especially if someone is at risk of severe disease, such as a child under 1 year of age or a pregnant woman in her third trimester.

Pertussis is usually prevented by routine immunization, starting at 2 months of age. The vaccine prevents disease in most children who have had the required number of doses for their age. Those who get pertussis despite receiving the vaccine will have much milder symptoms than those who have never been vaccinated.

Transmission

Pertussis is very contagious, spreading easily from person to person in households or group settings. The bacteria are present in mucus and droplets expelled from the nose or throat when an infected child coughs or sneezes. These droplets reach the nose or throat of persons nearby (within 1 m [3 ft.]). Indirect spread through contaminated toys or other objects occurs very rarely, if at all. Pertussis incubates for at least 7 to 10 days, and a child with pertussis can spread the germs from the beginning of the illness, which resembles a common cold, for as long as 3 weeks after the start of coughing spells.

What to do

1. Advise the parents to have their child seen by a doctor as soon as possible. If pertussis is diagnosed, contact your local public health unit immediately for guidance on how to manage exposed children and staff. Children who are not completely immunized may need to be vaccinated. Prophylactic antibiotics may be mandated for those at risk of severe disease, as well as for children and staff who are in contact with high-risk peers or household members.
2. Have the immunization records for all children and staff ready for review by public health authorities.
3. Watch other children for signs or symptoms of pertussis for up to 3 weeks after contact with a sick child.
4. A fact sheet is available at www.caringforkids.cps.ca and can be downloaded and distributed to the **parents of all children** in your program. Usually, public health authorities will also provide a letter for you to send to families.

Exclusion and reporting

- Exclusion is no longer considered effective. The decision to exclude is now made by public health authorities and may be mandated if high-risk persons are present (i.e., children under 1 year of age or pregnant women in their third trimester). If so, a child with pertussis should be excluded from child care until an appropriate antibiotic has been taken for 5 full days. If no treatment is given, the child must be excluded for 3 weeks from the start of the coughing spells.
- Pertussis is reportable to local public health authorities by the treating physician and testing laboratory.

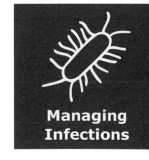

Managing Infections

Mumps

Mumps, a viral infection of the salivary glands, is now uncommon in Canada because almost all children receive routine immunization. Most outbreaks of mumps occur in adolescents and young adults, many of whom have received only one dose of the vaccine, or in unvaccinated children coming to Canada from countries where mumps vaccine is not routinely given.

This illness is not severe in most children. Children with mumps usually have swollen glands at the jaw line on one or both sides of the face. The infection may also have a mild effect on the lining of the child's brain, testicles and pancreas. Very rarely, mumps causes deafness. However, mumps is more severe in adults.

Mumps vaccine is given at 1 year of age, with a second dose at either 18 months or 4 to 6 years of age, depending on where you live in Canada. In vaccinated children, an infection of the salivary glands is usually not due to mumps but to a different virus.

Transmission

Mumps is a contagious disease, spreading easily from person to person in households or group settings through saliva or droplets from the mouth or nose of an infected person. It is spread through sneezing, coughing, kissing, and sharing food, drinks, water bottles or musical instruments. Mumps incubates for 14 to 25 days, which means a child with mumps can spread the germs even before showing any signs or symptoms.

What to do

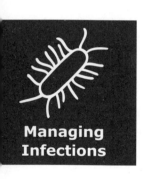

Managing Infections

1. Advise the parents to have their child seen by a doctor as soon as possible. If mumps is diagnosed, contact your local public health unit immediately for guidance on how to manage exposed children and staff. Immunization may be mandated. Non-immune children and caregivers may require immediate vaccination. As the vaccine is a live vaccine, it should not be given to people with weakened immune systems or to pregnant women.
2. Have the immunization records for all children and staff ready for review by public health authorities.
3. Watch other children for signs or symptoms of mumps for up to 25 days after contact with a sick child.

Exclusion and reporting

- Children with mumps should be excluded until 9 days after the onset of swelling.
- Mumps is reportable to local public health authorities by the treating physician and testing laboratory.

Cytomegalovirus (CMV)

CMV is a common virus that causes mild or no symptoms in healthy children but can have serious effects for women in the early stages of pregnancy or for people with a weakened immune system. Children enrolled in child care programs are more likely to become infected with CMV than children cared for at home, with as many as 80 per cent of toddlers becoming infected in a child care setting. The virus can become dormant (inactive) after the first infection, but the virus remains in the body for life. CMV has no disabling effect on children, but if a woman acquires CMV for the first time during pregnancy, her unborn child may develop deafness and/or a developmental delay. (See also Chapter 15, *Caregivers' Physical Health*.)

Transmission

CMV transmission requires direct contact with an infected person or objects contaminated with urine and saliva, fluids that can continue to excrete the virus for several years. CMV can also pass from mother to child in the womb, during birth or by breastfeeding. It spreads between toddlers at the age when toys and other objects are frequently mouthed and shared. Transmission from child to child care practitioners and to parents at home is very common.

What to do

1. Many children in child care have CMV and are never diagnosed. No extra measures are required for care of the occasional child in whom CMV is diagnosed.
2. Review and reinforce routine practices with all staff, especially hand hygiene, and the proper handling and disposal of soiled diapers.
3. Avoid oral contact with children's mouth secretions (e.g., kissing on the mouth).

Exclusion and reporting

- CMV excretion is so prevalent and the rate of unrecognized infection among young children is so high that exclusion is both impractical and inappropriate.
- CMV doesn't need to be reported to your local public health unit.

Diphtheria

Diphtheria is a severe bacterial disease that can be fatal. Fortunately, this infection is now very rare in Canada because almost all children are routinely immunized against it, starting at 2 months of age. Diphtheria persists in parts of the world where the vaccine is less available, and it is still occasionally diagnosed in unvaccinated children new to Canada. An infection of the throat that blocks breathing, diphtheria may be complicated by heart failure and nerve damage. Diphtheria bacteria sometimes cause infections of the nose, skin or ears.

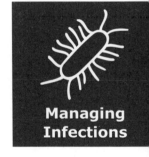

Managing Infections

If diphtheria is diagnosed in a child in your program, exposed children and staff will be required by public health authorities to see a doctor, have throat cultures done, and receive vaccine and antibiotic treatment, and they will be closely watched for signs of illness.

Exclusion and reporting

- A child with diphtheria must be excluded until antibiotic treatment has been completed and 2 cultures from the nose and throat (or skin if there's a skin infection) are negative.
- Diphtheria is reportable to local public health authorities by the treating physician and testing laboratory.

Gastrointestinal infections

Diarrhea

Diarrhea is a very common symptom in childhood, and is usually mild and brief. A child has diarrhea when she has more bowel movements and the stools are less formed and more watery than usual. Mild diarrhea, with a few loose stools on a single day and no other symptoms, may be due to dietary changes or other causes unrelated to infection. When bouts of diarrhea aren't mild or brief, they're usually called either "acute" (commonly caused by infection, also known as gastroenteritis or "stomach flu") or "chronic" (when diarrhea lasts longer than 2 weeks). Chronic diarrhea is less likely to be caused by infection than by diet. Managing acute diarrhea properly will help a child get better more quickly.

Apart from diarrhea, the signs of gastroenteritis are:

- fever,
- loss of appetite,
- nausea and/or vomiting,
- stomach cramps, and/or
- blood and/or mucus in the bowel movement.

Parents should let you know when their child has had one unusually unformed or watery bowel movement.
Assure them that you'll be alert through the day for diarrhea and other signs of infection (e.g., fever or vomiting). The child's doctor will decide whether a stool sample needs to be taken and tested.

Gastroenteritis can be particularly serious in babies because it can quickly lead to dehydration. **Dehydration** occurs when the loss of body fluids, made up of water, sugars and salts, exceeds fluid intake. It happens more rapidly if a child is also vomiting. Severe dehydration can result in shock and even death.

Viruses of different types are by far the most common cause of gastroenteritis in children, although bacteria or parasites are other possible causes. Viral gastroenteritis cannot be cured with antibiotics.

Rotavirus is the leading cause of acute diarrhea in babies and young children. Rotavirus infection usually begins with a high fever and vomiting. Within 12 to 24 hours, profuse and watery diarrhea appears, and vomiting becomes less frequent. If fluids aren't given, rotavirus diarrhea can lead to rapid dehydration, making it a more severe illness than that caused by other viruses. A rotavirus vaccine is available for babies under 6 months old, to protect them at the age when rotavirus infection is most dangerous. When older children and adults contract rotavirus, they have a milder illness and are less likely to become dehydrated.

Diarrhea may also be caused by several different bacteria, such as *Shigella*, *Escherichia coli* O157, other *E. coli* strains, *Salmonella*, *Campylobacter* and *Yersinia*. *Clostridium difficile* is a bacterium normally present in the stools of babies and young children that

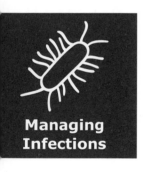

Managing Infections

only rarely causes illness. Bacterial diarrhea can be more severe than viral diarrhea, and stools may contain blood or mucus. Some bacterial diarrhea may be treated with antibiotics and, for some infections, treatment reduces spread. However, for other bacteria, antibiotics are not effective and may actually prolong infection and increase the likelihood of spread.

Giardia is a parasite that causes an intestinal infection called giardiasis. *Giardia* infections occur often in child care, and many children who have them have no symptoms at all. Some children experience diarrhea, with pale and greasy stools, or severe gas, with bloating, stomach cramps, and loss of appetite and/or weight. A *Giardia* infection can incubate (live in the system without causing illness) for 1 to 4 weeks, then cause illness for 2 to 6 weeks. Occasionally, symptoms last longer. Usually, *Giardia* infections go away on their own, and only children who feel ill are treated with medication. There are exceptions. If a child doesn't have diarrhea but tests positive for *Giardia* and is experiencing nausea, fatigue, weight loss or poor appetite, treatment is also required.

Other parasites (e.g., *Entamoeba histolytica, Endolimax nana, Iodamoeba, Dientamoeba* and *Cryptosporidium*) may sometimes cause diarrhea, but are often present in the intestinal tract without causing illness.

Transmission

Germs causing infectious diarrhea spread easily by direct and indirect contact in any group setting, and especially among children still in diapers. Spread accelerates when child care staff aren't thoroughly and routinely washing hands (both their own and the children's) with soap and water after changing diapers, after helping children with toilet or potty use, after using the toilet themselves, and before eating or preparing food. Fecal contamination of hands or objects that then touch the mouth accounts for the spread of most diarrheal infections.

What to do

1. Notify the parents right away and ask for an early pick-up if their child has diarrhea twice in one day, or diarrhea with fever, vomiting or blood in the bowel movement.
2. Advise them to have their child seen by a doctor as soon as possible.
3. Tell them to seek **immediate medical attention** if the child:
   - has bloody, mucousy or black stools,
   - is vomiting **and** showing any signs of dehydration:
     - ➤ no tears when crying,
     - ➤ dry skin, mouth and tongue,
     - ➤ fewer than 4 wet diapers in 24 hours,
     - ➤ sunken eyes or fontanel (the soft spot on the head of children younger than 18 months),
     - ➤ grayish skin, or
     - ➤ rapid breathing.
4. If possible, move a child with diarrhea to a separate area to prevent exposure to other children while you're waiting for an early pick-up.

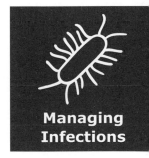

Managing Infections

5. Don't allow other children to use toys handled by an infected child until they've been cleaned and disinfected.
6. Review and reinforce proper hand-hygiene and diapering/toileting routines for all children and staff.
7. Clean and disinfect toys and equipment often.
8. Don't permit staff who are diapering and toileting children to prepare food or handle dishes/utensils on the same day. If these tasks are unavoidable, reinforce hand-hygiene routines.
9. Provided that you have written parental consent, start giving a child with diarrhea an oral rehydration solution (ORS), which contains an exact mixture of water, salts and sugar for preventing dehydration. The body can absorb these solutions, even when the child is vomiting. Give small amounts often, gradually increasing intake until the child can drink normally.
10. If the child isn't vomiting, continue to offer breast milk, formula or regular foods in small, frequent feedings. If the child vomits, you may need to stop food and drink but continue to give ORS.
11. Watch other children and staff for signs of diarrhea. Contact your local public health unit for advice if you suspect an outbreak (i.e., if several children and staff are ill at the same time). The definition of an outbreak varies among jurisdictions, but is usually defined as 2 to 3 or more children at a facility having diarrhea within the previous 48 hours.
12. A fact sheet on *Giardia* is available at www.caringforkids.ca. Public health authorities will often provide a letter for you to distribute to the **parents of all children** in your program.

Exclusion and reporting

- A child with diarrhea should be excluded from your facility if:
  - ➤ diarrheal stool cannot be contained in a diaper or a toilet-trained child cannot control bowel movements,
  - ➤ there's blood or mucus in the stool (unless bacterial infection has been ruled out by a doctor),
  - ➤ the child is also vomiting (unless infection has been ruled out), or
  - ➤ local public health authorities require it (e.g., if it is a symptomatic, confirmed *Giardia*, *E. coli*, *Shigella* or *Salmonella* infection).
- For certain gastrointestinal infections, the child should be excluded until 2 (for *Shigella* or *E. coli* O157) or 3 (for *Salmonella* typhi) stool tests, taken at least 24 hours apart, are negative. Consult your local public health authorities, as provincial/territorial regulations vary.
- Usually, children with a *Giardia* infection may return to child care once the diarrhea has resolved. If you have an outbreak of *Giardia* at your facility, screening and treating children who have no obvious symptoms may become necessary, and asymptomatic children with *Giardia* may need to be excluded until 2 stool specimens, taken at least 24 hours apart, test negative.

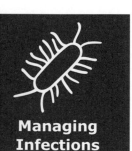

Managing Infections

- Giardiasis and bacterial gastroenteritis are reportable to local public health authorities by the treating physician and testing laboratory. As this information may not be linked to child care attendance, be sure to report any case of bloody or diagnosed bacterial diarrhea or giardiasis to your local public health unit.

Hepatitis A virus (HAV)

Hepatitis A is an infection of the liver caused by a virus. Many infants and young children infected with HAV don't get sick or have any symptoms. If illness does occur, it's very mild and brief, with fever only. However, even without symptoms, children are contagious and can spread the virus to others. Often, the first signal of an HAV outbreak in a child care facility is the diagnosis of the infection in a staff member or parent. A blood test is required to diagnose HAV.

Adolescents and adults are much more likely to become ill when infected with HAV. Symptoms include fever, fatigue, loss of appetite, nausea, vomiting, abdominal pain and—because the liver isn't working properly—yellowing of the skin and the whites of the eyes (jaundice), and tea-coloured urine. The illness may last several weeks, but most people recover completely. Permanent damage to the liver is rare, and immunity after infection lasts for life. No specific treatment is available for this infection.

Transmission

HAV is found in the stools of infected people and is spread by close contact with those who are infected, or through food or water that has become contaminated with stool containing HAV. As most children infected with HAV have no symptoms, adhering to and enforcing proper hand-hygiene and diapering/toileting routines for all children and staff are essential to prevent spread.

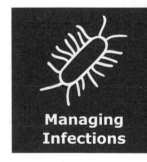

Managing Infections

HAV can be prevented in people who have been in close contact with an infected person by giving hepatitis A vaccine or immune globulin (Ig). Ig is a product made from blood donations containing protective antibodies against HAV. Although the vaccine is not administered routinely in all jurisdictions, it should be given to children 1 year of age and older when exposure is suspected. Families visiting a country where the disease is endemic should be immunized before departure. Hepatitis A vaccine and/or Ig is also given to:

- protect selected high-risk children and adults (e.g., those living in rural or remote areas lacking adequate sanitation),
- control outbreaks of HAV in child care centres, kindergartens, schools or communities,
- prevent infection after exposure (e.g., to household or other close contacts), and
- prevent infection in people travelling to or adopting a child from a country where HAV is common.

The vaccine is effective if given within a week of exposure, but can only be given to children over 1 year of age. If more than a week but less than 2 has elapsed since exposure, or if the exposed person has a weakened immune system, Ig is also given because the vaccine alone may not be effective. Exposed children under 1 year of age are given Ig only. Ig is not effective if more than 2 weeks have passed since exposure.

What to do

1. If a child looks jaundiced, advise the parents to have him seen by a doctor as soon as possible. Getting a prompt diagnosis of HAV is important because of the short time after exposure when treatment is effective.
2. If HAV is diagnosed, contact your local public health unit immediately for advice on how to manage exposed children and staff. Public health authorities will coordinate vaccination and/or treatment. Vaccination and/or treatment with Ig may be mandated.
3. Have the immunization records for all children and staff ready for review by public health authorities.
4. Review and reinforce proper hand-hygiene, diapering/toileting and food-handling routines with all children and staff. These routines are essential to prevent transmission.
5. Ensure there is no sharing of towels and facecloths.
6. Watch other children and staff for jaundice and/or any other signs and symptoms of HAV. Ask parents to tell you or to report directly to public health authorities if they or any household members also develop these signs and symptoms.
7. A fact sheet is available at www.caringforkids.cps.ca and can be downloaded and distributed to the **parents of all children** in your program. Public health authorities may also provide a letter for you to send to families.

Exclusion and reporting

- Children infected with HAV should be excluded from child care for a full week after the onset of the illness, unless all other children and staff in the program have received prophylaxis with Ig and/or HAV vaccine. Exclusion also applies to parents or staff members with HAV.
- HAV is reportable to local public health authorities by the treating physician and testing laboratory.

Pinworms

Pinworms are tiny, white thread-like worms that live in the rectum. The worms crawl out of the anus at night and lay their eggs on nearby skin. Infestations of pinworms are very common in preschoolers and spread easily among children and staff in child care settings. Control is difficult because the rate of reinfestation is high. Most children with pinworms do not have any symptoms apart from itching around the anus and, if the infection is severe, disturbed sleep and irritability.

Pinworms are a nuisance, not a serious disease, and are treated with medication prescribed by a doctor, usually in single doses 2 weeks apart. However, treatment does not prevent a new infestation if the child is re-exposed to other infested children. If an outbreak persists, it may be necessary to treat all members of the child care facility at once, and possibly their families.

Transmission

Pinworms can be spread directly (when an infected child scratches the itchy area and transfers eggs to her own or another child's mouth), or indirectly (by contaminated hands or objects, such as shared toys). Eggs are picked up on the hands of others and ingested.

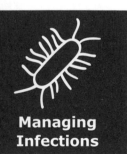

Managing Infections

Pinworm eggs can be found under the fingernails when children scratch and in the clothes or bed linens shared with an infected child or adult. These eggs survive for up to 3 weeks outside the body, on clothing, bedding or other objects.

What to do

1. Advise the parents to have their child seen by a doctor for diagnosis and treatment. Other family members may need to be treated at the same time to avoid reinfestation.
2. Review and reinforce proper hand-hygiene, diapering/toileting, food-handling and bedding routines for all children and staff.
3. Change the bed linens and underclothes of infected children, handle them without shaking (which can scatter eggs) and launder them promptly. If a child's laundry is being sent home, keep the bedding, clothing and towels in sealed plastic bags.
4. Ask the parents to bathe an infected child in the morning, to minimize the presence of eggs.
5. Watch other children and staff for signs of a pinworm infestation (e.g., anal scratching).
6. Advise all staff to keep their fingernails short and avoid nail-biting.
7. Because the eggs are sensitive to sunlight, open blinds or curtains in bedrooms/ sleeping areas during the day when children aren't sleeping.
8. A fact sheet is available at www.caringforkids.cps.ca and can be downloaded and distributed to the **parents of all children** in your program.

Exclusion and reporting

- Children with pinworms can continue to attend child care.
- Pinworms do not need to be reported to your local public health unit unless an outbreak cannot be controlled and guidance is needed.

Infections of the skin and scalp

Head lice

Head lice are tiny insects that live on the scalp, where they lay their eggs (or "nits"). Head lice spread easily in groups of children and are very common in child care settings.

Many children with head lice have no symptoms apart from an itchy scalp. To diagnose a case of head lice, a live louse must be seen, which can be difficult. Finding nits suggests that a child may have head lice, but it isn't conclusive. Head lice are found on the hair very close to the scalp, the bottom of the neck and behind the ears. If you see lice, the child needs to be treated. On average, children with head lice carry no more than 10 to 20 live lice, which are only the size of a sesame seed, move very fast and are hard to see. Easier to spot are the nits. They appear as whitish-grey ovals, about the size of a grain of sand, and stick to hair very close to the

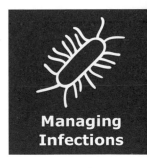

**Managing
Infections**

Common infestations of the skin and scalp, such as head lice and scabies, are not diseases—nor do they spread disease. They are a nuisance, but having them is in no way linked to lack of cleanliness.

scalp. Unlike dandruff, nits are so firmly attached to the hair that they can't be removed easily. A child can have a few nits without having live lice—the nits may be empty shells.

Transmission

While head lice do not transmit disease, they do spread through direct contact among children or through indirect contact from items such as shared hats, combs, hairbrushes, hair ornaments and headphones. They don't fly or hop, but they crawl very quickly. Nits hatch in 6 to 10 days, and lice survive for only 1 or 2 days away from the scalp. Head lice can't live on pets, such as cats and dogs.

What to do

1. Notify the parents and ask them to verify whether their child has lice and to consult a doctor or pharmacist about treatment, which is available without a prescription. Only children with a confirmed case of head lice should be treated. A child's age, allergies or certain medical conditions will affect the treatment choice, and other family members should be examined and treated at the same time **if infested**.
2. Don't remove nits after treatment, as it is not necessary to prevent spread.
3. Since lice don't live long off the scalp, there's no need for extensive cleaning. To get rid of lice or nits from specific items, like pillowcases or hats, wash them in hot water and dry them in a hot dryer. Dry-clean items that cannot be washed, such as stuffed animals, or simply store them in an airtight plastic bag for 2 weeks.
4. Teach children to avoid head-to-head contact with other children until the lice are gone. Combs, hairbrushes, caps, hats and hair ornaments should not be shared.
5. Watch for signs of lice (itchy scalp) in other children and staff.
6. A fact sheet is available at www.caringforkids.cps.ca and can be downloaded and distributed to the **parents of all children** in your program (or group, if you're working in a large facility).

Exclusion and reporting

- Children with head lice should be treated and can attend child care as usual. Although exclusion was common in the past, it's ineffective and unnecessary.
- Head lice do not need to be reported to your local public health unit unless an outbreak cannot be controlled and guidance is needed.

Scabies

Scabies is caused by mites, which are tiny insects that live only on the skin of people. Mites burrow under the skin and lay their eggs, causing a rash that is very itchy and red. Itchiness is usually worse at night. The rash usually appears between the fingers, in the groin area, between the toes, or around the wrists or elbows, but it may be found anywhere on the body. In children under 2 years of age, the rash may appear on the head, face, neck, chest, abdomen and back as white, curvy, thread-like lines, tiny red bumps or scratch marks. Scabies is a common condition in children and is easy to treat, but it is often confused with other skin conditions.

Once a doctor has made the diagnosis, scabies is treated with a prescription medication applied as a lotion or cream. To prevent recurrence, all members of a child's household may

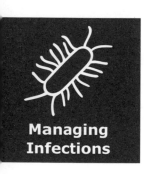

Managing Infections

need to be treated at once, and all clothes and bedding washed at the same time. Itchiness may continue for a few weeks after treatment even if no scabies is present.

Transmission

Scabies is spread by prolonged, close and intimate contact. Mites cannot live away from human skin for more than 3 days. Mites on clothing die immediately when the clothing is washed in hot water and dried in a hot dryer.

What to do

1. Advise the parents to have their child seen by a doctor for diagnosis and treatment.
2. Notify the parents of all children in your program and ask them to examine their child for scabies rash.
3. Wash an infected child's bed linen and the facility's towels and dress-up clothes in hot water, and dry them on the dryer's hottest setting. Send the child's special blanket, clothes, and other personal items home with the parents to be washed and dried in the same way. Items that cannot be washed can be stored in an airtight plastic bag for 1 week to kill the mites.
4. Watch for signs of scabies, such as itching and scratching, in other children.
5. A fact sheet is available at www.caringforkids.cps.ca and can be downloaded and distributed to the **parents of all children** in the same program.

Exclusion and reporting

- Children with scabies can return to the child care facility the day after the initial treatment has been applied.
- Scabies does not need to be reported to your local public health unit unless an outbreak cannot be controlled and guidance is needed.

Cold sores

Cold sores (or fever blisters) are blisters on the lips or in the mouth, caused by a virus called herpes simplex type 1. Infection is very common. Some children get an acute illness with many painful ulcers in their mouth and a high fever, while others have a simple cold sore or asymptomatic infection. The illness usually lasts for a week or more. The ulcers may be so painful that the child is unable to eat or drink and requires hospitalization. Once a person is infected with the herpes simplex virus, the virus remains in the body, and infections can recur over a lifetime. These recurrences are usually brief and mild. The frequency and pain of flare-ups vary widely from person to person.

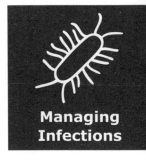

Managing Infections

Transmission

The risk of the herpes simplex virus spreading in child care is not known, although spread is common within families. Transmission usually happens through direct contact with infected lesions or mouth secretions such as saliva or drool. Most infections are asymptomatic, but young children with extensive infection who drool can pass the virus to other children. Immunocompromised children or those with open skin lesions (e.g., severe eczema) may be at increased risk. You can prevent infection by using proper hand hygiene, especially after contact with saliva, and by avoiding oral contact with a child's mouth secretions (i.e., holding hands instead of kissing).

What to do

1. Advise the parents to have their child seen by a doctor for diagnosis and treatment.
2. Review and reinforce mealtime and cleaning routines to minimize the sharing of cups, baby bottles and toys that are mouthed. Clean and disinfect all toys and equipment often.
3. Review and reinforce proper hand-hygiene routines with all children and staff.

Exclusion and reporting

- Children with simple cold sores don't need to be excluded from child care.
- Children who have extensive mouth lesions and are drooling should be excluded until they can eat comfortably and are well enough to participate in all program activities.
- Cold sores do not need to be reported to your local public health unit.

Impetigo and other bacterial skin infections

Impetigo is a very common infection of the skin caused by *Staphylococcus aureus* or Group A *Streptococcus* bacteria. These bacteria can cause skin infections that occur when the skin has been injured by a scrape or insect bite, most often in the summer. Impetigo is also common after chickenpox. Having impetigo is not linked to a lack of cleanliness, but it often affects school-aged children who live in crowded conditions, play contact sports, or have other skin problems or irritations.

Infection usually appears around a child's mouth or nose, or on exposed skin of the face or limbs as a cluster of red bumps or blisters, which may then ooze a clear fluid or become covered by an itchy honey-coloured crust. Many germs live under this crust. A severe skin infection occasionally develops, accompanied by fever, pain, general weakness and swelling.

A doctor usually diagnoses impetigo by sight. A skin swab may be used to identify the type of bacteria causing the infection, but this test usually isn't necessary.

***Streptococcus pyogenes* or Group A *Streptococcus* bacteria** are occasionally found on the skin and in the throat. (See *Streptococcal pharyngitis*, pages 181-82.) Streptococcal impetigo is treated with antibiotics, given orally or applied as an ointment to the skin. Some strains of Group A *Streptococcus* may cause severe invasive infections (see pages 211-12).

***Staphylococcus aureus* bacteria** are commonly found in the nose and on the skin. About 20 to 30 per cent of people carry them, most often with no ill effect on health. In the past, *Staphylococcus* could be treated with many different antibiotics. When strains resistant to penicillin-type antibiotics were first seen, they were called "methicillin-resistant *Staphylococcus aureus*" or MRSA. Resistant strains are found most often in health care facilities, but new strains have been identified in community settings, including child care facilities. **Community-associated methicillin-resistant *Staphylococcus aureus* (CA-MRSA)** is the term used for these strains. In Canada, CA-MRSA, although rare, is increasing and is more common in children than in adults. It sometimes causes skin infections and may require special antibiotic therapy. Minor skin infections don't always require antibiotic treatment.

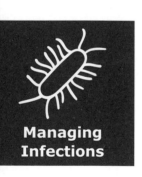

Managing Infections

Transmission

The bacteria that cause impetigo and other skin infections are spread by direct and indirect contact with infected, draining skin lesions. Keeping lesions covered and following proper hand-hygiene practices, especially after touching infected skin, help to prevent spread. Impetigo can be spread from one part of the body to another by scratching with contaminated fingers. It can also be spread on bed linens, towels or clothing that have been in contact with infected skin. Treatment with topical or oral antibiotics may prevent spread of Group A *Streptococcus* or *Staphylococcus aureus* bacteria.

What to do

1. Advise the parents to have their child seen by a doctor for diagnosis and treatment.
2. Review and reinforce proper hand-hygiene routines with all children and staff.
3. If possible, cover any draining lesions or wounds with a dressing.
4. Wash your hands after touching any skin lesions or contaminated materials (e.g., a soiled bandage or gauze skin dressing). Wear gloves if the dressing is visibly soiled.
5. Dispose of used dressings in a plastic-lined garbage container with a sealed lid immediately after they're removed.
6. Clean and disinfect all toys, equipment and frequently touched surfaces often.
7. Make sure that skin care products (e.g., creams, lotions and soaps), toothbrushes and unwashed towels are not shared.
8. Monitor all children and staff in your program for skin lesions.
9. Contact your local public health unit for advice if you suspect an outbreak. The definition of an outbreak varies, but it usually means more than one case in the same room within a month. Exposed children may need treatment to prevent further spread.
10. Inform the parents of other children in your program if there's an outbreak of impetigo in your facility and advise them to see their doctor if their child develops a skin infection.

Exclusion and reporting

- Children with impetigo or any other skin infection caused by Group A *Streptococcus* should be excluded until antibiotic treatment has been given for 24 hours and they are well enough to participate comfortably in all program activities.
- For other skin infections, children should be excluded only if they have a draining wound or lesions that can't be kept covered.
- In some jurisdictions, a case of CA-MRSA must be reported to the local public health unit by the testing laboratory. Regulations vary.

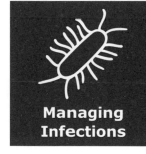

Managing Infections

Ringworm

Ringworm is an infection of the skin caused by a fungus. The infection causes a rash that may be ring-shaped, with a raised edge and scaly patches that blister and ooze. The rash is usually quite itchy and flaky, and may occur on a child's scalp, body, groin or feet. When the scalp is infected, an area of baldness often appears. Fungal infections on the feet are usually very itchy and cause cracking between the toes.

Once a doctor has made the diagnosis, ringworm is treated with a prescription medication, to be taken orally or applied as an ointment.

Transmission

Ringworm is contagious. It can be passed from one person to another by direct skin-to-skin contact or by contact with contaminated items such as combs or unwashed clothing, or shower or pool surfaces. You can also catch ringworm from pets that carry the fungus. Cats are common carriers.

What to do

1. Advise the parents to have their child seen by a doctor for diagnosis and treatment.
2. Make sure the child's hands and your own hands are washed carefully after touching infected skin.
3. Review and reinforce proper hand-hygiene routines with all children and staff.
4. Make sure children do not share combs, hairbrushes, hair ornaments, hats, clothing, towels and other personal items.
5. Examine other children in your program for ringworm.
6. Wear sandals or shoes at gyms, lockers and pools.
7. Avoid touching pets with bald spots.
8. A fact sheet is available at www.caringforkids.cps.ca and can be downloaded and distributed to the **parents of all children** in the same program.

Exclusion and reporting

- Children with ringworm may return to child care as soon as treatment has started.
- Ringworm does not need to be reported to your local public health unit.

Thrush and *Candida* diaper rash

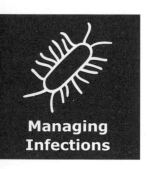

Managing Infections

Thrush is a common mouth infection in young children. It's caused by a fungus called *Candida*. The same fungus causes a specific type of diaper rash and other skin or vaginal infections. *Candida* is usually present in the large bowel, without causing illness. Infections are more likely to occur after treatment with antibiotics. Antibiotics destroy many of the bacteria in the intestinal tract, resulting in an overgrowth of *Candida*. Steroids also enhance the growth of *Candida*. Children using inhaled steroids for asthma management can get thrush if they aren't diligent about rinsing their mouth.

Thrush appears as whitish-grey patches on the inside of the cheek or on the tongue. Although the patches may look like milk, they cannot be rubbed off. In rare cases, a baby's mouth may be so sore that it becomes painful to suck, but most babies don't have mouth pain.

Candida diaper rash occurs most often in the deepest part of the creases in the groin and buttocks, where skin is more prone to stay moist. This rash consists of large bright-red patches with sharply defined borders surrounded by small red spots. It may be painful and/or itchy. The rash may also occur in other moist skin folds (e.g., around the neck in a plump baby).

Milder cases of thrush often disappear naturally, but treatment with medication prescribed by a doctor is usually required. *Candida* diaper rash is treated with antifungal creams or ointments.

Transmission

Candida is spread through direct contact. It may be transmitted to an infant from the mother at birth or from the mother's breast. Bottle nipples or soothers that have been contaminated with the fungus also spread it. Boiling bottle nipples and soothers may help to prevent thrush.

What to do

1. Advise the parents to have their child seen by a doctor for diagnosis and treatment.
2. Don't rub the rash. (For more about treating diaper rash, see Chapter 7, *Common Conditions*.)
3. Fact sheets on thrush and *Candida* diaper rash are available at www.caringforkids. cps.ca, and can be downloaded and given to the parents of a child with either condition.

Exclusion and reporting

- Children with thrush or *Candida* diaper rash can continue in child care provided they are well enough to participate comfortably in all program activities.
- Thrush and *Candida* diaper rash do not need to be reported to your local public health unit.

Molluscum contagiosum

Molluscum contagiosum is a common, mild skin disease caused by a pox virus. Although molluscum can occur at any age, it's most common in children 1 to 10 years of age. Tiny "pinpoints" appear on the skin 1 to 6 months after exposure. These turn into pinkish-white bumps that are smooth and shiny, have a dip in the middle and have a milky-white cheesy material inside. Bumps can appear anywhere on the child's body. Molluscum is harmless and will disappear after several months without treatment. If the growths are especially bothersome, a doctor will prescribe a topical medication or remove them by scraping or freezing.

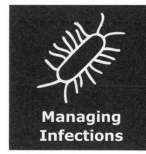

Managing Infections

Transmission

Molluscum can be transmitted by direct contact with the skin of an infected person. Scratching can also spread the infection. But it doesn't spread easily from person to person and outbreaks are rare.

What to do

1. Advise the parents to have their child seen by a doctor for diagnosis.
2. Wash hands frequently and properly. This is essential for preventing direct contact transmission.
3. Make sure the child does not share towels with others.
4. No other measures are usually required. Covering the lesions may not be necessary or practical. There may be many lesions on the face or other exposed skin areas and keeping these tightly covered for prolonged periods may lead to maceration, bacterial infection and scarring. If the child picks at exposed lesions, cover them with a loose gauze dressing. Persistent picking may be a signal for the parents to have the growths removed.

Exclusion and reporting

- Children with molluscum can continue to attend child care.
- Molluscum does not need to be reported to your public health unit.

Other viral infections with rash

Chickenpox (varicella)

Chickenpox is a very common childhood infection caused by the varicella-zoster virus. The infection typically begins with a fever, followed in 1 or 2 days by a rash. The rash usually starts as red spots, which turn into fluid-filled blisters that crust over within a few days. This rash may be very itchy, and new spots continue to appear over the next 2 to 3 days. Chickenpox is usually mild, but this infection can be accompanied by a high fever and severe rash.

Chickenpox is a more serious illness for adolescents and adults than for younger children. Most adults have already had the disease and will not get chickenpox again. However, the virus remains dormant in the nervous system and can be reactivated later in life to cause shingles (zoster).

The most common complication of chickenpox is a bacterial skin infection, which can be mild or severe. A dangerous though rare complication is a Group A *Streptococcus* invasive infection called necrotizing fasciitis (flesh-eating disease). (See *Other severe bacterial infections*, below.) Other (also rare) complications include pneumonia and encephalitis (inflammation of the brain). Chickenpox is a much more serious illness for people with immune deficiencies.

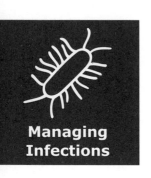

Managing Infections

Chickenpox vaccine is given routinely to all children at 1 year of age and is also recommended for older children, teens, and adults who haven't had chickenpox. It can also prevent the infection in susceptible contacts if it's given within 3 to 5 days after the first day of exposure. It's a live vaccine, so it isn't given to people with a weakened immune system or to women who are pregnant.

For susceptible people who cannot be vaccinated and are at high risk for severe chickenpox, including newborns of infected mothers, immunocompromised people or women who are pregnant, an immune globulin (Ig) preparation with a high concentration of antibody against chickenpox (varicella-zoster Ig) is used to prevent the disease or make it less severe. It must be given within 4 days of initial contact to be effective.

Transmission

Viruses in the throat and from scratched skin lesions spread very easily from person to person through the air, as well as by direct contact with the infected blister fluid. It can be spread through the air from 2 days before the rash starts until the last blister has crusted over (usually about 5 days after the rash appears). Spread is most likely to occur before the rash develops, when a child who is not known to be infected continues to be in contact with others. Because the same virus causes both chickenpox and shingles, a person who has never had chickenpox may get this infection from someone with shingles if their skin lesions are not covered. You cannot get shingles from someone who has shingles.

What to do

1. Advise the parents to have their child seen by a doctor as soon as possible.
2. If chickenpox is confirmed, notify everyone connected with your program (children, parents and staff) who may have come into contact with the infected child, as they may require vaccine or immune globulin (Ig). At risk are babies under 1 year of age, other children, their parents, and staff who haven't had chickenpox and haven't been vaccinated, particularly contacts who are immunocompromised or pregnant. Advise anyone who might be at risk to consult their doctor as soon as possible.
3. Recommend to the parents of all children over 1 year of age who are non-immune that they have their children vaccinated against chickenpox as soon as possible.
4. Advise the parents of all children in your program to watch for signs of chickenpox.
5. Watch for signs of chickenpox in children and staff.
6. Because chickenpox lesions are easily infected, keep the infected child's skin clean and discourage scratching.
7. Watch for signs of severe illness in a child with or recovering from chickenpox. Advise the parents to seek immediate medical attention if:
   • the child's fever lasts longer than 48 hours and is 39°C (102°F) or higher,
   • the fever subsides and then returns to 39°C (102°F) or higher in a day or two,
   • any chickenpox spots become enlarged, red or very sore, or
   • the child seems very ill.
8. Acetaminophen (e.g., Tylenol, Tempra, Panadol and others) may be given to reduce the child's discomfort. Follow your facility's policy for administering medication. Be sure to record giving medication on the *Medication consent form and record sheet*. (See Appendix 7.1, pages 139–40.)
9. If varicella is not reportable in your jurisdiction, contact your local public health unit if you suspect an outbreak in your facility and need advice about how to manage it.
10. A fact sheet is available at www.caringforkids.cps.ca and can be downloaded and distributed to the **parents of all children** in your program.

ALERT

Never give a child with chickenpox a medication that contains acetylsalicylic acid (ASA) (aspirin). This increases the risk of Reye's syndrome, a severe illness that can damage the liver and brain.

Exclusion and reporting

• Exclusion is not a very effective way to prevent the spread of chickenpox in child care facilities, because it is contagious 1 to 2 days before the rash appears.
• Children with mild chickenpox can continue to attend child care regardless of the state of their rash, provided they are well enough to take part comfortably in all program activities, including going outside. A child with a high fever or enough spots to be uncomfortable, or who is feeling unwell, should be excluded until he feels well enough to participate.
• In some jurisdictions, a case of chickenpox must be reported to the local public health unit by the treating physician or testing laboratory. Regulations vary.

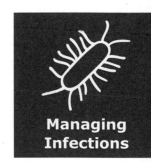

Managing Infections

Hand-foot-and-mouth disease

Hand-foot-and-mouth disease is a viral infection that most often affects young children, but it can occur at any age. It may cause fever, headache, a sore throat and mouth, loss of appetite, lack of energy and a characteristic rash. Red spots, often with small blisters on top, appear on the hands and feet and sometimes elsewhere on the body. Small, painful ulcers may also develop in the mouth. This illness usually lasts for 7 to 10 days. Because a virus causes it, antibiotics do not help. Outbreaks of hand-foot-and-mouth disease are most likely to occur in the summer and fall.

Transmission

Hand-foot-and-mouth disease spreads from person to person through direct or indirect contact with the virus present in an infected person's saliva or stool. This virus may remain in the stool for 4 weeks after the onset of illness.

What to do

1. Advise the parents to have their child seen by a doctor for diagnosis and treatment.
2. Review and reinforce proper hand-hygiene and diaper-changing routines with all children and staff.
3. Clean and disinfect any items soiled with nasal and/or throat discharges.

Exclusion and reporting

- Children with hand-foot-and-mouth disease can attend child care as long as they feel well enough to participate comfortably in all program activities.
- Hand-foot-and-mouth disease does not need to be reported to your local public health unit.

Measles

Measles is a serious viral disease that is now rare in Canada because almost all children are immunized against it. However, measles may still be seen in people new to Canada and in visitors from other countries where the disease hasn't been as closely controlled. Measles can make children very ill. Many children become so sick that they must be hospitalized.

Children with measles usually have a high fever, cough, runny nose and red eyes for a few days before the rash starts. The rash begins on the face as small red spots, which enlarge and clump together and then spread over the entire body. Many other illnesses resemble measles, and a child must see a doctor immediately for laboratory testing to confirm the diagnosis.

Complications, such as ear infections and pneumonia, occur in 10 to 15 per cent of cases, and more often in people who are poorly nourished or chronically ill, and in babies under 1 year of age. In about 1 in every 1,000 cases, encephalitis (inflammation of the brain) develops. About a third of the cases of measles encephalitis result in severe brain damage. Adults with measles can have a more serious illness than children and often develop complications such as pneumonia.

Children in Canada now routinely receive two doses of measles vaccine starting at 1 year of age, with the second dose given at either 18 months or 4 to 6 years of age. The spread

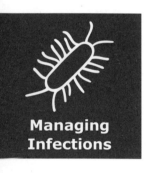

Managing Infections

of measles may be prevented by giving the vaccine or immune globulin (Ig) to children who haven't yet had the disease. Measles vaccine must be given within 72 hours of the first day of contact. Because it's a live vaccine, it can't be given to anyone who has weakened immunity or is pregnant, and it doesn't work in children under 6 months old. If measles vaccine can't be given, or if more than 72 hours have elapsed since the first contact, Ig is given to those who are non-immune. Antibiotics have no effect on measles.

Transmission

Measles spreads very easily from person to person through particles in the air. People with measles are infectious from 3 to 5 days before to 4 days after the rash appears. Almost all children who haven't been vaccinated will get measles if they're in the same household or child care facility as someone who has the disease. It takes about 2 weeks to get measles after being exposed to someone who has the disease. Quick action is essential for limiting an outbreak of measles.

What to do

1. Measles exposure in Canada is a medical emergency. Advise the parents of infected or susceptible children to have them seen by a doctor immediately for diagnosis and treatment. Measles is highly contagious, so they should inform their doctor of the suspected diagnosis before going to the office so that arrangements can be made to avoid any contact with other patients. All suspected cases of measles must be confirmed by blood testing.
2. Contact your local public health unit immediately upon confirmation that a child in your program has measles. The unit will direct and arrange for treatment of exposed children and staff. Vaccine or Ig may be urgently needed.
3. Be prepared to provide public health authorities with immunization records for all children and staff and contact information for all parents.
4. Consult public health authorities before distributing information about measles to the **parents of all children** in your program. Usually, the public health unit will provide a letter for you to send to families.

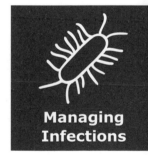

Managing Infections

Exclusion and reporting

*   Children with measles should be excluded for **at least** 4 days after the onset of the rash and only return once they are well enough to participate comfortably in all program activities, including going outside.
*   Unless they can be immunized within 72 hours of the first exposure, non-immune children and staff must be excluded until the incubation period for measles is past (for 2 weeks after the onset of a rash in the last case in the facility).
*   Measles is reportable to local public health authorities by the treating physician and testing laboratory.

Parvovirus B19 (also, fifth disease, erythema infectiosum, or "slapped cheek" syndrome)

A common infection, parvovirus B19 usually appears as a very red rash on a child's cheeks, giving a "slapped cheek" look. After 1 to 4 days, a red, lace-like rash develops, first on the child's torso and arms, then over the rest of the body. Occasionally, the rash may itch. The child is usually not very ill, but may have a low-grade fever, general malaise or a mild cold a few days before the rash breaks out. The rash may come and go over the next 1 to 3 weeks, fluctuating with environmental changes such as temperature and exposure to sun. Most outbreaks of parvovirus infection occur in school-aged children rather than in preschoolers.

Parvovirus B19 can also infect adults, who may experience fever and joint pain. If a pregnant woman becomes infected, there's a small risk that her unborn child will be infected. (See also Chapter 15, *Caregivers' Physical Health.*) About half of women of childbearing age have had parvovirus B19 and won't get it again if they're re-exposed. If a person with weakened immunity, sickle cell disease or some other chronic form of anemia is infected, severe anemia may occur. There's no treatment for parvovirus infection, and no vaccine is yet available.

Transmission

Parvovirus B19 has been found in the respiratory secretions (e.g., saliva, sputum or nasal mucus) of infected persons before the onset of the rash, when they appear to have a mild cold. The virus is probably spread from person to person by direct contact with those secretions, such as sharing drinking cups or utensils. It can also be transmitted from mother to fetus. Children are most infectious for several days before the rash starts. Once the rash appears, a child is no longer infectious unless she has a weakened immune system, in which case chronic infection may occur.

What to do

1. Advise the parents to have their child seen by a doctor.
2. Inform the parents of all children in your care if a parvovirus infection is diagnosed.
3. Watch for signs of rash in other children.
4. Remind children and staff that items such as utensils and drinking cups shouldn't be shared.
5. Advise exposed pregnant staff and parents to contact their doctor.
6. Laboratory diagnosis is not routine and may be necessary only when a pregnant staff member may have been exposed or if there's an outbreak at your facility.
7. A fact sheet is available at www.caringforkids.cps.ca and can be downloaded and given to the parents of a child who has parvovirus B19.

Exclusion and reporting

*   Children with a parvovirus infection can continue to attend child care. Unlike other infections with rash, by the time children have the characteristic "slapped cheek" rash, they are no longer contagious.
*   Excluding a pregnant child care practitioner from a workplace where there is a parvovirus infection is not recommended, because outbreaks in school or child care settings often indicate wider spread in the community. (See also Chapter 15, *Caregivers' Physical Health.*)
*   Parvovirus infection does not need to be reported to your local public health unit.

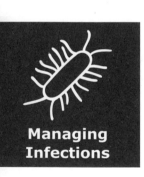

Managing Infections

Roseola

Roseola is a common infection in young children, caused by human herpes virus 6. It occurs most often in children between 6 and 24 months old. It is rare in infants under 4 months and children over 4 years of age. Children with roseola generally have a high fever and are cranky for several days without being very ill, although they may have febrile seizures. The fever can last for 3 to 5 days. When the fever goes away, a rash of small red spots appears on the face and body and lasts for anywhere from a few hours to 2 days. It's difficult to diagnose roseola until the rash appears. Roseola gets better without any treatment, and complications are very rare.

Transmission

Roseola is contagious even if there's no rash. It probably spreads from person to person through close contact with saliva, as the virus can be found in the saliva of many people even when no symptoms are present. Outbreaks are uncommon, but do happen.

What to do

1. Advise the parents to have their child seen by a doctor for diagnosis and treatment.
2. Follow your facility's policy for administering medication. Given as directed, acetaminophen (e.g., Tylenol, Tempra, Panadol and others) may reduce a child's discomfort. Be sure to record every dose on the child's *Medication Consent Form and Record Sheet*.
3. A fact sheet is available at www.caringforkids.cps.ca and can be downloaded and given to the parents of a child who has roseola.

Exclusion and reporting

- Children with roseola can continue to attend child care as long as they are well enough to participate comfortably in all program activities.
- Roseola doesn't need to be reported to your local public health unit.

Rubella (German measles)

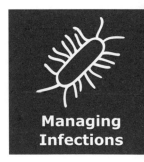

Managing Infections

Rubella (or German measles) is a viral disease that's now very uncommon in Canada, as a result of immunization. It isn't usually serious in children. Rubella may cause a mild illness with a low fever, swelling of the glands in the neck and behind the ears, and a rash with small red spots.

Adults with rubella usually get sicker than children. Some people may have aches and pains and swelling of the joints. Rubella is much more serious for susceptible (non-immune) pregnant women. If a mother is infected during the first 3 months of pregnancy, the unborn child may die or develop serious birth defects, including malformations of the brain, eyes, heart and/or other organs, and deafness. (See also Chapter 15, *Caregivers' Physical Health*.)

There are no antibiotics or other medicines that cure rubella.

Rubella vaccine is given routinely—combined with measles and mumps vaccine—starting at 1 year of age, with a second dose at either 18 months or 4 to 6 years of age, depending on where you live in Canada. It's a live vaccine and should not be given to people with a weakened immune system or to pregnant women.

Transmission

Rubella is spread by direct contact with the nose or mouth secretions of an infected person or through coughing or sneezing. People with rubella are considered infectious from 7 days before to 7 days after the rash first appears. It takes about 2 to 3 weeks for a person to develop rubella after being in contact with someone who has the disease.

Babies with congenital rubella syndrome (CRS), acquired in the womb from an infected mother, may excrete the virus in saliva and urine for a year or longer. They're considered to be infectious during this time, until saliva and urine cultures are negative. The number of babies born with CRS is extremely small, due to routine immunization.

What to do

1. Notify parents immediately if their child develops a rash, so they can have him seen by a doctor for diagnosis and treatment. All suspected cases of rubella must be confirmed by a blood test.
2. Rubella exposure in Canada is a medical emergency. Contact your local public health unit immediately upon confirmation that a child in your program has rubella.
3. Be prepared to provide public health authorities with immunization records for all children and staff and contact information for all parents.
4. Notify the parents of all children in your care that there has been a case of rubella at your facility and that immunization may be required. Exposed, non-immune children, staff and parents may need immunization right away.
5. Unvaccinated children with symptoms should be seen by a doctor, who may do a blood test for rubella.
6. Advise pregnant women within your child care community—staff, parents or other known contacts—to consult their doctor immediately. A fact sheet is available at www.caringforkids.cps.ca and can be downloaded and distributed to the **parents of all children** in your program.
7. As a preventive measure, encourage all susceptible child care staff and parents of children new to Canada to be vaccinated against rubella.

Exclusion and reporting

- Children with rubella should be excluded from child care until at least 7 days after the rash is first noticed.
- If a baby is diagnosed with CRS, the issue of exclusion should be referred to the treating physician and decided on a case-by-case basis.
- Rubella is reportable to local public health authorities by the treating physician and testing laboratory.

Meningitis

Meningitis is an infection of the membranes and fluid covering the brain and spinal cord. It can be caused by either a bacterium or a virus. Symptoms of meningitis include fever, headache, vomiting, a stiff neck, and pain when flexing the neck and back.

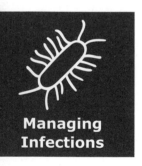

Managing Infections

Bacterial meningitis: Routine immunization (against *Haemophilus influenzae* type b [Hib], pneumococcal and meningococcal disease) has made cases of bacterial meningitis very rare, but it is a severe illness and a medical emergency. Despite prompt diagnosis and treatment, 5 to 10 per cent of infected children die of bacterial meningitis and 15 to 30 per cent have permanent brain damage. Bacterial meningitis is usually caused by *Streptococcus pneumoniae* (pneumococcus), Hib or *Neisseria meningitidis* (meningococcus). Vaccines provide protection from most meningitis-causing bacteria.

Bacterial meningitis usually begins with a fever and progresses very rapidly. Signs and symptoms include:

- lethargy (unusual sleepiness) or unresponsiveness, caused by increasing pressure on the brain,
- extreme irritability or fussiness, due to headache and pain from the inflammation around the brain,
- vomiting,
- a stiff neck, and
- a bulging fontanel (the soft spot on the head of children younger than 18 months of age).

In infants, the latter two signs may appear late in the illness. Seizures (convulsions) may also occur, as well as a rash, which starts as tiny red spots and progresses to purple spots and bruises.

Viral meningitis occurs most often in the late summer and fall, and is a milder illness. Enteroviruses (germs that usually infect the intestinal tract) are the most common cause. Viruses causing respiratory infections (especially influenza) may also occasionally cause meningitis. Complications of viral meningitis, including brain damage, are rare. Outbreaks of viral meningitis have been reported in child care centres only rarely.

Transmission

Bacterial meningitis doesn't spread very easily from person to person. The bacteria are found in mouth and nose secretions, and droplets produced when an infected child coughs or sneezes can reach the nose or mouth of another child who is nearby (within 1 m [3 ft.]), especially when exposure is prolonged. Bacterial meningitis can spread within households or child care facilities. Outbreaks of some types of meningitis (e.g., *Neisseria meningitidis*) are controlled using antibiotics and vaccines.

Enteroviruses causing meningitis are found in the saliva and stool and spread by direct or indirect contact with these substances.

What to do

1. **Call 911 first** (or emergency services where 911 service is unavailable), **then notify the parents**, if their child with fever also:
   - seems limp, less responsive or much more withdrawn than usual,
   - loses consciousness,
   - has poor colour (i.e., skin that is bluish, purple, greyish or very pale),

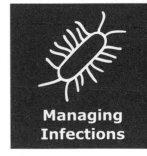

Managing Infections

- has a stiff neck,
- cries inconsolably with high-pitched screams or cries, or cries very weakly, or
- has a quickly spreading purple or deep red rash.

2. Ask the parents to notify your facility as soon as the doctor has made a diagnosis. Diagnosing meningitis is based on clinical symptoms and a lumbar puncture (spinal tap) to examine fluid around the spinal cord.

3. If bacterial meningitis is diagnosed, notify your local public health unit immediately. Antibiotic treatment may be needed for some or all of the children in your facility, depending on their age and immunization status.

4. Be prepared to provide public health authorities with immunization records for all children in your care. Children who have not received the appropriate number of doses for their age should be vaccinated as soon as possible.

5. Watch all other children in your care for fever and the signs of illness listed above.

Exclusion and reporting

- Children who have had meningitis can return to child care once a doctor has determined that they have recovered and are well enough to participate comfortably in all program activities.
- A child with bacterial meningitis is no longer contagious after receiving 24 hours of appropriate antibiotic therapy.
- Bacterial meningitis is reportable to local public health authorities by the treating physician and testing laboratory.

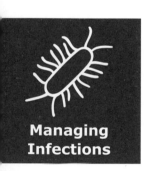

Managing Infections

Other severe bacterial infections

Haemophilus influenzae type b (Hib) disease

Because children are routinely vaccinated starting at 2 months of age, Hib infections are now extremely rare (fewer than 10 cases in Canada per year). Hib is a type of bacteria that can cause very severe illnesses in children under 5 years of age, including meningitis, epiglottitis, pneumonia, and infections of the blood, joints and bones. Epiglottitis is a rare but life-threatening infection of tissue at the back of the throat, which can swell and block the airway, making it impossible for a child to breathe. Early signs are severe sore throat, excessive drooling, inability to swallow, and difficulty breathing which worsens when the child lies down. The infection progresses very rapidly over 4 to 8 hours.

Hib infections require admission to hospital and treatment with intravenous antibiotics.

Transmission

Hib bacteria are not transmitted easily from person to person: spread involves a close and prolonged exposure. The bacteria are found in mouth and nose secretions. Droplets produced when an infected child coughs or sneezes can reach the nose or mouth of another child who is nearby (within 1 m [3 ft.]).

The spread of Hib infections after one child gets the disease can often be prevented by treating all members of a household or child care program with an antibiotic. Decisions about whether or not to use an antibiotic will be made by a treating physician and local public health authorities.

What to do

1. Keep a child showing signs of epiglottitis sitting up. **Call 911** (or emergency services where 911 service is unavailable). (For more about how to manage respiratory distress, see Chapter 11, *Emergencies*.)
2. Notify your local public health unit. Depending on the infection, the ages of the children in your program and their immunization status, antibiotic treatment may be needed.
3. Be prepared to provide public health authorities with immunization records for all children in your care. Children who haven't received the appropriate number of doses for their age should be vaccinated as soon as possible.
4. Notify the parents of all children in your care and advise them to seek immediate medical attention if their child has a fever and any one of the following behaviours or signs:
   - seems limp, less responsive or much more withdrawn than usual,
   - loses consciousness,
   - cries inconsolably with high-pitched screams or cries, or cries very weakly,
   - poor colour (i.e., skin that is bluish, purple, grayish or very pale),
   - a stiff neck,
   - a quickly spreading purple or deep red rash,
   - rapid or very difficult breathing,
   - pain on swallowing or refusal to swallow,
   - inability to swallow saliva, or
   - painful or swollen joints or refusal to use an arm or leg.
5. Watch for fever or signs of illness among other children in your care. The risk of a new case greatly diminishes if children have been immunized and/or received antibiotic prophylaxis. If fever and any of the symptoms listed in point 4 (above) occur while a child is in care, **call 911 first** (or emergency services where 911 service is unavailable), *then* **notify the parents**.

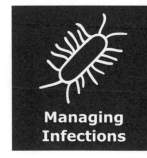

Managing Infections

Exclusion and reporting

- Children who have had a Hib infection can return to child care once a doctor has determined that they have recovered and are well enough to participate comfortably in all program activities.
- A child is no longer infectious after receiving **at least** 24 hours of appropriate antibiotic therapy.
- A Hib infection is reportable to local public health authorities by the treating physician and testing laboratory.

Meningococcal disease

Meningococcus is a type of bacteria (*Neisseria meningitidis*) that can cause very severe infections in children, including meningitis and sepsis (infection of the blood). Meningococcal infections can progress very rapidly, causing shock (inadequate blood flow and loss of consciousness) and damage to many organs in the body. Death from overwhelming shock can occur within 6 to 12 hours after the first sign of illness in about 10 per cent of cases, even with treatment and intensive care.

A distinctive rash is the most specific and noticeable sign of meningococcal disease. This rash begins as small red spots anywhere on the body. The rash may spread rapidly to all parts of the body, turn from deep red to a purple colour, and develop into large spots that look like bruises. Early signs of meningococcal infection may be similar to those of influenza and other viral infections, which can make early diagnosis difficult. These signs include fever, aches and pains, nausea, loss of appetite and general malaise. The characteristic rash usually appears within a few hours of the start of the fever.

Meningococcal infections require admission to hospital and treatment with intravenous antibiotics.

There are different types of meningococcal bacteria, and different vaccines protect against most of them. Vaccination against type C, the type causing the most serious disease in Canada at present, is routine for all infants. Another vaccine against all four preventable types of meningococcal germ is used to protect high-risk children over 2 years of age but isn't yet routine. A third vaccine protects children 5 years of age and older, teenagers and adults. A vaccine against Group B meningococcus has not yet been developed. Group B causes most of the infections in children under 2 years of age.

Transmission

Meningococcal infections spread from person to person through close, direct contact with nose and throat secretions transmitted by kissing, coughing, sneezing, and sharing items like water bottles, cans, drinking straws, or eating utensils, toothbrushes and toys. Fortunately, meningococcal bacteria are so fragile that these infections are not highly contagious.

Most spread occurs via healthy carriers, who don't develop any signs of illness but can still transmit infection. Although the risk of spread is small, it's higher in communal settings (e.g., families and child care) than in the general population. Spread may be prevented by treating all of an infected child's family members, child care providers and other close contacts with an antibiotic and, for some types of the bacteria, vaccination.

What to do

1. Notify your local public health unit. Preventive antibiotic treatment and vaccination may be needed for some or all children and staff at your facility, depending on their age and immunization status. If a report is made by a treating physician or testing laboratory, public health authorities will contact your facility if post-exposure prophylaxis is necessary.
2. Be prepared to provide public health authorities with immunization records for all children in your care. Children who have not received the appropriate number of doses for their age should be vaccinated as soon as possible.
3. Notify the parents of all children in your care and advise them to seek immediate medical attention if their child has a fever and any one of the following behaviours or signs:

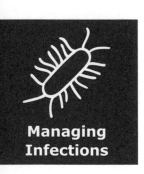

Managing Infections

- seems limp, less responsive or much more withdrawn than usual,
- poor colour (i.e., skin that is bluish, purple, greyish or very pale),
- rapid or very difficult breathing,
- a stiff neck,
- cries inconsolably with high-pitched screams or cries, or cries very weakly, or
- a quickly spreading purple or deep red rash.

4. Watch all other children in your care for fever or signs of illness. If fever and any of the symptoms listed in point 3 (above) occur, **call 911 first** (or emergency services where 911 service is unavailable), **_then_ notify the child's parents.**

Exclusion and reporting

- Children who have had a meningococcal infection can return to child care once a doctor has determined that they have recovered and are well enough to participate comfortably in all program activities.
- Children are no longer infectious after receiving 24 hours of appropriate antibiotic treatment.
- A meningococcal infection is reportable to local public health authorities by the treating physician and testing laboratory.

Pneumococcal disease

Pneumococcus is a bacterium that frequently causes infections in children. More than 90 strains of pneumococci exist and almost half of all children carry the bacteria, which live in the back of the nose and throat without causing illness. Children develop immunity to some strains of pneumococcal bacteria but not to others. When they come into contact with a strain of the bacteria they're not immune to, children may get ill, particularly if their system is already weakened from a viral infection such as a cold.

Pneumococci cause infections somewhere along the respiratory tract, usually in the ears. These germs are also the most common cause of acute sinusitis. The most serious respiratory infection caused by pneumococcal bacteria is pneumonia. Pneumococcal infections can also be very severe (invasive) if the bacteria spread to the blood, causing sepsis, or to the brain and spinal cord, causing meningitis, both of which are serious and possibly fatal. Infection may also spread to the bones or joints.

Invasive pneumococcal infections require admission to hospital and treatment with intravenous antibiotics. Until recently, all pneumococcal infections were cured with penicillin. However, some strains are becoming resistant to "first-line" antibiotics and must be treated with other antibiotics. Fortunately, a conjugate vaccine against pneumococcal infections is now available routinely for all infants, beginning at 2 months of age. This vaccine protects against the 7 most common types of pneumococci, which cause over 90 per cent of pneumococcal infections in young children. A vaccine against 23 types of pneumococci is also available and is recommended for certain high-risk children over 2 years of age, but it is not very effective in young children. Newer vaccines for children under 2 years of age are being developed. Children with spleen problems are likely to get very sick with pneumococcal disease and may be required to take antibiotics daily to prevent infection.

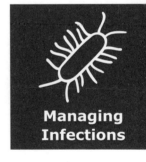

Managing Infections

Transmission

Pneumococci are very commonly found in the nose and throat, and up to 40 per cent of children and adults are healthy carriers. It's not known why one child shows no symptoms or develops only a mild infection while another develops a serious illness. The bacteria are spread from person to person through close direct contact such as kissing, or by coughing or sneezing. Many children become infected with the bacteria but only a very few become ill. Outbreaks of invasive pneumococcal infection are extremely rare.

What to do

1. Although invasive pneumococcal infections are not considered communicable and no prophylaxis is required, parents who learn about the case may be anxious and need reassurance. Consult your local public health unit for advice.
2. Review the immunization records for all children in your care. Advise parents of children who have not received the appropriate number of doses for their age to arrange for vaccination.
3. Inform all staff. Review and reinforce routine practices.

Exclusion and reporting

*   Exclusion is not required for a child with a minor illness (e.g., otitis media or sinusitis). A child with a more serious illness may return to child care once the treating physician has determined that he is well enough to participate comfortably in all program activities.
*   An invasive pneumococcal infection is reportable to local public health authorities by the treating physician and testing laboratory.

Tuberculosis (TB)

Tuberculosis is an infection caused by *Mycobacterium tuberculosis*. Most TB infections don't cause symptoms. When disease occurs, it usually affects the lungs, causing pneumonia or enlarged lymph nodes. TB germs can also travel in the bloodstream to other parts of the body, affecting the brain, bone and joints, abdominal lymph nodes or kidneys. If TB occurs in the lungs or larynx, it becomes contagious. Infection elsewhere in the body isn't contagious.

Young babies are more vulnerable to pulmonary (lung) TB than toddlers and preschoolers and can get very sick. However, they're less likely than adults to spread TB because they can't cough deeply. Children are more likely than adults to have non-pulmonary, non-infectious TB infection. Most children who test positive for TB do not get sick.

Symptoms include fever, difficulty breathing, poor appetite, weight loss, slow growth, night sweats and chills. A cough may or may not be present. Diagnosis is often so delayed that children have had a prolonged fever by the time TB is confirmed.

While TB is uncommon in most of Canada, it's still diagnosed in children who:

*   live in areas where adult TB is still common,
*   have a weakened immune system, or
*   are new to Canada, travelling from countries where TB is still common.

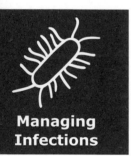

Managing Infections

Testing positive for TB isn't the same as having the disease. Infection can be detected by an immune system response using a skin test 2 to 12 weeks after exposure or by a blood test. A vaccine is available, but it isn't very effective and is used only in exceptional circumstances.

Transmission

TB germs are found in secretions from the lungs of people with active pulmonary disease. Bacteria get into the air when the infected person coughs and are then inhaled by others. Transmission usually requires close and prolonged contact. Children most often get the infection from an infected family member or other adult living in close quarters. Young children rarely transmit the infection, but they may acquire the disease in a child care facility from a worker or a parent of another child.

What to do

1. The treating physician or testing laboratory will notify public health authorities, who then try to determine whether the child acquired TB from an adult or from another child at your facility.
2. If the child has infectious TB, all other children and adults exposed to the child will need to be tested for TB and assessed for disease. Antibiotic treatment may be required.
3. Notify the parents of all children in your program. Public health authorities will notify your facility about any necessary follow-up for TB contacts.

Exclusion and reporting

- Children with infectious TB should be excluded until the treating physician or local public health authorities confirm that they are non-infectious, usually at least 2 weeks after starting appropriate antibiotic treatment. Treatment is required for as long as 6 to 9 months.
- TB is reportable to local public health authorities by the treating physician and testing laboratory.

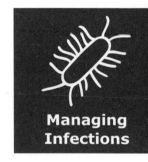

Managing Infections

Group A *Streptococcus* invasive diseases

Some strains of Group A *Streptococcus* (GAS) can cause invasive diseases such as toxic shock syndrome or necrotizing fasciitis (flesh-eating disease). In children, these infections can occur as a complication of chickenpox, though they are rare.

While non-invasive GAS infections (e.g., strep throat, impetigo) are common and spread easily in child care settings, outbreaks of invasive strains are extremely rare in Canada and should become rarer with routine implementation of chickenpox vaccine for all children 1 year of age. Early medical care and aggressive treatment with antibiotics are critical in cases of invasive GAS.

Early signs of toxic shock syndrome include fever, dizziness, confusion, abdominal pain and low blood pressure (feeling faint). Early symptoms of necrotizing fasciitis include fever, severe localized swelling and a rapidly spreading red rash (up to 2.5 cm [1 in.] an hour).

Transmission

Streptococci bacteria spread from person to person by respiratory particles or droplets, or by direct contact with infected skin. The risk of contracting invasive GAS is highest during the 2-week period after the onset of chickenpox, and may be triggered by a breakdown in the skin barrier, infection through lesions in the mouth or respiratory tract, or a weakened immune system.

What to do

1. Notify the parents of all children in your facility if a case of invasive GAS is diagnosed. Advise them to see their doctor immediately if their child develops fever or a skin infection.
2. Contact your local public health unit **immediately** if invasive GAS is diagnosed in a child or caregiver. Exposed children and staff may need antibiotic treatment to prevent infection.
3. Be prepared to provide public health authorities with chickenpox vaccination or immunity records for all children and staff.
4. Notify public health authorities about other children or staff in your program who have had non-invasive GAS infections, such as impetigo or pharyngitis, or who have had chickenpox within the previous 2 weeks.
5. Watch for signs of fever, sore throat or skin infection in other children and staff.
6. Review and reinforce proper hand-hygiene routines and wound treatment protocols with all staff.
7. Ensure skin cleanliness for all children in your program. Check for signs of infection, such as redness, swelling, pus or pain at any wound site.
8. Recommend that all family members of children in your program be immunized against chickenpox as soon as possible, if they aren't already immune.

Exclusion and reporting

- Children who have had an invasive GAS infection can return to child care once a doctor has determined that they have recovered and are well enough to participate comfortably in all program activities.
- Children are no longer infectious after receiving 24 hours of appropriate antibiotic treatment.
- An invasive GAS infection is reportable to local public health authorities by the treating physician and testing laboratory.

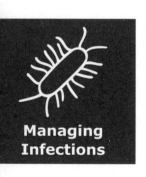

Managing Infections

Blood-borne viral infections

Hepatitis B virus (HBV)

Hepatitis B (HBV) is a virus that causes an infection of the liver. The virus is found in blood and certain other body fluids. Illness can range from an infection with no symptoms or acute hepatitis that gets better, to death from chronic liver disease or cancer of the liver. Newborn infants who get HBV from their mothers are most vulnerable to chronic HBV infection. Chronic liver disease eventually develops in 90 per cent of these infants, but only in about 10 per cent of older babies, children and adults who get HBV infection. With chronic infection, the virus persists in the blood and body fluids. As children with chronic infection usually remain well for many years, they're often not known to be infected.

The diagnosis of HBV is made by a blood test. Antiviral treatment is available, but its effectiveness is limited.

Vaccination prevents HBV. In provinces and territories where children are routinely vaccinated in infancy, most children in child care are immune. In some provinces and territories, the vaccine is routinely given at school.

Transmission

HBV is spread by direct contact with blood or body fluids containing the virus. For infection to occur, an open skin wound or mucous membrane must be directly exposed to sufficient quantities of infected blood, saliva or genital secretion. In the general population, the virus spreads mainly through sexual intercourse, transmission from an infected woman to her baby during pregnancy or delivery, the sharing of needles by intravenous drug users, or blood transfusions in countries where donated blood is not screened for HBV. Children living with a family member or caregiver who is HBV-positive may contract the infection, but this isn't common.

Rare cases of infection have been reported as a result of exposure in child care settings, and those few appear to be the result of biting. For transmission to occur, the bite must break the skin. Bites occur frequently among toddlers in child care settings, but the vast majority of children's bites cause bruising only. The biting child is more likely to be exposed to blood than the child who has been bitten.

The risk of spreading blood-borne viruses such as hepatitis B in a child care setting is so low that routine screening of children or staff is not recommended. Routine practices effectively prevent spread. Parents are **not** required to disclose their child's health status but may choose to do so, often in consultation with their doctor and taking into consideration their child's overall health and behaviour. Parents of other children should **not** be informed about the identity or presence in your program of a child with HBV. This policy is also true for other blood-borne viral infections, such as HIV and hepatitis C. **Excluding children with these infections is unacceptable.**

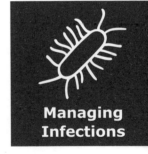

Managing Infections

Essential steps for cleaning up a large blood or body fluid spill:

- wear gloves,
- turn your face away to avoid possible splashing,
- wipe up the spill with paper towels, wash the area with detergent and water, then disinfect it with a strong (1:10) bleach solution,
- discard paper towels, bleach-soaked cloths and disposable gloves in a foot-activated, plastic-lined and tightly covered garbage container,
- disinfect reusable household rubber gloves in a mild (1:100) bleach solution and hang them to air dry,
- wash your hands.

For detailed protocol, see pages 159-60, and Table 8.1, page 154, for bleach solutions.

What to do

1. Parents of other children should **not** be informed about the identity or presence of a child with HBV in your program. However, general information about blood-borne viruses should be shared with parents and staff in a sensitive manner, to ensure acceptance if an infected child's identity becomes known.
2. Make all decisions for care of a child who is known to have HBV in consultation with the parents, the treating physician, a local medical officer of health and your facility's director (if applicable).
3. Caring for any child who frequently and aggressively bites, regardless of whether or not they have an infection, may be easier in a home setting, where the child can be closely supervised.
4. Review and reinforce routine practices for all contact with blood and body fluids. All staff should be adequately trained and regularly updated in the proper care of blood exposure or bite wounds. (See *Bite management*, below.)
5. All staff should be immunized against HBV.
6. Advise parents of any child known to have chronic HBV to have their child vaccinated against hepatitis A.

Exclusion and reporting

- Children with HBV should never be excluded from child care based solely on their HBV status.
- Any HBV infection is reportable to local public health authorities by the treating physician and testing laboratory.

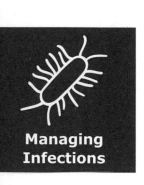

Managing Infections

Bite management

If a child is bitten and the skin is not broken, clean the wound with soap and water, apply a cold compress and soothe the child gently.

If a bite breaks the skin, these are the steps to follow:

1. Allow the wound to bleed gently, without squeezing.
2. Clean the wound carefully with soap and water.
3. Apply a mild antiseptic.
4. Review the hepatitis B immunization records for both the biter and the person bitten.
5. Check the personal medical record of the child (or staff member) who has been bitten for the date of their last tetanus shot.
6. Contact your local public health unit about **any** bite that breaks the skin. They may require referral to a physician and, possibly, blood tests, depending on the circumstances.
7. Notify the parents of both the biter and the child who has been bitten as soon as possible.
8. Write and file an *Injury report* (see pages 97–99), preferably within 2 hours of the incident.
9. Observe the bite wound over the next few days. Advise the child's parents to see a doctor if redness or swelling develops.
10. A fact sheet about bites in child care is available at www.caringforkids.cps.ca and can be downloaded and given to the parents of both children involved in a biting incident.

Human immunodeficiency virus (HIV)

HIV is the virus that causes AIDS (acquired immune deficiency syndrome). The time lag between becoming infected with HIV and the development of AIDS may be many years. HIV causes disease by weakening the immune system, leaving the infected person vulnerable to life-threatening infections and unusual forms of cancer. Treatment can prevent the progression of HIV infection to AIDS.

Most young children with HIV have no signs of infection. When AIDS develops, signs in young children include failure to gain weight normally, enlargement of the liver, spleen and lymph nodes throughout the body, persistent thrush and *Candida* skin infections, chronic diarrhea, frequent bacterial infections and pneumonia, and unusual infections that don't occur in healthy people.

The diagnosis of HIV infection is made by a blood test.

Transmission

There have been no reports of HIV infection as a result of exposure in child care. HIV is not very infectious and doesn't spread from everyday contacts in the home, child care setting or school. It can be spread:

- through transfusion with unscreened blood products,
- from an infected pregnant woman to her baby before or during birth, or by breastfeeding,
- through sexual intercourse, and
- through direct injection of contaminated blood when needles are shared by intravenous drug users.

The risk of HIV spreading in a child care setting is so low that routine screening of children or staff is not recommended, and parents are **not** required to disclose their child's HIV status. The decision to do so should be made by the parents in consultation with their child's doctor, taking into consideration the child's health status, behaviour and possibly an increased vulnerability to other common childhood illnesses.

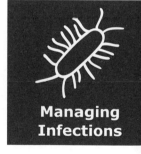

Managing Infections

What to do

1. Parents of other children should **not** be informed about the identity or presence in the program of a child with HIV. However, general information about blood-borne viruses should be shared with parents and staff in a sensitive manner, to ensure acceptance if an infected child's identity becomes known.
2. Make all decisions for care of a child who is known to have HIV in consultation with the parents, the treating physician, a local medical officer of health and your facility's director (if applicable).
3. Review and reinforce routine practices for contact with blood and body fluids. All staff should be adequately trained and regularly updated in the proper care of blood exposure or bite wounds. (See *Bite management*, opposite.)

Exclusion and reporting

- The exclusion of children with HIV is not acceptable.

- Any HIV infection is reportable to local public health authorities by the treating physician and testing laboratory.

Hepatitis C virus (HCV)

Like hepatitis B, HCV is a virus that infects the liver. HCV infection persists in more than half the children who contract it and has the potential to cause permanent liver damage, cirrhosis or liver cancer later in life. However, HCV is very uncommon in young children in Canada.

Like hepatitis B, HCV is found in blood and certain body fluids containing blood. Children with HCV often have no symptoms. For example, fewer than 20 per cent of children infected with HCV get jaundice. However, children can carry this infection for a long period and are considered to be infectious the whole time.

The diagnosis of HCV is made by a blood test. There is no vaccine against HCV at this time. Children tend to respond better than adults to antiviral treatments for HCV, but therapies can be complicated, problematic and have limited effect.

Transmission

There have been no reports of HCV infection as a result of exposure in child care. Children may get HCV from an infected mother before birth, or from blood transfusions in countries where blood is not routinely screened for HCV. HCV can also be spread by shared needles for intravenous drugs.

Parents are **not** required to disclose their child's HCV status, and the risk of infection via body fluids is extremely low. Routine practices are considered sufficient to prevent the spread of this illness in a child care setting.

What to do

1. Parents of other children should **not** be informed about the identity or presence in your program of a child with HCV. However, general information about blood-borne viruses should be shared with parents and staff in a sensitive manner, to ensure acceptance if an infected child's identity becomes known.
2. Make all decisions for care of a child who is known to have HCV in consultation with the parents, the treating physician, a local medical officer of health and your facility's director (if applicable).
3. Review and reinforce routine practices for contact with blood and body fluids. All staff should be adequately trained and regularly updated in the proper care of blood exposure or bite wounds. (See *Bite management*, above.)
4. Advise the parents of a child diagnosed with HCV to have their child vaccinated against hepatitis A and B.

Exclusion and reporting

- The exclusion of children with HCV is not acceptable.
- Any HCV infection is reportable to local public health authorities by the treating physician and testing laboratory.

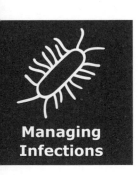

Managing Infections

Sexually transmitted infections (STIs)

It is extremely unlikely that an STI would pose an infection control problem in a child care facility. Nevertheless, child care staff should have some knowledge of STIs. The presence of an STI in a young child may be evidence of sexual abuse. (See Chapter 14, *Protecting Children from Maltreatment*.)

Signs that suggest an STI in a young child and require diagnosis by a doctor include discharge from the urethra or the vagina, and ulcers or warts in the genital or anal areas.

Germs causing sexually transmitted infections include:

- *Chlamydia trachomatis*,
- *Neisseria gonorrhoeae* (gonorrhea),
- genital herpes,
- human papillomavirus (e.g., genital warts),
- *Trichomonas vaginalis*, and
- *Treponema pallidum* (syphilis).

Other vaccine-preventable diseases

Although tetanus and polio are vaccine-preventable diseases and are extremely rare in Canada, there's still a risk of infection in non- or under-vaccinated children from other countries. The children of people new to Canada and newly adopted children need to be screened by their doctor and immunized against several diseases that have been almost eliminated in Canada because of universal immunization programs.

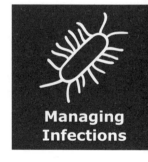

Managing Infections

Tetanus

Tetanus, also called lockjaw, is caused when tetanus bacteria get into an injury or cut. Although the germ that causes tetanus is common in soil and dust everywhere, the disease is very rare in Canada because almost everyone has been vaccinated against it. It's very common in parts of the world where the vaccine isn't used. Tetanus kills 6 out of every 10 people who get it. Tetanus can occur after even minor cuts or wounds in people who have not been immunized. It can also be acquired from animal bites, because breaking of the intact skin potentially exposes the wound to soil, street dust, or animal or human feces.

Tetanus vaccine is given routinely starting at 2 months of age. Tetanus cannot be transmitted from person to person. There is no reason to exclude a child who has had tetanus and who is well enough to return to child care. The treating physician and testing laboratory are responsible for reporting cases of tetanus to public health authorities.

Polio

Polio is caused by the poliomyelitis virus. It can produce permanent paralysis, because the virus can damage nerve cells in the spinal cord. Polio is very rare in Canada today because most people have been immunized against it. Polio vaccine is given routinely starting at 2 months of age. However, polio is still common in some other parts of the world, and can be imported into Canada by unvaccinated people from those areas. The virus is found in saliva and stool, and may remain in the stool for several weeks after the initial infection. It spreads from person to person through direct contact with throat secretions or unwashed hands, and indirectly, from contaminated water or food.

Polio exposure in Canada is a medical emergency. Cases are reportable to local public health authorities by the treating physician and testing laboratory. Your local public health unit will direct and arrange for the treatment of exposed children and staff. Children with polio cannot return to child care until public health authorities have determined that they are non-infectious.

Know the steps

Infection control means knowing what to do and when. Routine practices are always the first and best protection against the spread of infection. But being sensitive to how a child feels or looks at drop-off time, sharing this information with parents, and responding promptly and appropriately to a new sign or behaviour can mean the difference between one case of infection and an outbreak. Recognizing when a child needs an early pick-up or should stay at home can mean the difference between that child's absence from your program for 2 days or a whole week. Knowing when to alert the parents of other children in your program to the presence of infection and when to protect confidentiality can mean the difference between perspective and panic. And, finally, knowing when to consult or notify public health authorities can be the difference between one case of serious illness and a public health emergency.

Selected resources

See the *Selected resources* for Chapter 8, *Preventing Infections*.

Fact sheets

The Canadian Paediatric Society's website for parents and caregivers, Caring for Kids, has parent notes and information about the infections and infection control strategies discussed in this chapter. These can be downloaded at www.caringforkids.cps.ca and shared with families and child care staff. Brochures on the following topics are also available.

———. 2008. Common infections and your child.

———. 2006. Diarrhea in children: Prevention and treatment.

———. 2006. Fever and temperature taking.

———. 3rd ed., 2006. *Your Child's Best Shot: A Parent's Guide to Vaccination*. Ottawa, Ont.: Canadian Paediatric Society.

American Academy of Pediatrics. www.aap.org

Centers for Disease Control and Prevention (CDC, U.S.). Diseases and conditions. www.cdc.gov

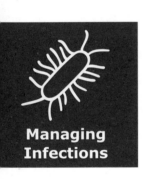

Managing Infections

Government of Quebec. 2002. *Prévention et contrôle des infections dans les centres de la petite enfance : Guide d'intervention*. Sainte-Foy, QC: Les publications du Québec.

Health Canada. Diseases and conditions. www.hc-sc.gc.ca

Public Health Agency of Canada. Infectious diseases. www.phac-aspc.gc.ca

Region of Peel (Ont.) Public Health. See free educational resources on respiratory infection control at www.peelregion.ca

Provincial/territorial public health information

Aboriginal Canada Portal. www.aboriginalcanada.gc.ca

Alberta Health and Wellness, Diseases and conditions. www.health.alberta.ca

British Columbia Centre for Disease Control (B.C. CDC). www.bccdc.org

Manitoba Health, Communicable Disease Control (CDC). www.gov.mb.ca

New Brunswick Department of Health, Public Health Services. www.gnb.ca

Newfoundland and Labrador, Health and Community Services. www.health.gov.nl.ca

Northwest Territories Department of Health and Social Services. www.hlthss.gov.nt.ca

Nova Scotia Department of Health, Health promotion and protection. www.gov.ns.ca

Nunavut Health and Social Services. www.gov.nu.ca/health

Ontario Ministry of Health Promotion. www.healthyontario.com

Prince Edward Island Department of Health. www.gov.pe.ca/health

Quebec Health and Social Services. www.msss.gouv.qc.ca

Saskatchewan Health, Disease prevention. www.health.gov.sk.ca

Yukon Health and Social Services. www.hss.gov.yk.ca

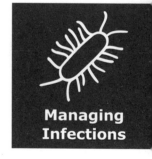

Managing Infections

Appendix 9.1: Administering medication

When giving medication to a child in your care, make sure to:

- comply with child care regulations for your jurisdiction,
- follow your facility's policy, and
- follow all doctor's or pharmacist's directions.

Your responsibilities also include obtaining written parental and/or physician consents and keeping proper records. A separate, signed consent form and record sheet is required for **each** prescription and **every** "over-the-counter" (OTC) medication or product (e.g., vitamins, sunscreen) that are administered for health reasons. (See the *Medication consent form and record sheet*, pages 139-40.) Every time a medication is given, you must note the dosage, the date and time it was given, and by whom, on this record sheet.

You may wish to include a special consent form in your program's orientation booklet or information package that a parent or guardian can choose to sign when their child is first enrolled. If signed, this consent form would allow you to give a child specified medication when appropriate and without necessarily notifying a parent or an emergency contact beforehand. However, be sure to offer parents the option of withholding their consent to your giving medication unless they're notified beforehand.

Explain your facility's general guidelines for giving medication in the orientation handbook or information package. These may minimize your facility's responsibility for administering medication by requiring parents to:

- request a treatment schedule that allows all medications to be given at home, and
- give vitamins at home—they are considered to be medications.

Your facility's policy should also require families to:

- supply all medications for their child (with the possible exceptions of fever reducers and oral rehydration solutions) to lessen the risk of cross-contamination,
- have a prescription filled in two bottles so that child care staff and parents don't have to pass the medication back and forth every day,
- administer a new prescription or OTC medication at home for the first 24 hours so that they're available to handle any adverse reactions,
- keep you informed of any prescription or OTC medication they give the child at home so that you're aware of possible side effects (e.g., drowsiness) and double-dosing is avoided,
- renew their written permission to give medication at least once a year and whenever the prescription is changed, and
- provide a doctor's prescription for any OTC medication other than acetaminophen or ibuprofen.

Any new medication must be in its original container, marked with the child's name. A prescription medication should also include the pharmacist's label, marked with the child's name, the name of the medication, dosage, the date it was dispensed, any special

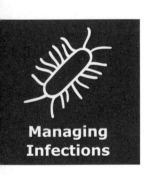

Managing Infections

instructions for storage or administration, and an expiry date. Any prescription or OTC medication that has expired or appears to have been dispensed in the past or prescribed for another child should not be administered.

Ask the parents (or the doctor or pharmacist if the parents don't know) what should be done if their child spits out a medication or vomits within 15 minutes of taking it.

Consult a pharmacist or the child's doctor if your general questions about medications cannot be answered by the parents.

Storing medication

- Store medication out of the reach of children, preferably in a locked cupboard.
- Refrigerate it when required, in a locked plastic container if children have access to the refrigerator.
- Ask parents to deliver the medication directly to a staff member at drop-off time, rather than handing it over in a lunch bag (for example).
- Return any unused medication directly to a parent to dispose of at home or return it to a pharmacy for disposal. Never keep medications that aren't being used.

Who should give medication?

A child care practitioner whom the child knows and trusts should give medication. To avoid mix-ups:

- one person should be responsible for giving medication to all the children on a given day, **or**
- one person should be responsible for giving medication to a particular child.

Ideally, a second child care practitioner would help in both scenarios.

Extra training may be needed when a device is used to administer medications (e.g., epinephrine, glucagon). Often, a parent or public health nurse will demonstrate the use of common medical devices to all child care staff in a workshop. Your local public health unit can also advise you about training options.

If a child requires regular injections, the parents may request that the same child care practitioner administer the medication each time. However, all staff will need to be trained for times when this person isn't available.

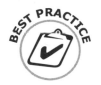

Consult your provincial/territorial child care office if you have questions about liability relating to medications.
Stay informed about medications in the news—especially when they are administered to children—and tell your co-workers of any changes that might affect children in your program.

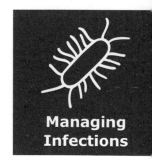

Managing Infections

Helping children to take medication

- Make sure the parents have let their child know beforehand that you will be giving her medication, so that she won't be surprised.

- Ask the parents how they give the medication at home and what might make the process easier for you or the child.
- Give the child a few minutes' notice, so that she can complete an activity or prepare to leave it for a few moments.
- Try to give medication away from other children, in a quiet and comfortable place.
- Be matter-of-fact. Let the child know what you're doing just before you do it, and share how a medication might taste or feel—but only if you know. If the child asks about the medication or why she is taking it, keep things simple and straightforward.
- **Never refer to the medication as food or candy.** To make it easier for the child to swallow, you might say that the medication has a fruit flavour—but only if that is true.
- Give the child some sense of control over the process. Invite her to hold the medication cup or to choose whether to stand, sit or be on your lap while taking it. Hold an infant or toddler in your arms in an upright position, and encourage a young child to hold a special blanket or stuffed toy.
- Praise children for taking their medication.
- If a child refuses medication, try again in 15 minutes. If she refuses again, don't force the issue. Record the refusal on the *Medication consent form and record sheet*, and inform the parents so that they can follow up at home.

Routine steps for administering medication

Prepare to give medication in a quiet place, away from activity areas. Ideally, two people should work together—one to prepare and administer the dose and the other to double-check procedures. Read the medication's label (with the child's name, the medication's name and dosage information) at three points in the process:

Check the **"Five Rights"** whenever you give medication. Make sure you give

1. The right medication,
2. To the right child,
3. In the right dose,
4. At the right time,
5. By the right route (e.g., by mouth).

1. When the medication is removed from the storage space,
2. Before the medication is poured out of the container, and
3. When the medication is returned to the storage space.

What to do when there is a problem

Double-check with a parent or co-worker if a child says she no longer needs the medication or has already taken it that day. A parent may have forgotten to tell you that the medication was changed or stopped, or the message may not have been relayed.

Notify your facility's director (if applicable) or a child's parents immediately if you make an error in any of the "Five Rights" (e.g., giving the wrong medication or the wrong dose), and note the mistake on the *Medication consent form and record sheet* and in the child's file. If you've given a child medication designated for another child, both families need to be notified and—depending on the circumstances—their doctors may also need to be informed.

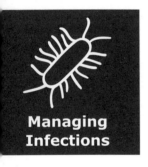

Managing Infections

Report to the parents immediately any side effects a child experiences after taking medication. Also record them on the *Medication consent form and record sheet* and in the child's personal file. The parents will need to consult a doctor before the medicine is given again.

If you accidentally spill liquid medication, note this on the *Medication consent form and record sheet*. Prepare a replacement dose for the child and be sure to let the parents know, in case an extra dose is needed from the pharmacist to replace the spilled amount.

10 steps for giving medication correctly

1. Check the *Medication consent form and record sheet* to confirm that medication is required.

2. Have everything you need to give the medication (e.g., the measuring container, a drink the child might have afterward, tissues) ready beforehand.

3. Wash your hands.

4. Remove the medication from its storage space and read the label. The label should always specify:

   - the child's name,
   - the name of the medication,
   - dosage information,
   - the prescription date (if applicable) and an expiry date, and
   - directions for use (e.g., to shake it well, not to mix it with certain foods or fluids, or not to administer it within a certain time before or after a meal). Follow all instructions.

5. Reconfirm the "**Five Rights**" (opposite), checking once more against information on the *Medication consent form and record sheet*. Then, measure the medication accurately, using a proper measuring spoon, syringe, dropper or cup. Don't use household teaspoons, which vary in size. Don't use the dropper that comes with bottled medications to administer a dose directly into a child's mouth. It can be contaminated and become an infection risk if the medication is shared (e.g., acetaminophen). Measure the dosage with the dropper into a spoon, and give it to the child that way.

6. Give the medication to the child.

7. Check the label once again and put the medication safely away, out of the reach of children.

8. Record the date, time and dosage with your initials on the *Medication consent form and record sheet*.

9. Wash the measuring spoon or dropper in warm soapy water and rinse well before allowing the spoon to air dry or returning the dropper to the bottle.

10. Wash your hands.

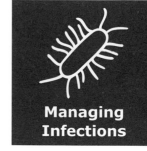

Managing Infections

Tablets and capsules

- Wash your hands before and after giving a child a tablet (pill) or capsule.
- Shake out the required number of tablets into a serving container. Try not to touch the tablets.
- Give the tablets to the child with a glass of water or other liquid to make swallowing easier. (If the child asks for a certain drink, check the label to be sure it's appropriate. Some medications, for example, cannot be taken with milk.)

Ear drops

You may need to administer ear drops to a child with an ear infection. Here are a few tips:

- Depending on the child's age, it may be easier for two people to administer ear drops—one to hold and speak with the child and the other to prepare and give the dose.
- **Wash your hands before and after giving the medication.**
- Invite the child to lie down with her head in your lap, but allow her to choose an alternative spot.
- Gently turn the child's head to the side and pull the middle of the outer ear back slightly to help the liquid enter the ear canal more easily.
- To avoid contamination, try not to touch the ear with the dropper tip.
- Remove any visible leftover medication from the outer ear with a tissue and dispose of it right away.
- Wash the dropper in warm soapy water and rinse it well before returning it to the bottle.

Eye drops or ointment

You may need to give eye drops or ointment to a child with an eye infection. Here are a few tips:

- Depending on the child's age, it may be easier for two people to administer eye drops or ointment—one to hold and speak with the child and the other to prepare and give the dose.
- **Wash your hands before and after giving the medication.**
- Invite the child to lie down with his head in your lap, but allow him to choose an alternative spot.
- Gently pull down the lower eyelid to make a pocket and put the drops or ointment into it rather than directly into the eye.
- To avoid contamination, try not to touch the eye with the dropper or tube tip.
- Remove any visible leftover medication from the outer eye with a tissue and dispose of it right away.
- Wash the dropper or tube tip in warm soapy water and rinse it well before returning it to the container.

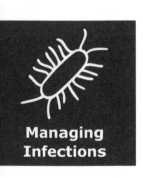

**Managing
Infections**

Ointments and creams

- **Wash your hands before and after applying ointment or cream.**
- Either remove the medication from its container with a clean tongue depressor and apply it to a tissue, or squeeze it from a tube onto a tissue (being careful not to touch the end of the tube).
- Use the tissue to apply the ointment or cream to the child's skin.
- Discard used tissues and/or tongue depressors right away, using fresh ones if more ointment or cream is needed.

Appendix 9.2. Managing infections

Requirements for reporting vary across Canada. Find out which infections are reportable in your province/territory by contacting your local public health unit.

Illness	Transmission	Signs/symptoms	Infectious period	Exclusion	Reporting and notification
Viral respiratory infections					
Viruses include: respiratory syncytial virus, parainfluenza virus, influenza, adenovirus, rhinovirus, coronavirus, metapneumovirus. See page 175 for additional information.	Viruses in the nose and throat spread by: **direct contact** with respiratory secretions or contaminated hands, **indirect contact** with toys, tissues, or other objects contaminated with respiratory secretions, or **droplets** from coughs and sneezes.	**Common cold:** Runny nose, cough, sneezing, sore throat, headache, possibly fever. **Bronchiolitis:** Cough, laboured breathing, wheezing, fever. **Croup:** Hoarseness, barking cough, rapid, laboured or noisy breathing, fever. **Influenza:** Fever, chills, cough, headache and muscle pains. **Pneumonia:** Fever, cough, rapid or laboured breathing, poor skin colour.	Depends on the virus but usually 3 to 8 days (longer for children with a weakened immune system). Most infectious while symptoms are present.	**Common cold:** No, unless the child is too ill to participate in all program activities. **Bronchiolitis, croup, influenza, pneumonia:** Yes, until the child is well enough to participate in all program activities.	No. No, unless you suspect an outbreak.
Bacterial pneumonia See pages 206, 209 for additional information.	Bacteria usually present in the nose and throat and can cause disease if they get into the lungs.	Fever, cough, rapid or laboured breathing, poor skin colour.	Usually not considered contagious.	Yes, until the child is well enough to participate in all program activities.	No, unless pneumococcus or *Haemophilus influenzae* type B is isolated during blood testing.
Gastrointestinal infections					
Can be viral or bacterial. See page 186 for additional information.	Germs in stool spread by: **direct contact** (hand to mouth), or **indirect contact** with toys, other objects or surfaces contaminated with stool.				
Campylobacter	Bacteria usually ingested in contaminated **food** (e.g., improperly cooked poultry, unpasteurized milk) or water. Person-to-person spread by **direct or indirect contact with stool** can occur, especially among young children.	Fever, diarrhea (often with blood and/or or mucus in stool), cramps.	Bacteria excreted in stool for 2 to 3 weeks. Most contagious during the acute illness.	Yes, if a child's diarrhea can't be contained in a diaper, or a toilet-trained child can't control his bowel movements.	Yes, by the testing laboratory. Contact your local public health unit if a child at your facility is diagnosed with *Campylobacter* gastroenteritis.

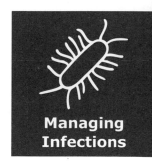

Managing Infections

Illness	Transmission	Signs/symptoms	Infectious period	Exclusion	Reporting and notification
Clostridium difficile (*C. difficile*)	Bacteria are normally found in soil and in the intestinal tract. Antibiotic treatment permits overgrowth of *C. difficile* in the gut and may trigger disease. Person-to-person spread by **direct or indirect contact with stool** can occur.	Diarrhea (sometimes with blood and/or mucus in stool), cramps, fever. Most children under 1 year of age have no symptoms, and most older children have a very mild illness.	Infectious as long as diarrhea lasts.	Yes, if a child's diarrhea can't be contained in a diaper, or a toilet-trained child can't control his bowel movements.	No.
Escherichia coli O157 (*E. coli*)	Bacteria usually ingested in contaminated **food** (e.g., poultry, beef, milk, unpasteurized apple juice, raw vegetables), or **water** contaminated with animal or human feces. Also spread from person to person by **direct or indirect contact with stool**.	Starts as non-bloody diarrhea, usually progressing to visibly bloody stools, with severe abdominal pain.	Bacteria excreted in stool for about a week. Infectious as long as diarrhea lasts.	Yes, until diarrhea subsides **and** 2 stool cultures (taken when the child is no longer receiving antibiotics) test negative.	Yes, by the testing laboratory. Contact your local public health unit if a child in your facility is diagnosed with *E. coli* O157 gastroenteritis.
Giardia See page 187 for additional information.	Parasites in the stool are spread from person to person by **direct or indirect contact with stool** or are ingested in **contaminated food or water**.	Watery diarrhea, recurrent abdominal pain. Some children experience chronic diarrhea with foul-smelling stools, a distended stomach and weight loss. Many infected children have no symptoms.	Infectious as long as cysts are in the stool, which can be for months.	Yes, until diarrhea subsides.	Yes, by the testing laboratory. Contact your local public health unit if a child at your facility is diagnosed with *Giardia* gastroenteritis. In the case of an outbreak, authorities may screen and/or treat all children and staff, with or without symptoms.
Rotavirus See page 186 for additional information.	Viruses in the stool spread easily from person to person by: **Direct or indirect contact with stool and contaminated toys.**	High fever, vomiting, followed within 12 to 24 hours by profuse, watery diarrhea.	Infectious just before onset of symptoms and as long as 3 weeks later.	Yes, if a child's diarrhea can't be contained in a diaper or a toilet-trained child can't control her bowel movements.	No. Contact your local public health unit if you suspect an outbreak (i.e., 2 to 3 or more children have diarrhea within 48 hours).
Salmonella typhi (gastroenteritis or typhoid fever)	Bacteria in the stool are spread from person to person by **direct or indirect contact with stool**, or are ingested in **contaminated food**.	Diarrhea, cramps, fever.	Infectious as long as bacteria are in the stool, which can be many weeks.	Yes, until diarrhea subsides **and** 3 stool cultures (taken when the child is no longer receiving antibiotics) test negative.	Yes, by the treating physician and testing laboratory. Inform your local public health unit **immediately** if a child or adult at your facility is diagnosed with *S. typhi* infection. Stool cultures for other children and staff may be required.

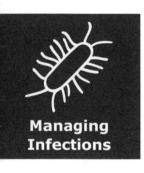

Managing Infections

Illness	Transmission	Signs/symptoms	Infectious period	Exclusion	Reporting and notification
Salmonella **gastroenteritis (non-typhi)**	Bacteria are usually ingested in **contaminated food** (e.g., meat, poultry, eggs, unpasteurized dairy products, vegetables and fruit). Person-to-person spread **may occur from direct or indirect contact with stool**. **Reptiles and amphibians** are also sources of infection.	Diarrhea, cramps, fever.	Infectious as long as bacteria are in the stool, which can be many weeks.	Yes, until the child is well enough to participate in all program activities.	Yes, by the testing laboratory. Contact your local public health unit if a child at your facility is diagnosed with *Salmonella* gastroenteritis.
Shigella **gastroenteritis**	Bacteria in stool spread from person to person **by direct or indirect contact with stool**.	Watery diarrhea, with or without blood and/or mucus, fever, cramps.	Infectious as long as bacteria are in the stool, which can be up to 4 weeks.	Yes, until diarrhea subsides **and** 2 stool cultures (taken when the child is no longer receiving antibiotics) test negative.	Yes, by the testing laboratory. Contact your local public health unit if a child at your facility is diagnosed with *Shigella* gastroenteritis. Other children, staff or household contacts with symptoms may need testing.
Yersinia **gastroenteritis**	Bacteria are ingested in **contaminated food** (e.g., raw or undercooked pork, unpasteurized milk) or **water**. Person-to-person spread is rare.	Fever, diarrhea (often with blood and/or mucus in stool).	Infectious as long as bacteria are in the stool, which can be up to 2 to 3 weeks.	Yes, if a child's diarrhea can't be contained in a diaper, or a toilet-trained child can't control his bowel movements.	Yes, by the testing laboratory. Contact your public health unit if a child at your facility is diagnosed with *Yersinia* gastroenteritis.

Other illnesses

Illness	Transmission	Signs/symptoms	Infectious period	Exclusion	Reporting and notification
Chickenpox (varicella) For more information and important requirements, see pages 198–99 and 375.	Viruses in the throat and from skin lesions spread easily from person to person **through the air**, and can travel large distances. Viruses in skin lesions spread **by contact with fluid from blisters**. Virus persists in the body for life and may recur as shingles. **Viruses can spread by contact with shingles if lesions are not covered.**	Fever and itchy rash. Crops of small red spots turn into fluid-filled blisters that crust over within a few days and become itchy.	Infectious for 2 days before rash starts until all blisters have crusted over and dried (usually about 5 days after start of rash).	No. Children with mild chickenpox can attend child care regardless of the state of their rash, as long as they feel well enough to participate in all program activities.	Yes, in some jurisdictions, by the treating physician and testing laboratory. Contact your local public health unit if there is an outbreak at your facility. Non-immune children and staff may need to see a doctor right away. Preventive treatment (vaccine or immune globulin) may be needed. **Notify all parents and staff immediately.**

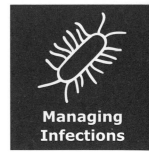

Managing Infections

Illness	Transmission	Signs/symptoms	Infectious period	Exclusion	Reporting and notification
Cold sores (herpes simplex type 1 virus) See page 193 for additional information.	Viruses spread from person to person by **direct contact** of mucous membranes (mouth, nose, eyes) with cold sores or saliva. Virus persists in the body for life and infections may recur.	Range from no symptoms to a simple cold sore or many painful ulcers in mouth and a high fever.	Infectious for at least a week during the first infection. Recurrences are less contagious for a shorter time.	No, for a child with simple cold sores. Yes, for a child with mouth ulcers who is drooling, until she is well enough to eat and participate comfortably in all program activities.	No.
Conjunctivitis (pinkeye) See page 180 for additional information.	Bacterial or viral. Germs spread easily by: **direct and indirect contact with eye secretions**, or **droplets** from coughs and sneezes when associated with a respiratory virus. It can also be caused by an allergy or eye irritation.	Scratchy, painful or itchy red eyes, light sensitivity, tearing with purulent (pus) or mucousy discharge.	**Bacterial**: Infectious until 24 hours of appropriate antibiotic treatment received. **Viral**: Infectious as long as there is eye discharge.	Yes, until seen by a doctor. If bacterial, child can return to the program after 24 hours of appropriate antibiotic treatment. If viral, child can return with doctor's approval. No need to exclude if there is no eye discharge, unless there is an outbreak.	No. Contact your local public health unit if you suspect an outbreak.
Cytomegalovirus (CMV infection) See pages 184 and 380 for additional information.	Viruses in saliva and urine spread by **direct contact**. Virus persists in the body for life and infections may recur.	Children usually have no symptoms. Can infect a fetus if the mother is infected or re-exposed during pregnancy.	Infectious as long as virus is in the urine and saliva, which can be for months in many healthy infants.	No.	No.
Group A *Streptococcus* (GAS) invasive diseases (e.g., toxic shock syndrome, necrotizing fasciitis [flesh-eating disease]) For more information and important requirements, see page 211.	Some strains of GAS cause invasive disease. Bacteria spread from person to person by: **direct contact with skin lesions**, or **respiratory droplets**. Children are at highest risk of infection within 2 weeks of having chickenpox.	**Toxic shock syndome:** Fever, dizziness, confusion and abdominal pain. **Necrotizing fasciitis**: Fever, severe, painful localized swelling, and a rapidly spreading red rash.	Infectious until 24 hours of appropriate antibiotic treatment received.	Yes. A child can return to the program once she has received **at least** 24 hours of appropriate antibiotic therapy, and a doctor has determined she is recovered and well enough to participate in all program activities.	Yes, by the treating physician and testing laboratory. **Notify your local public health unit immediately if a child or adult at your facility is diagnosed with invasive GAS.** Antibiotic treatment may be required for all exposed contacts, especially if chickenpox is also present. Inform public health authorities if a child or staff member in your program has had a non-invasive GAS infection (e.g., impetigo or pharyngytis) or chickenpox within the previous 2 weeks.

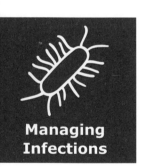

Managing Infections

Illness	Transmission	Signs/symptoms	Infectious period	Exclusion	Reporting and notification
Haemophilus influenzae type b (Hib) disease For more information and important requirements, see page 206.	Bacteria in mouth and nose are spread by: **direct contact** and respiratory droplets. Does not spread easily, and requires prolonged close contact.	Causes fever and pneumonia, meningitis, epiglottitis, blood, bone and joint infections. Symptoms develop rapidly.	Infectious until **at least 24 hours** of appropriate antibiotic therapy received.	Yes. A child can return to the program once she has received at least 24 hours of appropriate antibiotic therapy and a doctor has determined she is well enough to participate in all program activities.	Yes, by the treating physician and testing laboratory. **Inform your local public health unit immediately if a child at your center is diagnosed with a Hib infection.** Antibiotic treatment or vaccine may be required for exposed children. Notify all parents.
Hand-foot-and-mouth disease See page 200 for additional information.	Intestinal viruses spread from person to person by: **direct or indirect contact with stool or saliva**.	Fever, headache, sore throat, small, painful mouth ulcers and a rash (small red spots or small blisters), usually on the hands and feet.	Virus in saliva for a few days only but can remain in stool for 4 weeks after onset of illness.	No. Children can attend child care as long as they feel well enough to participate in all program activities.	No.
Head lice See pages 191–92 for additional information.	Spread from person to person by: **direct contact** (head to head), or **indirect contact** (e.g., shared hats, hairbrushes, headphones).	Itchy scalp.	Infectious as long as left untreated.	No. Exclusion is ineffective and unnecessary.	No. Contact your local public health unit for guidance if an outbreak cannot be controlled.
Hepatitis A virus (HAV) For more information and important requirements, see pages 189–90 and 380–81.	Virus in stool spreads from person to person by: **direct or indirect contact with stool**, or **contaminated food or water**.	Tea-coloured urine, jaundice and fever. Most young children do not get sick but can still spread the virus to others. Older children and adults are more likely to have symptoms.	Most infectious 1 to 2 weeks before onset of illness until 1 week after onset of jaundice.	Yes, for 1 week after onset of illness (unless all other children and staff have received preventive treatment).	Yes, by the treating physician and testing laboratory. **Inform your local public health unit immediately if a child or adult at your facility is diagnosed with HAV.** Contacts may need vaccine or immune globulin. **Notify all parents and staff.**
Hepatitis B virus (HBV) For more information and important requirements, see pagess 212–14 and 377–78.	Virus in blood and other body fluids (e.g., saliva, genital secretions). Mainly transmitted through sexual intercourse, from mother to newborn, by sharing contaminated injection equipment or by transfusion of unscreened blood. May be transmitted if an open cut or the mucous membranes (eyes or mouth) are exposed to blood.	Young children almost always have no symptoms. Older children and adults may have fever, fatigue, jaundice.	Infectious as long as the virus is in the blood and body fluids. May persist for life, especially in infants infected at birth.	No. A child with HBV can participate in all program activities.	Yes, by the treating physician and testing laboratory. Contact your local public health unit about **any** bite that breaks the skin. Blood tests may be required.

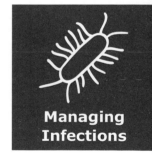

Managing Infections

Illness	Transmission	Signs/symptoms	Infectious period	Exclusion	Reporting and notification
Hepatitis C virus (HCV) For more information and important requirements, see page 216 and 378.	Virus in blood. Mainly transmitted from mother to newborn. Also by sharing contaminated injection equipment or by transfusion of unscreened blood. May be transmitted if an open cut or the mucous membranes (eyes or mouth) are exposed to blood.	Young children almost always have no symptoms. Older children and adults may have fever, fatigue, jaundice.	Infectious as long as the virus is in the blood. May persist for life.	No. A child with HCV can participate in all program activities.	Yes, by the treating physician and testing laboratory Contact your local public health unit about **any** bite that breaks the skin. Blood tests may be required.
Human immuno-deficiency virus (HIV) For more information and important requirements, see pages 215–16 and 378–79.	Virus in blood, genital secretions and breast milk. Children usually acquire HIV from their mothers before, during or after birth (by breastfeeding). Otherwise, transmitted through sexual intercourse, by sharing contaminated injection equipment or by transfusion of unscreened blood. May be transmitted if an open cut or the mucous membranes (eyes or mouth) are exposed to a large amount of blood.	Children usually have no symptoms. If AIDS develops, they may have persistent thrush, *Candida* dermatitis, chronic diarrhea, and failure to gain weight.	Infectious as long as the virus is in the blood and body fluids, presumably for life.	No. A child with HIV can participate in all program activities.	Yes, by the treating physician and testing laboratory. Contact your local public health unit about **any** bite that breaks the skin. Blood tests may be required.
Impetigo For more information and important requirements, see pages 194–95.	Caused by Group A *Streptococcus* or *Staphylococcus aureus* bacteria. Both spread from person to person by: **direct contact** (e.g., by touching skin lesions), or **indirect contact** (e.g., via contaminated bed linens or clothing).	Fluid-filled blisters, usually around the mouth or nose, but may occur elsewhere. Blisters break, ooze, and become covered by a honey-coloured crust.	Infectious until lesions have dried up. If Group A *Streptococcus*, until 24 hours after first dose of an appropriate antibiotic.	Yes, if draining lesions cannot be kept covered. For Group A *Streptococcus* infections, until 24 hours of appropriate antibiotic treatment received.	No (but community-associated methicillin-resistant *S. aureus* [CA-MRSA] is reportable by the testing laboratory in some jurisdictions). Contact your local public health unit for advice if you suspect an outbreak (e.g., more than one child in the same room has impetigo within a month).

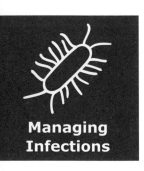

Managing Infections

Illness	Transmission	Signs/symptoms	Infectious period	Exclusion	Reporting and notification
Measles For more information and important requirements, see pages 200–01 and 377.	Viruses in respiratory secretions **spread easily from person to person through the air**.	High fever, cough, runny nose and red eyes 2 to 4 days before a rash appears, first on the face, then over entire body.	Highly infectious from 3 to 5 days before and up to 4 days after the rash appears.	Yes. A child with measles cannot return to child care until **at least 4 days after onset of rash**. Non-immune children and staff must be excluded for 2 weeks after the onset of rash in the child diagnosed with measles, unless they have been vaccinated within 72 hours of first exposure	Yes, by the treating physician and testing laboratory. **Measles exposure is a medical emergency. Notify your local public health unit immediately if a child or adult at your facility is diagnosed with measles.** Exposed susceptible children and staff may require vaccine or immune globulin within 72 hours of the first contact. **Notify all staff and parents immediately.**
Meningitis (bacterial or enteroviral) For more information and important requirements, see pages 204–06.	Not all forms of meningitis are contagious. **Bacterial:** See Meningococcal disease and *Haemophilus influenzae* type b disease. **Enteroviruses** in saliva and stool are spread by **direct or indirect contact**.	**Bacterial:** Fever, lethargy, headache, extreme irritability, vomiting, stiff neck, seizures, a bulging fontanel in babies under 18 months old. Usually progresses rapidly. Child may have a rapidly spreading, bruise-like rash. **Viral:** Usually milder, often fever and irritability only.	**Bacterial** meningitis is infectious until 24 hours of appropriate antibiotic therapy received. **Enteroviruses** are found in saliva for only a few days but can remain in stool for 4 weeks after onset of illness.	Yes. A child can return to the program once she has received **at least** 24 hours of appropriate antibiotic therapy, and a doctor has determined she has recovered and feels well enough to participate in all program activities.	**Bacterial** meningitis: Yes, by the treating physician and testing laboratory. **Notify your local public health unit immediately if a child or adult at your facility is diagnosed with bacterial meningitis.** Antibiotic treatment or vaccine may be mandated for some or all exposed children and staff. **Notify all parents and staff immediately.**
Meningococcal disease For more information and important requirements, see pages 207–09.	Meningococcus is a bacterium found in the mouth and respiratory secretions. Does not spread easily but can be transmitted by: **close, direct contact** (e.g. with saliva), or **respiratory droplets**.	Usually causes sepsis or meningitis, with high fever and rapid progression to shock (decreased responsiveness, poor skin colour). Child may have a distinctive rash that starts as small red spots but rapidly progresses to large red-purple bruises.	Infectious until after 24 hours of appropriate antibiotic treatment received.	Yes. A child can return to child care once he has received **at least** 24 hours of appropriate antibiotic therapy, and a doctor has determined he has recovered and feels well enough to participate in all program activities.	Yes, by the treating physician and testing laboratory. **Inform your local public health unit immediately if a child or adult at your facility is diagnosed with meningococcal disease.** Public health authorities may mandate antibiotic treatment and/or vaccination for exposed children and staff. **Notify all parents and staff immediately.**

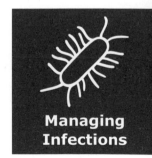

Managing Infections

Illness	Transmission	Signs/symptoms	Infectious period	Exclusion	Reporting and notification
Molluscum contagiosum See page 197 for additional information.	Virus spreads from person to person by **direct (skin-to-skin) contact with lesions**, or **indirect contact (e.g., with bed linens contaminated with material from the lesions**. Not very contagious.	Smooth, shiny pinkish-white bumps with a dip in the middle and a cheesy material inside, anywhere on the body.	Unknown. Molluscum disappears after several months without treatment.	No.	No.
Mumps For more information and important requirements, see pages 184 and 376–77.	Virus in saliva and respiratory secretions spreads easily from person to person by: **direct contact** (e.g. kissing), or **respiratory droplets**.	Fever, swollen glands at the jaw line or on the face, headache.	Infectious from 2 days before onset of swelling until 9 days after.	Yes, for 9 days after onset of swelling.	Yes, by treating physician and testing laboratory. **Notify your local public health unit immediately if a child or adult at your facility is diagnosed with mumps.** The authorities may mandate vaccination for non-immune contacts.
Otitis media (middle ear infections) See page 178 for additional information.	Viral or bacterial, usually a complication of the common cold. Non-contagious.	Earache, irritability, possibly fluid draining from ears. Child may have fever or cold symptoms.	Non-contagious.	No, unless child is too ill to participate in program activities.	No.
Parvovirus B19 infection (fifth disease, erythema infectiosum, or "slapped cheek" syndrome) For more information and important requirements, see pages 201–02 and 379–80.	Virus in respiratory secretions spreads by: **direct contact**, and (possibly) **respiratory droplets**. Can also be transmitted from mother to child before birth.	Red rash on the cheeks followed by a lace-like rash on the torso and arms that spreads to the rest of the body. Sometimes preceded by a low fever or cold symptoms 7 to 10 days before rash appears.	Infectious for several days before the rash, and non-infectious once rash appears.	No. Once rash appears, a child is no longer contagious.	No. Notify all parents and staff. Advise exposed pregnant staff and parents to contact their doctor.
Pertussis (whooping cough) For more information and important requirements, see pages 182–83 and 379.	Bacteria in respiratory secretions spread easily from person to person by **droplets from coughs and sneezes**.	Runny nose, frequent and severe coughing spells, sometimes followed by a whooping sound, gagging or vomiting. Babies may have serious difficulty breathing.	Infectious for up to 3 weeks from onset of illness if not treated, and for 5 days if appropriate antibiotic treatment is received.	Not routine but exclusion may be mandated by public health authorities if high-risk persons are present. Exclude until 5 days of appropriate antibiotic treatment received or for 3 weeks from onset of illness if not treated. Exclusion may be mandated if high-risk persons are present.	Yes, by the treating physician and testing laboratory. **Inform your local public health unit immediately if a child or adult at your facility is diagnosed with pertussis.** Antibiotic treatment and/or vaccination may be mandated. **Notify all parents and staff immediately.**

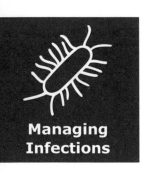

Managing Infections

Illness	Transmission	Signs/symptoms	Infectious period	Exclusion	Reporting and notification
Pinworms See pages 190–91 for additional information.	Worm eggs spread by: **direct contact** (e.g., contaminated fingers), or **indirect contact** (e.g., contaminated bed linens, clothing, toys).	Anal itching, disturbed sleep, irritability.	Infectious as long as eggs are being laid on skin. Eggs are infective for 2 to 3 weeks indoors.	No.	No.
Pneumococcal disease See pages 209–10 for additional information.	Bacteria are normally found in the nose and throat and usually do not cause infection. Possible person-to-person spread by: **close, direct contact with mouth secretions** (e.g., kissing), or **respiratory droplets**.	Usually an ear or sinus infection following a cold. Invasive infections include fever and pneumonia, meningitis, blood, bone and joint infections. Symptoms develop rapidly.	Not usually considered infectious. Probably not transmissible after 24 hours of appropriate antibiotic therapy.	No, for minor illness (e.g., otitis, sinusitis). A child with serious illness can return to child care once a doctor has determined he is well enough to participate in all program activities.	Yes (for invasive pneumococcal infections **only**), by the treating physician and testing laboratory.
Ringworm See pages 195–96 for additional information.	Fungus spreads from person to person by: **direct contact** (skin-to-skin), and **indirect contact** (e.g., shared combs, unwashed clothes, or shower or pool surfaces). Also acquired from **pets, especially cats**.	Ring-shaped itchy, scaly lesions on scalp, body or feet (Athlete's foot). Bald spots on the scalp.	Transmissible as long as rash is untreated and/or uncovered.	Yes, until the first treatment has been applied.	No.
Roseola See page 203 for additional information.	Virus probably spreads from person to person by **direct contact with saliva**. Often found in saliva of people with no symptoms.	High fever and crankiness for 3 to 5 days. When the fever subsides, a rash of small red spots appears on the face and body, lasting a few hours to 2 days.	Infectious while symptoms are present.	No. A child with roseola can continue to attend child care as long as she is well enough to participate in all program activities.	No.
Rubella (German measles) For more information and important requirements, see pages 203–04 and 376.	Virus spreads from person to person by: **direct contact with nose/mouth secretions**, or **respiratory droplets**.	Mild in children, with low fever, swollen glands in the neck and behind the ears, and a rash with small red spots. More severe in adults. If acquired in pregnancy, may seriously affect the fetus.	Infectious from 7 days before to 7 days after the rash appears.	Yes, for 7 days after the rash is first noticed.	Yes, by the treating physician and testing laboratory. **Rubella exposure is a medical emergency. Notify your local public health unit immediately if a child or adult at your facility is diagnosed with rubella.** Non-immune children and staff may need immunization. **Notify all parents and staff immediately.** Advise pregnant staff and parents who aren't sure of their immune status to see their doctor.

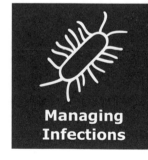

Managing Infections

Illness	Transmission	Signs/symptoms	Infectious period	Exclusion	Reporting and notification
Scabies See pages 192–93 for additional information.	Mites spread from person to person by **direct (prolonged, close and intimate) contact.**	Itchy red rash, usually between fingers and toes, or the wrists or in the groin, with thread-like lines and scratch marks. May be elsewhere on the body in children under 2 years of age.	Transmissible as long as infestation is untreated.	Yes, until the first treatment has been applied.	No. Contact your local public health unit for guidance if an outbreak cannot be controlled.
Streptococcal pharyngitis (strep throat) and **scarlet fever** See pages 181–82 for additional information.	Bacteria in throat spread from person to person by: **direct contact with saliva**, or **respiratory droplets.**	Sore throat, fever, swollen tender neck glands. Scarlet fever is strep throat with a red sunburn-like rash covering the entire body.	Infectious from onset of illness until 24 hours of appropriate antibiotic treatment received.	Yes. A child can return to the program once he has received at least 24 hours of appropriate antibiotic treatment, and the child is well enough to participate in all program activities.	Scarlet fever is reportable by the treating physician in some jurisdictions. Contact your public health unit if you suspect an outbreak at your facility (more than 2 cases in a month).
Thrush and *Candida* **diaper rash** See pages 196–97 for additional information.	Fungus is normally present in the body without causing illness, and rarely spreads from person to person. Thrush can be transmitted to an infant by contact with contaminated bottle nipples or soothers.	Thrush presents as whitish-gray patches on the inside of the cheek or on the tongue. *Candida* diaper rash is a painful bright-red rash in the deepest creases of a baby's groin, on the buttocks or in moist neck folds.	Usually not spread from person to person.	No.	No. Make sure bottle nipples and soothers aren't shared between children.
Tuberculosis (TB) For more information and important requirements, see pages 210–11 and 381.	Bacteria from the lungs **spread through the air in particles produced by coughing.**	For infectious TB: fever, cough, difficulty breathing. Young children rarely have infectious TB.	If infectious TB: As long as bacteria are in the respiratory secretions.	If infectious TB: Yes, for at least 2 weeks after starting appropriate antibiotic treatment and until the treating physician or local public health unit states that the child is no longer infectious.	Yes, by the treating physician and testing laboratory. **Notify your local public health unit immediately if a child or adult at your facility is diagnosed with TB.** Exposed children and adults may need testing and antibiotic treatment. **Notify all parents and staff immediately.**

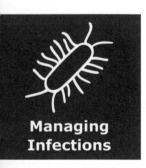

Managing Infections

chapter

10

Chronic Medical Conditions

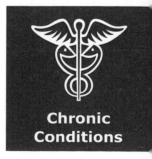

Chronic Conditions

Some children attending your child care program may have a chronic condition that requires medical care and regular monitoring. Providing quality child care for children with special health needs means learning about their condition, accommodating their needs, being observant and working closely with parents to ensure their child's health and well-being. It's also essential to have certified first aid and CPR skills and to be connected with health resources in your community. If a child experiences a medical crisis or is just having a bad day, you need to be able to respond in an effective, calm and supportive way. While caring for children with a chronic medical condition can be a challenge, it is also richly rewarding. Providing an inclusive environment benefits all the children in your care, not just those with special needs. (See Chapter 13, *Including Children with Special Needs*.)

When a child with an ongoing health issue is first enrolled, ask the parents to fill out a condition-specific medical form in consultation with their child's doctor. This form should outline the child's treatment and include detailed instructions for child care practitioners on aspects of care that might affect the child's day. The doctor may charge parents for reviewing this form periodically, as it is a health service that isn't usually covered by provincial health insurance plans.

Providing a condition-specific medical form is the parents' responsibility but is not mandatory under current privacy laws. However, requesting this information is best practice and most families are glad to comply. Once you have this form on file, check with the parents every 6 months or whenever there's a treatment change to make sure it remains current and correct. (See the appendices to this chapter for examples of condition-specific action plans.)

---

10 steps for meeting special health needs

1. Ask the child's parents to fill out a condition-specific medical form in consultation with their child's doctor.
2. Request that the form include specific instructions for managing the condition day-to-day.
3. Ask the parents to fill out and sign a *Medication consent form and record sheet* (see pages 139–40), if needed, and record every dose given while the child is in your care.
4. Review medical information with the parents every 6 months or whenever their child's treatment changes.
5. Know the early signs and symptoms indicating that the child is experiencing difficulties with her condition.
6. Document observations about the child's health and behaviour—this may help the child's family and/or doctor with treatment.
7. Work closely with the child's parents.
8. Attend education sessions for the management of a specific condition.
9. Ask parents to demonstrate the proper use of any treatment devices, if needed.
10. Keep first aid and CPR skills current.

Children whose chronic medical conditions make them more vulnerable to complications from common respiratory or other infections may be at less risk in smaller child care facilities or home settings, where their exposure to germs is minimized. Children who have a chronic medical condition that can worsen rapidly or be potentially life-threatening, such as a severe allergy, asthma, diabetes or epilepsy, should wear a MedicAlert bracelet or tag at all times. If a child doesn't wear one, speak with his parents about the importance of MedicAlert to their child's safety.

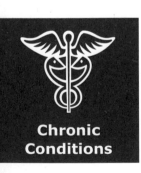

Chronic Conditions

Allergies

An allergy involves an immune system reaction that is triggered by a specific substance (the allergen). An allergen can be inhaled (e.g., dust or pollen), ingested as food (e.g., nuts, eggs or shellfish) or medication (e.g., penicillin), injected via an insect sting (e.g., bee or wasp venom) or absorbed through the skin (e.g., poison ivy). While foods and insect stings generally trigger more severe allergic reactions, very common trigger substances, such as dust mites, animal dander, pollens and moulds, pose more frequent problems for children. Strenuous exercise or exposure to cold can also cause an allergic reaction in susceptible children. Usually, an allergy develops gradually over repeated exposures to a trigger substance, but on rare occasions children can react immediately, with their first known exposure to an allergen. For example, a child may eat peanut butter several times before experiencing an allergic reaction to the protein in peanuts, or she may have a severe allergic reaction the first time she is stung by a bee.

Signs and symptoms of an allergic reaction can include:

Respiratory trouble,
such as:
- coughing
- wheezing
- shortness of breath
- voice changes
- choking

Nasal symptoms,
such as:
- sneezing
- blocked nose
- runny nose

Gastrointestinal trouble,
such as:
- diarrhea
- stomach cramps
- vomiting
- problems swallowing

Skin symptoms,
such as:
- hives
- swelling (of the face, lips or tongue)
- itching
- eczema

Eye problems,
such as:
- itchiness
- redness
- watery eyes
- swelling

Cardiovascular difficulties,
such as:
- pallor (pale skin)
- dizziness
- loss of consciousness

These symptoms can range from minor to life threatening. At its most severe, an allergic reaction can lead to anaphylaxis and even death.

Anaphylaxis is a rapid, extreme allergic response to a trigger substance. It can occur within minutes or hours of a susceptible child's exposure to an allergen. Anaphylaxis is a potentially life-threatening medical emergency requiring immediate recognition and treatment. (See Chapter 11, *Emergencies*, pages 277–78.) Your first aid training must include how to respond to a severe allergic reaction.

Your role

Familiarize yourself with the signs of an allergic reaction so that you recognize them right away. Remember, an allergic reaction can occur without prior warning. If you suspect an allergy, inform the child's parents as soon as possible. Your observations may help the child's doctor diagnose an allergy. Know the most common food allergens—peanuts, tree nuts, eggs, shellfish, fish, milk and soy—and don't offer these foods to children in your program before you're sure parents have served them at home.

When a child in your care has a diagnosed allergy, you need to protect her from exposure to the allergen. Having the information you need to protect her is key:

- Ask the parents to fill out a condition-specific medical form in consultation with their child's doctor. This form should outline the child's treatment and include detailed instructions about managing allergies that might affect the child's program day. (See Appendix 10.2 for a sample action plan.)

BEST PRACTICE

Some jurisdictions require that child care centres have an anaphylaxis policy for all children at risk. This policy may require you to:

- have annual staff training,
- implement a plan to minimize exposure to a certain allergen, and
- have an established emergency procedure.

Contact your provincial/ territorial ministry of health or child care for special health care planning requirements.

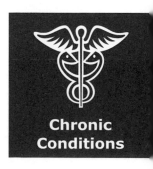

Chronic Conditions

- Post an Anaphylaxis Emergency Plan in appropriate locations (e.g., the kitchen and eating areas, in the case of a food allergy). The plan has two pages. The first is a form with the child's photo, emergency contact information, and allergy signs/symptoms to watch for, as well as emergency instructions and a signed consent to administer medication. The second page is the instruction sheet for either EpiPen or Twinject, whichever device has been prescribed for the child. The Anaphylaxis Emergency Plan can be downloaded at www.allergysafecommunities.ca. (See also Chapter 11, *Emergencies*, pages 277–78.)
- Review medical and contact information with the parents every 6 months or whenever their child's treatment changes.
- Ask what allergy medication the child is currently receiving and if giving it at home at all times is practical. If medication must also be available at your facility, you'll need to obtain a signed *Medication consent form and record sheet* (see pages 139–40) to keep on file and update as required. Some medications affect behaviour. For example, an antihistamine used to treat a seasonal ragweed allergy may make a child drowsy (or, less commonly, overactive).

If a child has a potentially severe allergy that requires the immediate availability of an epinephrine kit (e.g., EpiPen or Twinject), make sure his parents supply this medication. Some facilities require parents to sign a contract to this effect. Clearly label the medication with the child's name and the date received and store it in a location that's readily accessible by staff (i.e., **not** in a locked cupboard or drawer) but not by children. Everyone on staff should know where this medication is kept and how to administer it.

Avoiding exposure to a specific allergen is the key to allergy management. If a child in your care has a **food allergy**, always take the following precautions:

- Teach all children in your care not to trade or share food, food utensils or containers.
- Serve food to a child who has an allergy on a napkin or personal placemat so that the food doesn't touch the table or other shared surface.
- Make sure all children wash their hands before and after eating.
- Wash your own hands between preparing different foods to prevent cross-contamination.
- Wash surfaces such as tabletops, trays or toys clean of contaminating foods.
- Make sure that no trigger food is used in craft activities.
- Use non-food items (e.g., stickers) as rewards for special activities, rather than cookies.
- Closely supervise young children during meals and snacks.

ALERT

Allergies to peanuts, tree nuts and shellfish tend to be lifelong and are usually more severe than allergic reactions to other foods. A very small, even minute amount of a food allergen can trigger an allergic reaction if ingested. Inhaling airborne peanut protein (i.e., the smell of peanuts) can cause an allergic reaction but usually not anaphylaxis.

If the child has a potentially severe food allergy, you'll need to be vigilant:

- Post the Anaphylaxis Emergency Plan in the kitchen and eating areas so that staff preparing or serving food are reminded that a child in the program has an allergy and know how to manage a reaction.

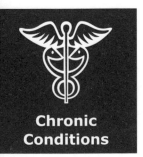

Chronic Conditions

- Read food labels carefully and don't buy foods that contain the allergen.
- Ask the child's parents to supply all of their child's meals and snacks from home.
- Store food with an allergy-causing ingredient (e.g., soy, milk or wheat) in a separate, clearly labelled container, away from an allergic child's food.

If a child in your care has a **peanut allergy,** remember that:

- Peanuts are the most common cause of food-induced anaphylaxis and are found throughout the food supply as whole or ground nuts, nut butter and nut oil.
- A minute amount of peanut or a derivative can cause a reaction. A skin rash or stomach upset can result from residual contact. Anaphylactic shock can result if peanuts are ingested inadvertently.

Implement a "peanut-sensitive" policy:

- Require the family of a child with a peanut allergy to prepare all meals and snacks at home.
- Don't allow **any** food in your facility that contains peanuts, peanut butter or peanut oil. Try to let all parents know at the time of enrolment. A sample letter of notification to send later, if a child joining your program has a peanut allergy, can be downloaded at www.allergysafecommunities.ca.
- Educate staff and parents about the dangers associated with a peanut allergy and advise them not to bring in food or special treats that contain peanuts, peanut butter or peanut oil.
- Review these precautions with children, parents and staff before any outing.

Make it clear to the parents of a child with a peanut allergy that, because peanuts are so prevalent in the food supply, even a "no peanut" policy cannot totally eliminate the risk of accidental exposure.

If a child in your care has an **allergy to insect stings**, you should:

- check for and remove insect nests found near your facility,
- store garbage in tightly covered containers,
- avoid wearing fragrant sunscreen or cosmetics, which can attract insects,
- drink soda pop or juice from cups—rather than cans or bottles—and use straws when serving children drinks outdoors.

If a child in your care has a severe **pollen allergy**, you should:

- try to stay indoors when the seasonal pollen count is known to be high, particularly on hot, dry, windy days, in the early morning, late afternoon and early evening,
- have the child wear a hat and wraparound sunglasses outdoors and wash these when she comes inside,
- try not to play under pollinating trees—most pollen will stay within 10 m (11 yds.) of its source,
- ensure that the child is taking the appropriate allergy medication.

See also **Asthma**, below.

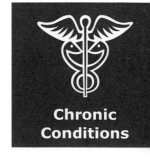

Chronic Conditions

In an emergency

If a child shows signs of anaphylaxis, you must:

1. **Call 911** (or emergency services where 911 service is unavailable).
2. Administer epinephrine (e.g., EpiPen or Twinject). (See Chapter 11, *Emergencies*, pages 277–78.)
3. Notify the child's parents.
4. Record the reaction in the child's file.

Anemia

The human body needs iron to make hemoglobin, which gives colour to red blood cells and carries oxygen to organs, muscles and tissue. When a child doesn't get enough iron, his red blood cells become small and pale, and he doesn't have enough oxygen circulating in his system. This condition is called anemia.

Signs of anemia can include:

* pale lips, palms or skin,
* fatigue and weakness,
* rapid heart beat,
* apathy, lack of interest or inattention during play, and
* irritability.

Anemia has several causes. The most common in children is a diet low in iron-rich foods. (See also Chapter 3, *Nutrition*.) Often, when a child drinks too much milk or juice, he doesn't eat enough nourishing solid food.

Anemia also has several medical causes, including two genetic diseases—sickle cell disease and thalassemia. Children with **sickle cell disease** are prone to bone problems, abdominal pain, damage to lungs and kidneys, worsening anemia and very serious bacterial infections. They require a daily oral antibiotic or a monthly intramuscular (injected) antibiotic to prevent infection. Sickle cell disease, although rare in most ethnic groups, is more prevalent in people of African descent. **Thalassemia**, which occurs in people of Mediterranean ancestry, can cause mild anemia in children who carry the gene from one parent and severe anemia in those carrying the gene from both parents. Children with severe thalassemia require regular blood transfusions and take medication to prevent iron build-up in their organs.

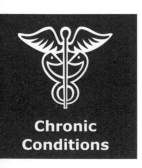

Chronic Conditions

Your role

Familiarize yourself with the signs of anemia and report any concerns to the child's parents. Your observations may help the child's parents and doctor to manage this condition. If you're caring for a child with severe anemia caused by a disease:

* Require that a condition-specific medical form be completed by the parents in consultation with their child's doctor. The form should outline the child's medical treatment and include detailed instructions for child care practitioners about managing this condition.

- Review this information with the parents every 6 months or whenever their child's treatment changes.

If you're caring for a child with anemia caused by a dietary iron deficiency, share nutrition information, menus and feeding strategies with the parents—preferably in consultation with their child's doctor or a registered nutritionist. Ask the parents to keep you updated after doctor's visits so you're aware of any changes, such as the need for additional iron supplements.

Asthma

Asthma is a chronic breathing disorder characterized by recurring attacks of wheezing, coughing and shortness of breath. About 1 in 10 children, and twice as many boys as girls, have asthma. Cases range from mild to severe. Between attacks, most children are well and can tolerate normal levels of exercise and activity. During an asthma attack, air passages to the lungs swell, become inflamed or go into spasm, and lung secretions (mucus) become thicker. As a result, the child must work harder to move air into and out of his lungs.

Signs of an asthma attack include:

- coughing,
- difficulty breathing,
- a wheezing or whistling sound when breathing out, and
- chest tightness.

Symptoms can come on very quickly (e.g., when the child is exposed to an allergen) or slowly, over days (e.g., when they are brought on by a common cold). In both scenarios, asthma attacks can be serious and, in rare cases, even result in death.

Triggers that cause asthma attacks include:

- cold viruses (the most common cause),
- smoke and smoking,
- allergies (e.g., dust, pollen, mould, feathers, animal dander),
- odours (e.g., paint fumes, aerosol sprays, cleaning materials, chemicals, perfumes),
- strenuous exercise,
- weather conditions (e.g., cold air, weather changes, windy or rainy days),
- vigorous crying or laughing.

Your role

Familiarize yourself with the signs of asthma and report any concerns to the child's parents. Your observations may help the child's parents and doctor to manage this condition. First aid training must include how to respond to a serious asthma attack.

When a child in your care has been diagnosed as asthmatic, you need to protect him from exposure to triggers wherever possible. Having the information you need to help manage this condition is key:

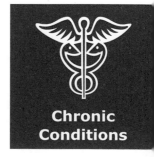

Chronic Conditions

- Require that a condition-specific medical form be completed by the parents in consultation with their child's doctor. The form should outline the child's medical treatment and include detailed instructions for child care practitioners about managing her asthma. (See Appendix 10.3 for a sample action plan.)
- Review this information with the parents every 6 months or whenever their child's treatment changes.
- Make sure that all staff know what triggers cause the child's asthma and what to do if an attack occurs.

A doctor may prescribe medications to relax the child's airways and/or to prevent or reduce inflammation. These medications may need to be administered every day or only during attacks and can include a liquid or pill, or a metered-dose inhaler and spacer (e.g., AeroChamber).

Follow your facility's policy for administering medication. At the time of enrolment, the parents of a child with asthma need to fill out and sign a *Medication consent form and record sheet* (see pages 139–40), outlining exactly what medication is to be given, by what method, when, and in what dosage. The child's parents must also demonstrate the proper use of any treatment devices. Each time you administer medication to a child, be sure to record the time, date and dosage, and initial the form.

It's part of your responsibility to protect children from substances or activities that may trigger an asthma attack. Here are some things you can do:

- Enforce a strict "no smoking" policy.
- Do not have pets on site.
- Vacuum daily and dust often.
- Remove feather pillows and down duvets, and launder all bed sheets and blankets in hot water once a week.
- Watch for and remove mould growth.
- When using bleach solutions, keep a child with asthma away from the fumes.
- Avoid carpeting. Use washable, low-pile throw rugs.
- Avoid heavily scented household cleaners, personal care products and air fresheners.
- Post a sign to discourage parents or delivery drivers from idling vehicle engines outside your facility.
- Avoid play outdoors when the seasonal pollen count is known to be very high (usually in hot, dry and/or windy weather).

If a child's asthma is triggered by exercise, monitor her activities and stop her if she begins to have breathing difficulties or starts to wheeze. This may happen more often in cold or damp weather. You may need to help a child use her inhalation medication 5 to 10 minutes before beginning the exercise, if that's part of her regimen. Also:

- Encourage a child with asthma to participate at her own pace and to rest if she feels like it.
- Don't initiate an activity if a child is showing signs of difficulty.
- Start with an easy warm-up before moving on to more vigorous activity.

Be sure to communicate with the child's parents well in advance of activities or outings that could trigger asthma, such as visiting a farm or a petting zoo.

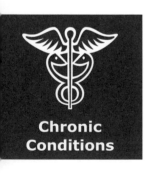

Chronic Conditions

If a child has an asthma attack:

1. Stop the child's activity or remove the trigger substance, if possible.
2. Calm the child.
3. Administer medication.
4. Contact the parents.

For details on responding to an asthma attack, see Chapter 11, *Emergencies*, pages 278–79.

In an emergency

If the child doesn't respond to medication or has difficulty breathing, or if the attack seems unusually severe or persistent, **call 911** (or emergency services where 911 service is unavailable).

Celiac disease

Celiac disease is a condition in which the surface of the small intestine is damaged by gluten, a protein found in wheat, rye, oats and barley. This damage makes the body less able to absorb nutrients, including vitamins and minerals, carbohydrates, protein and fat, which are necessary for health. Although its cause is unknown, celiac disease can run in families and is often associated with other conditions, such as type 1 diabetes mellitus and Down syndrome. About 1 child in 130 has celiac disease. While there is no cure and medication is usually not prescribed, the condition can be managed by following a gluten-free diet.

Common signs and symptoms of celiac disease are:

- anemia,
- chronic diarrhea,
- weight loss,
- fatigue,
- cramps and bloating, and
- irritability.

Your role

Familiarize yourself with the signs of celiac disease and report any concerns to the child's parents. Your observations may help the child's parents and doctor to manage this condition. If a child in your care is diagnosed with celiac disease, you'll need to work closely with the parents to ensure that he follows a gluten-free diet according to doctor's instructions.

- Require that a condition-specific medical form be completed by the parents in consultation with their child's doctor. The form should outline the child's medical treatment and include detailed instructions for child care practitioners about managing this condition.
- Review this information with the parents every 6 months or whenever their child's dietary regimen changes.

For information about a gluten-free diet, visit the Canadian Celiac Association website at www.celiac.ca. Since many prepared foods have ingredients that contain gluten, you must

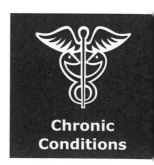

Chronic Conditions

read the ingredients on food labels, especially before purchasing soups, lunch meats and sausages.

Cystic fibrosis

Cystic fibrosis (CF) is a serious genetic illness that is present at birth but may not be recognized immediately. One in 2,000 Caucasian children is born with CF, and the disease is less common in other ethnic groups. Children with CF produce abnormal mucus in the respiratory and gastrointestinal tracts that obstructs and infects the lungs and causes poor digestion and food absorption. Because the pancreas doesn't function properly, children with CF also lack the digestive enzymes needed to absorb nutrients, which also results in poor nutrition. This condition is managed by pancreatic enzyme capsules, which almost all affected children must take daily. Children with CF tend to get frequent chest infections, some develop diabetes—insulin injections are added to their treatment regimen—and a few develop liver problems.

Signs of CF can include:

- lung infections,
- chronic coughing and spitting,
- poor weight gain and failure to thrive,
- diarrhea, or large, greasy or sticky stools that have a foul odour,
- recurrent and severe common colds,
- vomiting and abdominal pain, and
- abnormal loss of body salts while sweating.

Children with CF are treated with a combination of daily medications to replace missing enzymes, airway-relaxing medications in inhalers, and sometimes oxygen. Daily physiotherapy is often necessary to help with breathing.

Your role

If a child in your care has CF, you'll almost certainly be involved in daily treatment. Having the information you need to help manage this condition is key:

- Require that a condition-specific medical form be completed by the parents in consultation with their child's doctor. The form should outline the child's medical treatment and include detailed instructions for child care practitioners about managing CF. (See Appendix 10.4 for a sample action plan.)
- Review this information with the parents every 6 months or whenever their child's treatment changes.

Follow your facility's policy for administering medication. At the time of enrolment, the parents of a child with CF need to fill out and sign a *Medication consent form and record sheet* (see pages 139–40), outlining exactly what medication is to be given, by what method, when, and in what dosage. The parents must also demonstrate the proper use of any treatment devices. Each time you administer medication to a child, be sure to record the time, date and dosage, and initial the form.

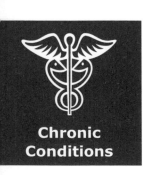

Chronic Conditions

In an emergency

If a child with CF is vomiting or has abdominal pain, you should:

1. Call the parents immediately.
2. If symptoms seem severe, **call 911** (or emergency services where 911 service is unavailable).
3. Record these symptoms and your response in the child's file.

Diabetes

Type 1 diabetes mellitus (formerly called juvenile diabetes or insulin-dependent diabetes) is a disease in which the pancreas produces little or no insulin. Insulin is a critical hormone that helps the body store and use glucose (sugar). All cells in the body need sugar to work properly, since it's their main fuel for energy. Without insulin, the sugar in the blood can't be used and builds up in the bloodstream even while the body is starved for energy. Cells are unable to process blood sugar and can't get enough nourishment. Type 1 diabetes affects about 1 in 600 children and can run in families. It is not clear what causes diabetes, and type 1 diabetes cannot be prevented.

The early signs of type 1 diabetes include feeling generally unwell, along with:

- frequent urination,
- bedwetting in a previously "dry" child
- excessive thirst,
- hunger,
- fatigue,
- weight loss,
- diaper rash.

These signs disappear with proper treatment, but if diabetes goes undetected and untreated, symptoms of increasing hyperglycemia (high blood sugar) can appear, including these serious symptoms:

- dry mouth and tongue (dehydration),
- a fruity or sweet breath odour,
- nausea and vomiting,
- drowsiness and lethargy,
- heavy, laboured breathing, and
- unconsciousness.

Left untreated, children with type 1 diabetes would die.

Type 2 diabetes (formerly called adult-onset diabetes) develops when the body either cannot produce enough insulin or doesn't use the insulin it makes properly. Although usually a disease of adulthood, type 2 diabetes is becoming more common in teens and in children who are seriously overweight.

Your role

Diabetes is controlled by carefully balancing three factors: food, exercise and insulin.

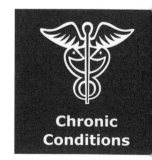

Chronic Conditions

Monitoring a child's blood sugar levels is the best tool for assessing this balance. Food makes blood sugar levels rise, while exercise and insulin make levels fall. A child with diabetes will have a meal plan that corresponds to his particular insulin regimen. For example, a child on 2 or 3 daily injections of insulin must eat at specific times and in specific amounts each day. Appropriate snacks include crackers with cheese, a mini bag of pretzels, fresh fruit, graham crackers, one cup of milk or one juice box.

If a child in your care has diabetes, you'll almost certainly be involved in daily treatment. The child's family and health care team are your best resources. The parents must demonstrate the proper use of treatment devices, usually an insulin syringe, pen, or pump for administering insulin, and a glucose meter for measuring blood sugar levels. You can learn more about treatment procedures and devices from a health professional, diabetes nurse educator or pharmacist. You'll need to know how to check a child's blood sugar levels, supervise the test, and record readings in a daily log book. This ongoing record is maintained both at home and in child care, and captures details about food intake and signs of low blood sugar and how these interact for the child in your program.

Program staff should be prepared to:

- attend educational sessions on children's diabetes to learn how diet and exercise affect insulin levels,
- monitor and record blood sugar readings in a daily log book, and check blood sugar levels if you suspect a child feels "low."
- make appropriate nutritional interventions (e.g., giving 125-200 mL [4 to 6 oz.] of juice or a soft drink containing sugar to treat low blood sugar symptoms),
- administer medication, including glucagon, and
- share meal plans with parents.

In addition, you should:

- Require that a condition-specific medical form be completed by the parents in consultation with their child's doctor. The form should outline the child's medical treatment and include detailed instructions for child care practitioners about managing diabetes. (See Appendix 10.5 for a sample action plan.)
- Review this information with the parents every 6 months or whenever their child's treatment changes.
- Follow your facility's policy for administering medication. At the time of enrolment, the parents of a child with diabetes need to fill out and sign a *Medication consent form and record sheet* (see pages 139–40), outlining exactly what medication

ALERT

The most common problem for children with diabetes is hypoglycemia (low blood sugar), caused by:

- eating too little food at meals,
- a delayed meal or snack,
- doing too much unplanned physical activity, or
- too much insulin.

Hyperglycemia (high blood sugar) is less common but can be caused by:

- eating too much food,
- doing too little physical activity,
- taking too little insulin, or
- having an illness or infection.

Hyperglycemia is not a cause for immediate concern unless a child also has high blood sugar symptoms. Notify parents immediately if the blood sugar reading is high **and** a child is vomiting.

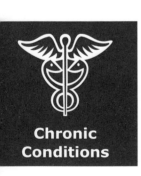

Chronic Conditions

is to be given, by what method, when, and in what dosage. Each time you administer medication to a child, be sure to record the time, date and dosage, and initial the form.

Working closely with the child's parents, you can help prevent the most common diabetes-related symptoms, both of hypoglycemia (low blood sugar) and hyperglycemia (high blood sugar).

While common signs of low blood sugar include trembling, hunger and blurred vision, each child reacts differently. Early symptoms may also include:

- headache,
- pallor (pale skin colour),
- fatigue/drowsiness,
- confusion/inattention,
- moist cold skin/sweating,
- irritability,
- dizziness/shakiness,
- rapid pulse rate, and
- loss of coordination.

Familiarize yourself with the specific signs or symptoms that a child in your care is likely to have. Encourage the child to tell you if she feels "low." All staff must be aware that the child has diabetes, be sensitive to the signs and symptoms of low blood sugar, and be ready to respond in a diabetic emergency. (See Chapter 11, *Emergencies*, pages 285–86.)

The child's parents should supply you with a glucagon kit to use in case of emergency. Glucagon is a natural hormone and a prescription medication that is injected to raise blood sugar levels quickly if a child with diabetes loses consciousness. You may request that the parents supply two glucagon kits, in case a mistake is made in preparing an emergency dose. Check the expiration date: glucagon kits need replacing every 1-1/2 to 2 years. Clearly label the medication with the child's name and the date received and store it in a location that's known to everyone and readily accessible by staff (i.e., **not** in a locked cupboard or drawer) but not by children.

Instructions on how to give a glucagon injection should be kept with the medication at all times, but only a trained or experienced person should give a glucagon shot. Optimally, everyone on staff should know where this medication is kept and be trained to administer it. Glucagon is safe. You cannot harm a child with glucagon.

In a low blood sugar emergency

If a child shows signs of low blood sugar and is unable to eat or drink, but still able to swallow:

1. Rub a fast-acting sugar (e.g., glucose gel, cake icing from a tube, jam or syrup) on the inside of her cheeks or gums with your finger.

If a child is unable to swallow, has a seizure or becomes unconscious:

- Roll her onto her side.
- **Call 911** (or emergency services where 911 service is unavailable).
- Disconnect the child's insulin pump.
- Inject glucagon, if you are trained to administer this shot.

2. Notify the child's parents.
3. Record the reaction in the child's daily log book.

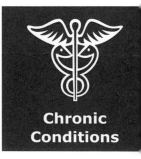

Chronic Conditions

Epilepsy

Epilepsy is a condition characterized by recurring seizures. It occurs in about 1 in 100 children. A seizure happens when there's a temporary, unusually high level of electrical activity in the brain.

Seizures can take many forms. The classic type is the generalized seizure, affecting the whole body. It starts with muscle stiffening and is usually followed by loss of consciousness, a fall and uncontrollable shaking. The child may drool and/or bite his lips, cheeks or tongue and/or lose control over his bladder and bowel functions. This type of seizure lasts only a few minutes and, while it can be frightening to onlookers, it generally passes without complications for the child. Deep sleep often follows an episode. It is uncommon for a child with epilepsy to have multiple generalized seizures in one day.

Another common form of seizure is the more subtle "absence" type. It lasts only seconds, and the child may appear momentarily blank, inattentive or lost in a daydream. However, unlike a child who is daydreaming, he cannot be aroused. There can be many of these episodes during a single day, and because the child hardly moves, this type of seizure often goes unnoticed.

Another form is the partial seizure, during which a child experiences unusual sensations, such as odours or visual or hearing abnormalities. Other characteristics of the partial seizure include sudden, restless movement, stomach discomfort and fear. In other partial seizures, a child might appear confused, with random walking, mumbling, head turning or clothes pulling, signalling an episode.

The signs of an epileptic seizure can be very subtle in infants and young children, and may include:

- staring,
- rolling of the eyes,
- drowsiness,
- inattention,
- lack of awareness, and
- twitching.

What causes epilepsy is largely unknown, and the condition can occur in otherwise healthy children. Children with certain brain disorders or injuries may also have epileptic seizures. For some children with epilepsy, particular stimulants or triggers will bring on a seizure. You can help identify these triggers over time by recognizing a seizure pattern.

ALERT

Common seizure triggers for children with epilepsy are:

- an infection,
- a rapidly rising fever,
- flashing or blinking lights (e.g., camera flashes),
- fatigue,
- a scary amusement park ride (e.g., roller coaster),
- particular sounds or odours,
- hyperventilation.

Your role

Familiarize yourself with seizure signs and report any concerns to the child's parents. Your observations may help the child's parents and doctor to manage this condition. Your first aid training must include how to respond to an epileptic seizure.

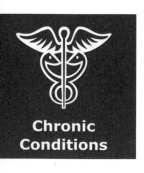

Chronic Conditions

When a child in your care has epilepsy, you need to protect him from exposure to triggers wherever possible and deal with seizures when they occur. Having the information you need to help manage this condition is key:

- Require that a condition-specific medical form be completed by the parents in consultation with their child's doctor. The form should outline the child's medical treatment and include detailed instructions for child care practitioners about managing epilepsy.
- Review this information with the parents every 6 months or whenever their child's treatment changes.
- Make sure that all staff know what triggers may cause a child's seizure and what to do if one occurs.
- Familiarize yourself with any side effects, such as drowsiness, that may be a result of anti-convulsant medications prescribed by the child's doctor.

Follow your facility's policy for administering medication. At the time of enrolment, the parents of a child with epilepsy need to fill out and sign a *Medication consent form and record sheet* (see pages 139–40), outlining exactly what medication is to be given, by what method, when, and in what dosage. Each time you administer medication to a child, be sure to record the time, date and dosage, and initial the form.

Witnessing a seizure can be frightening for other children. Try to remove them from the area during an episode, if possible. After the seizure, discuss what happened in a reassuring way.

In an emergency

If a seizure lasts longer than 5 minutes or if multiple seizures occur and the child doesn't wake up in between, **call 911** (or emergency services where 911 service is unavailable). (See Chapter 11, *Emergencies*, page 287.)

Heart conditions

Heart problems occur when one or more parts of this complex muscle—the pumping chambers (atriums or ventricles), the valves that separate the chambers, or the blood vessels leading to or from the heart—don't work properly. Most children with a heart condition have a congenital defect, which means they were born with it. About 8 in 1,000 children are born with some form of heart condition, ranging from the mild to the serious. Others develop a heart condition as a result of illness, although this is rare.

Symptoms of a heart condition can include:

- failure to thrive,
- limited exercise tolerance,
- breathlessness, with or without exertion,
- bluish lips,
- abnormal weight gain due to fluid retention, and
- lack of appetite.

Most children with a serious heart problem will have had surgery before they are enrolled in a child care program. Most who have undergone surgery are considered healthy and

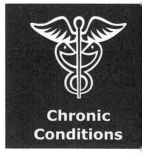

Chronic Conditions

shouldn't be treated differently from other children because of their heart problem. Some children may be on medication to control this condition.

Your role

If a child in your care has an ongoing heart condition, having the information you need to help manage his condition is key:

- Require that a condition-specific medical form be completed by the parents in consultation with their child's doctor. The form should outline the child's medical treatment and include detailed instructions for child care practitioners about managing this condition, including any dietary or activity restrictions (although these are rare). Be careful to respect the limits determined by the child's parents or treating physician.
- Review this information with the parents every 6 months or whenever their child's treatment changes.

Follow your facility's policy for administering medication. At the time of enrolment, the parents of a child with an ongoing heart condition need to fill out and sign a *Medication consent form and record sheet* (see pages 139–40), outlining exactly what medication is to be given, by what method, when, and in what dosage. Each time you administer medication to a child, be sure to record the time, date and dosage, and initial the form.

Hemophilia

Hemophilia is a rare genetic blood disorder in which the blood clots very slowly. It occurs in about 1 in 10,000 children, and the severity of the disease varies. Due to the way it is inherited, hemophilia is much more common in males than in females. Children with hemophilia bruise easily, and routine cuts and scrapes take longer to stop bleeding. Also, an injury can lead to serious internal bleeding, which may not become apparent until some time after the event.

Hemophilia can be detected in infancy, and most cases are diagnosed before a child turns 4 years of age. Signs of hemophilia are:

- easy and excessive bleeding,
- swelling of the joints after an injury (caused by internal bleeding),
- excessive bleeding after minor cuts and scrapes.

Your role

If a child in your care is diagnosed with hemophilia, your role is to prevent injury. Head injuries are particularly dangerous because they can cause serious bleeding into the brain. Any situation that might result in a head injury, such as rough play, **must** be avoided. Preventing injury to the child's joints is also important. Have the child's parents outline what activities he cannot participate in, as well as the ones requiring close supervision. Notify them well in advance of any special activity that might involve a risk of injury.

- Require that a condition-specific medical form be completed by the child's doctor. The form should outline the child's medical treatment and include detailed instructions for child care practitioners about managing bleeding.

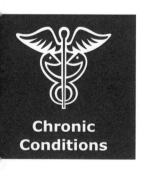

Chronic Conditions

- Review this information with the parents every 6 months or whenever their child's treatment changes.
- Make sure that all staff know that the child has hemophilia so his activities can be closely monitored.

In an emergency

If a child with hemophilia receives even a minor injury:

1. Contact his parents immediately.
2. If they are unavailable, contact the child's doctor.
3. **Call 911** (or emergency services where 911 service is unavailable) if the child vomits or shows signs of drowsiness after a fall or other injury.
4. If there is bleeding, follow routine practices to prevent contact with blood.
5. Record the injury in the child's file.

Special health needs

Most of the time, children with ongoing medical issues can be easily accommodated in child care programs. Staff training, adequate preparedness, appropriate precautions and good communication are usually enough to ensure a child's safety and full participation. For more about inclusion, see Chapter 13, *Including Children with Special Needs*.

Selected resources

Allergies/Asthma

Allergy/Asthma Information Association. www.aaia.ca

Allergy Safe Communities. www.allergysafecommunities.ca. An excellent downloadable Anaphylaxis Emergency Plan and sample letter of notification that a child in the program has a food allergy are available at this website.

Anaphylaxis Canada. www.anaphylaxis.ca

Asthma Society of Canada. www.asthma.ca

Canadian Society of Allergy and Clinical Immunology. 2007. *Anaphylaxis in schools and other settings*. Ottawa, Ont.: CSACI. www.csaci.medical.org or www.allergysafecommunities.ca

Children's Asthma Education Centre. www.asthma-education.com

Food Allergy and Anaphylaxis Network (U.S.). www.foodallergy.org

Gold, Milton, Ed. 2003. *The Complete Kid's Allergy and Asthma Guide: The Parent's Handbook for Children of All Ages*. Toronto, Ont.: Robert Rose.

Lung Association of Canada. Children and asthma. www.lung.ca

Public Health Agency of Canada. Asthma. www.phac-aspc.gc.ca

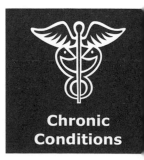

Chronic Conditions

Anemia

B.C. Health Guide. 2007. Iron-deficiency anemia. www.bchealthguide.org

Canadian Paediatric Society. 2007. Iron needs of babies and children. www.caringforkids.cps.ca

HealthyOntario.com. Sickle cell anemia. www.healthyontario.com

Hospital for Sick Children. Iron: Helping your child get enough. www.aboutkidshealth.ca

Celiac disease

Canadian Celiac Association. www.celiac.ca

HealthyOntario.com. Celiac disease. www.healthyontario.com

Cystic fibrosis

Canadian Cystic Fibrosis Foundation. 2003. *Your child and cystic fibrosis*. www.ccff.ca, www.cysticfibrosis.ca

Diabetes

Canadian Diabetes Association. 2004. *Kids with diabetes in your care: Resource kit*. Toronto, Ont.: CDA. www.diabetes.ca

Daneman, Denis, Marcia Frank and Kusiel Perlman. 2nd ed., 2002. *When a Child Has Diabetes*. Toronto, Ont.: Key Porter.

Diabetic Children's Foundation. www.diabetes-children.ca

Juvenile Diabetes Research Foundation. www.jdrf.ca

National Aboriginal Diabetes Association. www.nada.ca

Epilepsy

Epilepsy Canada. www.epilepsy.ca

Epilepsy Ontario. 2001. *Children living with epilepsy: Kit for parents, teachers and caregivers*. www.epilepsyontario.org

HealthyOntario.com. Epilepsy. www.healthyontario.com

Heart conditions

Canadian Cardiovascular Society. www.ccs.ca

Heart and Stroke Foundation of Canada. 2004. *Heart and Soul: A guide to congenital heart disease*. Toronto, Ont.: HSF. www.heartandstroke.com

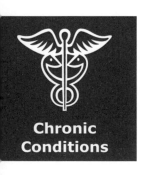

Chronic Conditions

Hospital for Sick Children. 2007. Congenital heart defects: Information for teachers. www.aboutkidshealth.ca

Variety Children's Heart Centre. Children's Hospital of Winnipeg. www.vchc.ca

Hemophilia

Canadian Hemophilia Society. 2001. *All About Hemophilia: A Guide for Families*. Montreal, Que.: CHS. www.hemophilia.ca

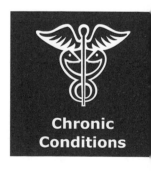

Chronic Conditions

Appendix 10.1: Sample cover page for condition-specific action plans

[Condition] _____ action plan

for: _____ [child's name]

> CHILD'S PHOTO

Date developed: _____

Review date(s): _____

Note: Review this information with the parents every 6 months or whenever their child's treatment changes.

Child's birth date: _____

Child's weight: _____

Designated staff member (if applicable):

_____

Contact information

Mother/guardian: _____

Tel: Home _____ Work _____ Cell_____

Father/guardian: _____

Tel: Home _____ Work _____ Cell_____

Child lives with: _____

Child's doctor's name: _____ Tel:_____

Allergy specialist's name (if applicable): _____ Tel:_____

Alternate emergency contact (if parents are unavailable): _____

Relationship to child: _____

Tel: Home _____ Work _____ Cell_____

Notify parents/guardians or emergency contact in the following situations:_____

_____

Note any other conditions that may affect the treatment of this child:_____

_____

Name, address and phone number for child care centre or home setting

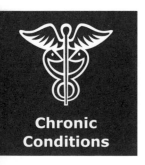

Chronic Conditions

Appendix 10.2: Sample anaphylaxis action plan

Emergency preparedness

Parent responsibilities:

❑ Provide epinephrine devices and replace them every 6 months or before the expiry date, whichever comes first.
❑ Complete and sign (with the child's doctor) an Anaphylaxis Emergency Plan, downloaded at www.allergysafecommunities.ca.
❑ Fill out and sign a *Medication consent form and record sheet*.
❑ Make sure the child wears a MedicAlert bracelet or tag.
❑ If the child has a food allergy, provide all meals and snacks from home.
❑ Discuss appropriate location for epinephrine devices.
❑ Be involved with staff training for emergency use of epinephrine devices.

Additional information: _____

_____

Program responsibilities:

❑ Provide allergy awareness education and emergency training for all staff.
❑ Post the Anaphylaxis Emergency Plan prominently in relevant areas (e.g., kitchen and eating areas for a child with a food allergy).
❑ Alert substitute or new staff to the child's Anaphylaxis Emergency Plan and the location of epinephrine devices.
❑ Implement "allergy-sensitive" policies.
❑ Have a back-up supply of "safe" foods in case a lunch or snack from home is forgotten, or the child's pick-up is delayed because of weather or another emergency.
❑ Take epinephrine devices and the child's *Emergency record* along on any outing or field trip.
❑ Ask a supervising adult to ride with this child in a bus or other vehicle.

Additional information: _____

_____

Typical signs or symptoms of this child's reaction (circle all that apply):

- swelling (eyes, lips, face, tongue)
- cold, clammy, sweating skin
- fainting or loss of consciousness
- stomach cramps
- choking
- voice changes

- diarrhea
- difficulty breathing or swallowing
- dizziness or confusion
- coughing
- wheezing
- vomiting

Other (please describe): _____

I give permission for my child's photo to be placed on the Anaphylaxis Emergency Plan, and for that plan to be posted appropriately.

_____   _____
Signature of parent/guardian   Date

Name, address and phone number for child care centre or home setting

Source: University of Victoria Child Care Services, *Anaphylaxis action plan* and *Anaphylaxis action form*. Adapted with permission.

Chronic Conditions

Appendix 10.3: Sample asthma action plan

Asthma episodes

Known triggers for this child's asthma (circle all that apply):

- cold viruses
- smoke and smoking
- allergies (e.g., dust, pollen, mould, feathers, animal dander, or other _____)
- odours (e.g., paint fumes, aerosol sprays, cleaning materials, chemicals, perfumes, or other [e.g., foods] _____)
- strenuous exercise
- weather conditions (e.g., cold air, weather changes, windy or rainy days)
- vigorous crying or laughing

Other (please specify): _____

Name of irritant/allergy (e.g., perfumes in cosmetics, soap, aftershave)	Reaction (e.g., wheezing, coughing)
_____	_____
_____	_____
_____	_____
_____	_____
_____	_____
_____	_____

Is there a time of year when this child seems to have more asthma episodes?
❑ Yes   ❑ No

If so, when? _____

Typical signs or symptoms of this child's asthma episodes (circle all that apply):

- coughing
- difficulty breathing
- a wheezing or whistling sound when breathing out
- chest tightness

Other (please describe): _____

Does this child tend to develop a very severe episode very quickly?

❑ Yes   ❑ No

Additional comments concerning episodes: _____
_____
_____
_____
_____
_____

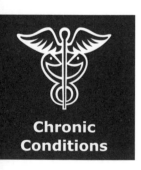

Chronic Conditions

Complete the following schedule

Medications for routine and emergency treatment of asthma for:			
Child's name			
Time	Medication name and dosage	Method (e.g., metered-dose inhaler and spacer)	How much
Morning			
Noon			
Afternoon			
Night			
Possible side effects, if any:			
Describe all other medications or products to be used when needed (e.g., ointments, antihistamines, sunscreens, etc.)	Name (e.g., salbutamol)	Reason used (e.g., to relieve symptoms)	How often (e.g., only as needed)
Parent's permission to follow this medication plan	Date:	Signature:	

Reminders

1. Administer medication as specified and record on the child's *Medication consent form and record sheet*.
2. If the episode seems unusually severe or persistent, **call 911** (or emergency services where 911 service is unavailable).
3. If the attack persists but is not severe, advise the parents to pick up their child early and see a doctor.

Questions or concerns to be discussed with the child's doctor:

_____

_____

_____

_____

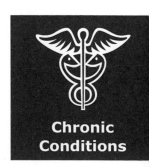

Chronic Conditions

Name, address and phone number for child care centre or home setting

Appendix 10.4: Sample cystic fibrosis action plan

Daily care plan

Parent responsibilities:

❑ Recognize when the child is not well enough to attend child care.
❑ Provide information about food allergies.
❑ Provide daily medications (e.g., enzymes, inhalers, antibiotics).
❑ Be involved in staff training for giving medications (e.g., digestive enzymes).
❑ Discuss side effects of medications (e.g., how antibiotics may affect the child's stool).
❑ Discuss appropriate location for storing medications.
❑ Inform child care staff of additional medications that are prescribed intermittently during the year.
❑ Provide child care staff with devices and instructions for airway clearance techniques.

Additional information: _____

_____

Program responsibilities:

❑ Encourage the child's participation in all physical activities.
❑ Provide plenty of fluids.
❑ Provide nutritious, high calorie meals and snacks.
❑ Give digestive enzymes as indicted in the child's individualized action plan.
❑ If the child has a cough, provide easy access to tissues and a means of disposing them.
❑ Provide opportunities for frequent hand hygiene.
❑ Help the child to feel comfortable during toileting routines, which may be more frequent than for other children.
❑ Minimize attention to giving medications.
❑ Minimize attention to a child's coughing.

Additional information: _____

_____

Signs or symptoms to bring to a parent's attention at the end of the program day:

- bulky stools
- gas
- stomach cramps
- abdominal swelling

- frequent visits to the bathroom to pass stool
- markedly decreased or increased appetite
- lower tolerance to activities
- increased coughing

Other (please describe): _____

Reminders

1. During vigorous activities or hot weather, a child with cystic fibrosis will need plenty of fluids and may be required to have salt supplements or salty snacks.
2. Some antibiotics cause photosensitity. Remember to use sunscreen and a hat.
3. Notify a parent if the child has eaten food without enzymes.

Call a parent immediately if: _____

_____

_____

Name, address and phone number for child care centre or home setting

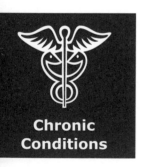

Chronic Conditions

Complete the following schedule

Medications for routine and emergency treatment of cystic fibrosis for:				
Child's name				
Time	Medication name and dosage	Method (eg: oral, metered dose inhaler)	Additional treatments (e.g., airway clearance)	Comments
Breakfast				
Morning snack				
Lunch				
Afternoon snack				
Dinner				
Possible side effects, if any:				
Describe all other medications or products to be used when needed (e.g., ointments, sunscreens).	Name	Reason used	How often	
Parent's permission to follow this medication plan	Date:	Signature:		

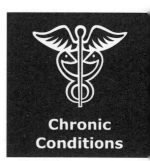

Chronic Conditions

Reminders

1. Administer medications only as specified.
2. Record every dose of any medication on the child's *Medication consent form and record sheet*.

Source: Lisa Semple, for the Canadian Cystic Fibrosis Nurses' Interest Group.

Name, address and phone number for child care centre or home setting

Appendix 10.5: Sample diabetes action plan

Diabetes management

Blood sugar (glucose) monitoring

Target range is: _____

* Note: Most preschoolers have a target range of 6 mmol/L to 12 mmol/L prior to meals.

Usual times to check blood sugar:_____

Other times to check blood sugar (e.g., before or after exercise, or if the child shows signs of feeling "low"): _____

Times when parents want to be notified immediately _____

Parent responsibilities:

❑ Provide glucose meters, test strips, lancing device and lancets, and batteries.

Program responsibilities:

❑ Help monitor levels by:

_____

_____

❑ Record blood sugar levels in the child's *Diabetes daily care record.*

Additional information: _____

_____

_____

Insulin injection

For a child using an insulin syringe/pen:

Parent responsibilities:

❑ Determine staff willingness to administer insulin injections and help with their training.
❑ Provide insulin vials and syringes, or insulin pen and supplies.
❑ Provide a container to dispose of sharps.

Other: _____

_____

Program responsibilities:

❑ Determine their role in giving insulin, in collaboration with the child's parents.
❑ Enlist support of a community nurse to ensure staff comfort and competance with giving injections.
❑ Help the child to administer an injection.
❑ Record the injection on the child's *Medication consent form and record sheet.*

Other: _____

_____

Name, address and phone number for child care centre or home setting

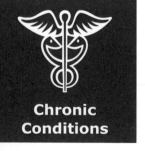

Chronic Conditions

For a child using an insulin pump:

Parent responsibilities:

❑ Help train program staff to administer insulin using a pump.
❑ Ensure that the pump is in good working condition.

Program responsibilities:

❑ Check the child's blood sugar levels at the times requested by parents.
❑ Administer the correct dose based on blood sugar level and carbohydrates provided.
❑ Record the dose on the child's *Medication consent form and record sheet.*
❑ Take some simple, problem-solving steps to ensure the pump is working if a blood sugar reading is unexpectedly high.
❑ Attend education sessions on managing children's diabetes.

Food management

Regular times for meals and snacks: _____

Parent responsibilities:

❑ Provide a daily snack containing carbohydrates (e.g., cheese and crackers).
❑ Provide program with a back-up supply of fast-acting sugar (e.g., glucose tablets or gel, honey).
❑ Label meals/snacks provided with their carbohydrate content, in grams, for children using a pump.

Other: _____
_____

Program responsibilities:

❑ Ensure that meals and snacks are offered on time.
❑ Share meal plans with parents in advance.
❑ Keep a back-up supply of fast-acting sugar on hand.
❑ Advise parents of special days involving food.

Other: _____
_____

Instructions for when food/treats are provided for the group for a special event: _____
_____
_____

Instructions for days involving extra activity: _____
_____
_____

Additional information: _____
_____
_____
_____

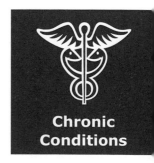

Chronic Conditions

Name, address and phone number for child care centre or home setting

Typical signs or symptoms of this child's hypoglycemia (circle all that apply):

- headache,
- pallor (pale skin colour),
- fatigue/drowsiness,
- confusion/inattention,
- moist cold skin/sweating,
- hunger,
- irritability,
- dizziness/ shakiness,
- rapid pulse rate, and
- loss of coordination.

Other (please describe): _____

_____

Can your child recognize his/her own low blood sugar signs?

❏ Yes   ❏ No

If so, how might she/he describe feeling "low"? _____

_____

_____

_____

What is usually given to treat low blood sugar? _____

_____

_____

_____

Reminders

If in doubt, treat a child's symptoms:

If child is conscious:

1. Check the child's blood sugar level, if possible.
2. If the child's blood sugar is under 6 mmol administer fast-acting sugars immediately. Repeat in 10 to 15 minutes if symptoms persist.
3. Once the reaction subsides, offer a snack of cheese and crackers. Don't change the time for the next scheduled meal or snack.
4. Stay with the child until you are sure that recovery is complete.

If the child is unable to swallow, unconscious or having a convulsion:

1. Turn the child on her side.
2. **Call 911** (or emergency services where 911 service is unavailable).
3. Don't attempt to give anything by mouth.
4. Only administer glucagon if you have been trained to do so.

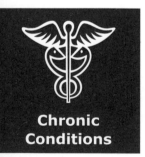

Chronic Conditions

Name, address and phone number for child care centre or home setting

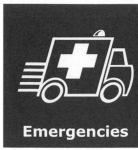
chapter

11

Emergencies

S erious emergencies don't happen often in child care settings. But when they do, being properly prepared can make the difference between a tragedy and a happy ending. Being trained and equipped to handle common medical and other emergency situations is critical for quality child care. Every centre and home-based program must:

- have a written emergency plan that outlines basic policies and procedures in case of emergencies (e.g., fire),
- regularly check and refresh all safety/medical equipment on site (e.g., testing fire alarms and making sure the first aid kit is complete), and
- ensure that all staff have first aid and cardiopulmonary resuscitation (CPR) training and regular practice in safety drills and procedures.

Knowing your responsibilities in an emergency and having the skills to respond effectively go a long way to ensuring the health and safety of children in your care. Being well prepared also helps you respond to children's fear or anxiety in a calm and comforting manner.

Your written emergency plan

Be familiar with the provincial/territorial child care regulations governing safety for your jurisdiction—including staff training requirements—before preparing your facility's

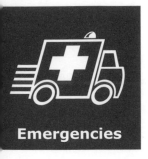

emergency plan. Your basic plan must comply with local regulations before you develop additional emergency procedures to meet the unique needs of your facility. Fire or the threat of fire is the most common reason to put an emergency plan into action, and the staff at your local fire department can help with developing the emergency plan for your program. Other dangers, such as a power failure or extreme weather, may require all or part of the plan to be implemented.

The emergency plan

Your written plan should cover the following topics:

1. Evacuation procedures, routes and where to gather safely while awaiting assistance from emergency services
2. Evacuation drills
3. Emergency telephone numbers
4. Staff emergency training in first aid and CPR
5. First aid supplies
6. Emergency records (i.e., key contacts/basic medical information)
7. Protocol for notifying parents
8. Emergency equipment
9. Emergency transportation
10. Planning for environmental hazards

---

1. Evacuation procedures, routes and where to gather safely while awaiting assistance from emergency services

In a fire or other emergency, you have two major responsibilities: first, to evacuate the children from the building safely; then, to notify the fire department. An evacuation procedure needs to be shared and practiced to be effective. Here's what to do:

- Prepare and post a floor plan of your facility or home setting, showing the evacuation routes and all possible exits.
- Post the floor plan and evacuation procedures in key locations (e.g., in each room of a child care centre or near all telephones in a home-based setting).
- Choose an alternate warning sound (e.g., a hand-held bell) to be used only if smoke detectors or other alarms do not go off in an emergency.
- Plan how you will get the children out of the building efficiently. Depending on staff-to-child ratios, those caring for infants and toddlers should know how each adult will carry three or four children out of the building. Some facilities use cribs to transport a few babies at once. Practitioners working alone in a home setting should know how to remove all children without assistance.
- Consult your local fire department or inspector for help with:
  - ➤ planning exit routes,
  - ➤ how best to physically remove children from the building,
  - ➤ using and maintaining safety equipment, and
  - ➤ teaching fire safety to staff and children.
- Designate a safe area for everyone to meet after evacuating. This area should be at least 15.5 m (50 ft.) from the building. Also arrange for an evacuation site (e.g., a nearby school or church) where everyone can go if you can't return to your facility.

- Make one person responsible for calling 911 or the fire department, but only after everyone is out of the building.
- Keep daily attendance records and parent contact information in a readily accessible, consistent place, such as near the exit.
- Make sure every staff member is thoroughly familiar with the plan and review it regularly, however often you practice.

Here's an example of an emergency procedure to post in your facility:

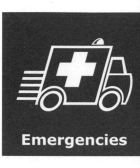

Emergency procedure

In case of fire:

- At the first sign of fire or smoke, sound the alarm.
- Calmly alert children and staff to evacuate the building. Do not shout "Fire!"—this can cause panic.
- Help children leave the building.
- Close all doors behind you to help prevent fire from spreading.
- If you run into flames and/or smoke when trying to leave the building, use another exit.
- Meet in the designated safe area.
- Make sure that everyone is safely accounted for.
- Telephone the fire department (911) from a safe location.

If you can't leave your room because of smoke, or you've had to return to a room:

- Close the door.
- Call 911 and tell them about your situation.
- Wave at the window to signal to firefighters.
- Seal the cracks around the door with blankets or clothes (wet them first, if possible).
- Crouch low to the floor if smoke enters the room.
- Open a window for ventilation, but close it if smoke enters.
- Wait to be rescued.
- Listen for instructions or information that authorized personnel may give over loudspeakers.
- Jump from the second or an upper storey **only** as a last resort.

Source: Region of Peel (Ont.) Public Health, *Keep on Track: A Health and Resource Guide for Child Care Providers in Peel*. Adapted with permission.

---

2. Evacuation drills

Conduct drills once a month, rain or shine, to help ensure that staff and children will respond appropriately in a true emergency. Your goal is to make the drill as real as possible and to train staff and children to react the same way they would in a real situation. This means **not** stopping to put on shoes, coats, clothes or to finish a diaper change. Remind parents who may be in the building at the time of your drill of all the steps, so their well-intentioned actions won't contradict facility policy. Incomplete or unrealistic drills can lead to repeating mistakes during a real fire, with tragic results.

To plan for any situation, do drills at different times of the day, including during naptime and when you are short staffed. Even in winter, practice getting out of the building. Keep shoes or boots in a basket during naptime so that they can be carried out during the drill. Have one staff member waiting outside with blankets and the basket. In extreme weather conditions, reschedule your drill to another day. Be sure to alert your fire department or alarm-monitoring company to any change of plan.

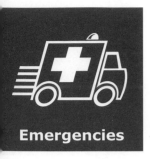

Train children and staff to be aware of all possible exits by painting pretend "flames" on the side of a box to simulate the presence of real fire during a drill. Place this box in front of an exit occasionally, so that staff have to choose another route.

Here's how to conduct an evacuation drill:

- Alert the fire department or alarm-monitoring company that a drill will be conducted.
- Sound the alarm.
- Help children exit the building.
- Meet with staff and children at a pre-planned safe area.
- Be sure that everyone is accounted for.
- Let staff and children know when they can re-enter the building.
- Notify the fire department or alarm-monitoring company when the drill is finished.
- Record the time it took for everyone to exit the building.
- Meet with staff and children after the drill to assess performance and get feedback.

Source: Region of Peel (Ont.) Public Health, *Keep on Track: A Health and Resource Guide for Child Care Providers in Peel.* Adapted with permission.

Teach children to crawl on hands and knees to the nearest exit if a room is smoky. Air is freshest near the floor.

Also teach them to:

1. **STOP** (not run) if your clothing catches fire.

2. **DROP** to the ground and cover your face with your hands.

3. **ROLL** over and over to put out the flames.

3. Emergency telephone numbers

Make sure every staff member knows how to make an emergency call—it means more than dialing 911.

- Stay on the line to receive instructions or relay them to a colleague to carry out.
- Don't hang up until told to do so by the emergency service operator. Staying on the line makes it possible to trace the call, so emergency personnel can be sent to your location.
- Use the speakerphone function if you're working alone, or leave the phone off its hook and shout information into the receiver while attending to a child in trouble.

Post emergency numbers next to all telephones, along with the address of your facility. Having the address right there is helpful in a stressful situation, especially for new staff, substitute staff or back-up caregivers.

Here are numbers you need to post next to all telephones:

- Emergency medical services: 911, where available.
- If 911 service is not available for your area, post telephone numbers for emergency services: ambulance, fire department and police department.
- Your local or provincial poison control centre.
- The name and telephone number of emergency back-up caregivers, in case you must leave (e.g., to accompany a child to hospital).
- Other phone numbers as required by provincial/local regulations.

You may also want to include the numbers for your local public health unit or medical officer of health, the nearest hospital or clinic, and taxi company.

4. Staff emergency training in first aid and CPR

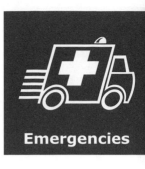

Emergencies

Being properly trained and prepared for emergency situations is essential to quality child care, and maintaining current paediatric certification in first aid and CPR is an employment requirement for child care practitioners in many jurisdictions. Those working with infants should also be certified in infant CPR. Where training isn't mandatory, centre supervisors must arrange staff schedules so that at least one child care practitioner with valid CPR certification is on the premises during working hours. Facilities with physically separate areas for different groups of children should have at least one trained staff member in each area (e.g., if infants and toddlers are on the first floor and preschoolers on the second, there should be an appropriately certified staff member on each floor). A child care practitioner with certification should always accompany children to the playground, outdoors and on all field trips. If some children remain at the facility, at least one person with certification should stay with them.

If you plan to run a child care program out of your home, obtaining certification in first aid and CPR for children is an essential first step. Check provincial/territorial regulations for staffing requirements in your area.

When choosing first aid and CPR training, take courses designed for child care situations or that emphasize techniques and situations specific to the care of young children. At a minimum, the course should cover techniques and skills required to prevent death or further injury.

TABLE 11.1

Recommended course content for certified first aid and CPR in child care (knowledge/skill requirements)

A. Principles and practices of first aid and CPR, including:
- priorities in the management of casualties
- ABC's of first aid
- resuscitation, including CPR for infants and young children
- getting assistance
- when and how to move an injured child

B. Prevention, recognition and management of:
- allergic reactions, including insect stings and use of epinephrine devices
- asthma, including use of a metred-dose inhaler (MDI) and a spacer
- choking
- wounds, bleeding, bruising and bites, including routine practices to prevent contact with blood and body fluids
- shock, loss of consciousness, fainting
- injuries, including head, eye, tooth, neck, chest, abdomen/pelvis, back and bone injuries
- seizures/convulsions
- insulin responses, including low blood sugar (hypoglycemia), giving a glucagon shot
- poisoning
- burns and scalds
- environmental injuries, including frostbite, heat stroke, electrical shock, gaseous exposure

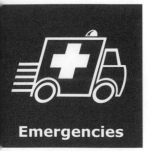

You should know how and when to administer potentially life-saving medications (e.g., EpiPen) or devices (e.g., an inhaler), especially if a child with a severe allergy or asthma is in your care. Check for workshops or other training opportunities in your area.

5. First aid supplies

Child care programs need at least two first aid kits: one to stay in the centre or home, and a second to be taken to the playground and on all field trips. Larger centres may need a kit for each area of the centre—for instance, one for each floor, or one for infants and toddlers and one for preschoolers.

Store first aid supplies in lightweight, waterproof containers (e.g., a plastic food bin that snaps closed). Label all kits and keep them in central, clearly marked locations, out of the reach of children. Check and refill their contents on a regular basis and before each field trip. One way to ensure that your first aid kit remains fully equipped is to place a seal (e.g., a sticky label that needs to be torn) onto the container. Check this seal daily and if it has been broken, count the supplies and refill, then reseal.

If you have a child in your care with a medical condition requiring special support, you'll need to have appropriate supplies on site and remember to take them along on outings (e.g., a current EpiPen for a child with a severe allergy or a sweet snack or insulin for a child with diabetes).

While required contents in first aid kits for child care programs vary regionally, the items in Table 11.2 are a recommended minimum. These supplies can be purchased at your local pharmacy or through local St. John Ambulance or Red Cross offices.

TABLE 11.2

Recommended minimum contents in first aid kits for child care programs

❑ pocket first aid reference book
❑ children's emergency records (1 complete set)
❑ bandage scissors (1 pair)
❑ blunt-nosed tweezers (splinter forceps) (1 pair)
❑ 10 individually wrapped sterile gauze dressings 5 cm x 5 cm (2 in. x 2 in.)
❑ 25 (5)* individually wrapped sterile gauze dressings 10 cm x 10 cm (4 in. x 4 in.)
❑ 25 (10)* individually wrapped plastic bandages
❑ 10 child-sized plastic bandages
❑ 5 individually wrapped sterile non-adhesive compresses 10 cm x 10 cm (4 in. x 4 in.)
❑ 6 (1)* slings or triangular bandages

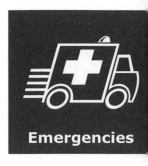

❑ 4 (1)* rolls sterile gauze bandage 8 cm (3 in.) + 4 (1)* rolls 10 cm (4 in.)
❑ 1 roll non-allergic adhesive tape 2.5 cm (1 in.) wide
❑ 1 elastic tensor bandage 8 cm (3 in.) wide
❑ 12 (5)* safety pins
❑ 1 digital thermometer
❑ 25 individually wrapped antiseptic pads
❑ 25 individually wrapped alcohol pads
❑ 1 needle
❑ 5 tongue depressors
❑ 4 eye bandages
❑ 1 tube petroleum jelly or other lubricant
❑ disposable non-latex or vinyl gloves (2 pairs)
❑ plastic eye bath

* The smaller quantity in brackets is recommended for home-based programs. Note: An extra epinephrine device (where needed) should be kept somewhere more accessible than your first aid kit.

Every child care program should have a supply of disposable gloves, tongue depressors, instant cold packs and woollen blankets. Additional supplies for field trips should include:

❑ a fully charged cell phone, if your facility has one,
❑ 8 quarters (25 cents) for a public telephone,
❑ a pad and pencil for jotting down information,
❑ an index card with your facility's phone number and address, and the phone numbers for emergency services in areas without 911 service, and
❑ a complete set of emergency records.

6. Emergency records (i.e., key contacts/basic medical information)

On index cards, record current information about children in your care, including:

* contact information for their parents, as well as for an alternate caregiver in case a parent cannot be reached (specify the alternate caregiver's relationship to the child, such as aunt or next-door neighbour),
* pertinent medical information (e.g., an allergy alert), and
* the child's doctor's name and phone number.

Keep these cards together in a box for quick and easy access in an emergency, and review with parents for accuracy every 6 to 12 months. Keep the box in an accessible spot, preferably near an exit. Keep another (duplicate) set of cards in each first aid kit and be sure they are taken on all field trips.

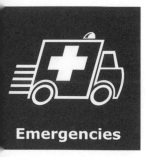

7. Protocol for notifying parents

Encourage parents to read and respond to your emergency plan. They need to be familiar and comfortable with policies, especially for notification and early pick-up. As well, parents must sign a consent form for emergency treatment and transportation. (See Appendix 11.1, page 292, for a sample.)

8. Emergency equipment

While the range and nature of required safety/ emergency equipment for child care programs may vary regionally, the items listed below are a recommended minimum. In all child care centres and home settings, required emergency equipment includes:

- working smoke detectors (alarms),
- fire alarms or a warning system (child care centres only),
- carbon monoxide detectors (alarms),
- blanket(s),
- large flashlight(s) and batteries sufficient to last 72 hours (keep these in designated areas in case of power failure),
- first aid kit(s), and
- fire extinguisher(s).

In home settings, smoke alarms should be located on each level of the house, in the hall outside each sleeping area and also in bedrooms where occupants sleep with the door shut. They should be tested monthly and the batteries changed every 6 months. Replace any alarm that is more than 10 years old with one that takes "long-life" batteries—these batteries can last up to 10 years. If your facility is in a newer home, one or more alarms may be hard-wired into the house wiring and connected to a private alarm-monitoring service.

Ensure the safety of all children in your care before using a fire extinguisher. Fire prevention authorities emphasize that trying to extinguish or control a fire is last on the list of priorities for handling a fire. In homes, extinguishers should be placed near the entrance to the kitchen. It is strongly recommended that each home be equipped with extinguishers that are:

- approved,
- annually serviced,
- portable (for putting out a small fire),

> **REMEMBER**
>
> When an emergency or injury happens, or any time first aid is required, you must:
>
> 1. Inform parents as soon as possible.
>
> 2. Make a detailed written record, including:
>   - what happened,
>   - preceding or precipitating events,
>   - the names of adult witnesses, and whether children were present,
>   - the staff-to-child ratio at the time of the incident,
>   - who called for help, and when.

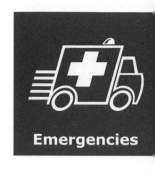

- easily accessible,
- multi-purpose, and
- dry-chemical.

Check the test window monthly (the marker should be in the green zone), and make sure it has not passed its expiry date. **All staff require training in the use and function of any fire extinguisher on site.** Contact your local fire department to arrange fire safety training and for information about your provincial/territorial fire code regulations.

Check all emergency equipment regularly to ensure that it is current, in working order and easily accessible. Make sure all staff know how to use all emergency equipment you have on site.

9. Emergency transportation

Most true medical emergencies will require calling 911 and safely transporting a child to hospital by ambulance. There may also be circumstances where you'll need to decide quickly whether to drive the child to the hospital, take her in a taxi or call an ambulance. Always err on the safe side. If you are transporting a child in an urgent situation, two adults must be in the vehicle: one to drive and one to care for the injured or ill child on the way to hospital.

For each child in your care, require parents to complete a consent form giving you permission to contact the child's doctor and to transport the child in an emergency. Keep the consent form in each child's file and the contact information with the child's emergency record. (See Chapter 6, *Transportation Safety*.)

BEST PRACTICE

Even if your facility's vehicle is only for emergency use, having an appropriate car or booster seat for the children in your care is best practice and may be required in your jurisdiction. All provinces and territories require the use of car seats for transporting children up to about 4 years of age, and most require booster seats for children age 4 to 8.

10. Planning for environmental hazards

Every child care facility needs a policy outlining procedures in case of a power outage, severe weather (e.g., a bad electrical storm, blizzard, or even a tornado if your area is along a storm corridor) or natural disaster (e.g., an earthquake, flood, or landslide if your area is vulnerable). A power outage may be caused by severe weather or happen on its own. Every facility should keep (at a minimum) a supply of bottled water, non-perishable food and a non-electric can opener on hand. For more information on specific recommendations and free resources, contact Public Safety Canada (PSC) at www.publicsafety.gc.ca. PSC has regional offices in each province and territory—look in the federal government listings in the telephone book for locations.

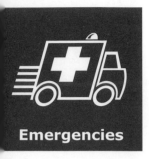

FIRST AID

First aid is the help given in an emergency until regular medical care is available. Taking a certified course in paediatric and/or infant first aid and CPR is required for employment in child care in many jurisdictions. All scenarios described below would require you to write a report and notify parents as soon as possible after the incident.

The following guidelines are no substitute for proper training. They are just here as reminders of essential steps you need to take in a medical emergency. Of all medical emergencies in child care, choking is by far the most common.

Choking

Choking occurs when a child's airway is blocked, preventing air from entering the lungs. The most common causes are liquids (in infants) and food or small objects (in babies, toddlers and preschoolers). The blockage may be mild or severe. If severe, the child is unable to make a sound. How choking is managed depends on the age of the child, whether the blockage is mild or severe, and whether or not the child is conscious.

Mild obstruction

When the airway is partially blocked, a child can still breathe. Breathing is difficult but crying, coughing or speaking is still possible. In such cases:

1. Stay with the child.
2. Encourage coughing and do not try to remove the object.
3. If the situation becomes more serious, have someone call 911 (or emergency services where 911 service is unavailable).

Severe obstruction

When a severe airway blockage occurs, a child:

- cannot cry, cough or talk,
- cannot breathe,
- turns blue,
- is limp, or
- loses (or has lost) consciousness.

For an infant under 1 year of age

If the infant is conscious:

1. Place the infant face-down over your arm so that his head is lower than his body. Rest your forearm on your thigh. Place a larger infant face-down across your lap.
2. Deliver up to 5 back blows (slaps), striking high between the infant's shoulder blades.
3. Turn the infant over if the blockage is not relieved. Cradle the infant face up across your lap. Using 2 fingers, give up to 5 rapid chest compressions ("thrusts") just below the inter-nipple line.

4. Repeat back blows and chest compressions until the blockage is removed, the infant loses consciousness or medical help arrives.

If the infant becomes unconscious:

1. **Shout** for help. Have someone **call 911** (or emergency services where 911 service is unavailable).

2. Place the infant flat on her back on a firm surface. Open her mouth and look for anything that might be blocking the airway. Remove any blocking matter with a hooked finger. If you don't see anything, don't sweep your finger round her mouth blindly—you may push blocking matter further down the airway.

3. Open the infant's airway by pressing down on her forehead with one hand and bringing her chin up with pressure from the index finger of your other hand, below the jaw.

4. Check to make sure that the infant is not breathing (no air entry) by placing your ear near her nose and mouth. Look, listen and feel for air movement. Take no more than 10 seconds.

5. If the infant is not breathing, place your mouth over the infant's nose and open mouth and give 2 rescue breaths. Ensure adequate

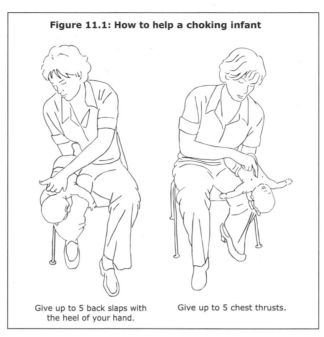

Figure 11.1: How to help a choking infant

Give up to 5 back slaps with the heel of your hand.

Give up to 5 chest thrusts.

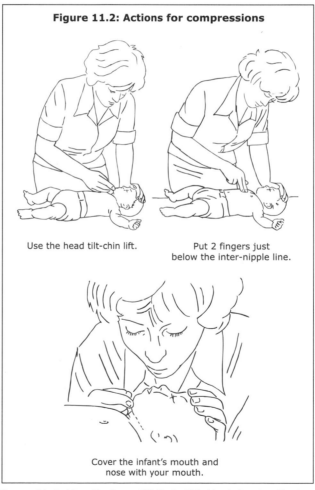

Figure 11.2: Actions for compressions

Use the head tilt-chin lift.

Put 2 fingers just below the inter-nipple line.

Cover the infant's mouth and nose with your mouth.

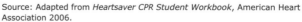

Source: Adapted from *Heartsaver CPR Student Workbook*, American Heart Association 2006.

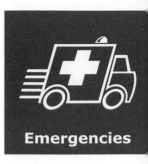

Emergencies

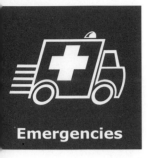
chest rise. If the chest does not rise or you feel an obstruction, reposition the head and try again. If air still does not enter, **begin CPR**.

6. Give 30 compressions (compress 1/3 to 1/2 the depth of the chest). Open the mouth and look for any obstruction. Give 2 rescue breaths for every 30 compressions.
7. Continue CPR until the blockage is removed or medical help arrives.

For a child over 1 year of age

If the child is conscious:

Perform the **Heimlich manoeuvre** (abdominal thrusts):

1. Grasp the child from behind, encircle the abdomen between the navel and breastbone, make a fist and press **firmly but gently** into the abdomen with inward and upward thrusts.
2. Repeat abdominal thrusts until the object is expelled, the child becomes unconscious or medical help arrives.

If the child becomes unconscious:

1. **Shout** for help. Have someone **call 911** (or emergency services where 911 service is unavailable).
2. Place the child flat on his back on a firm surface. Open his mouth and look for anything that might be blocking the airway. Remove any blocking matter with a hooked finger. If you don't see anything, don't sweep your finger round his mouth blindly—you may push blocking matter further down the airway.
3. Open the child's airway by pressing down on his forehead with one hand and bringing his chin up with pressure from the index finger of your other hand, below the jaw.
4. Check to make sure that the child is not breathing (no air entry) by placing your ear near his nose and mouth. Look, listen and feel for air movement. Take no more than 10 seconds.
5. If the child is not breathing, place your mouth over the child's open mouth and give 2 rescue breaths. Pinch the nose. Ensure adequate chest rise. If the chest does not rise or you feel an obstruction, reposition the head and try again. If air still does not enter, **begin CPR**.
6. Give 30 compressions (compress 1/3 to 1/2 the depth of the chest). Open the mouth and look for any obstruction. Give 2 rescue breaths for every 30 compressions.
7. Continue CPR until the blockage is removed or medical help arrives.

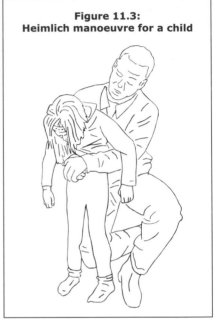

Figure 11.3:
Heimlich manoeuvre for a child

Source: Adapted from *Basic Life Support for the PALS Healthcare Provider*, American Heart Association 2005.

How to perform CPR

Perform CPR if you suspect a child's breathing or heartbeat has stopped. Taking a certified course in paediatric and/or infant first aid and CPR is the best way to learn how to handle emergencies.

The following guidelines are to remind you of the steps to take when children experience the most common emergencies. CPR is often required in cases of severe choking, near-drowning, electric shock and smoke inhalation.

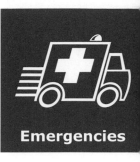

If a child is not moving (unresponsive):

1. **Shout** for help. Have someone **call 911** (or emergency services where 911 service is unavailable). **Start CPR.**
2. Place the child on her back on a firm surface.
3. Tilt the child's head and lift her chin to open the airway. Make sure that the child is not breathing (no air entry) by placing your ear near her nose and mouth. Look, listen and feel for air movement. **Take no more than 10 seconds and don't try to find a pulse.**
4. If the child is breathing and there is no evidence of trauma, turn the child onto her side.
5. If the child is not breathing or only gasps occasionally, give 2 breaths into an infant's nose and mouth or into an older child's mouth with nostrils pinched closed. Ensure adequate chest rise. If the chest does not rise or you feel an obstruction, reposition the head and try again.
6. If air still does not enter, **give 2 rescue breaths and begin chest compressions immediately**.

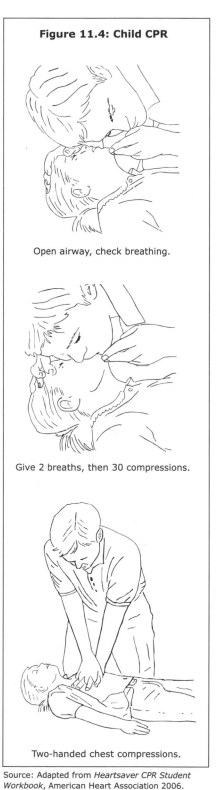

Figure 11.4: Child CPR

Open airway, check breathing.

Give 2 breaths, then 30 compressions.

Two-handed chest compressions.

Source: Adapted from *Heartsaver CPR Student Workbook*, American Heart Association 2006.

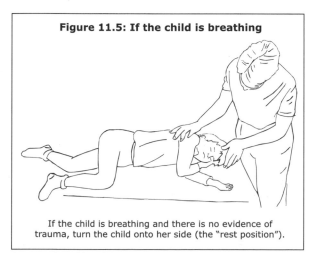

Figure 11.5: If the child is breathing

If the child is breathing and there is no evidence of trauma, turn the child onto her side (the "rest position").

Source: Adapted from "Pediatric basic life support, part 11," *Circulation*, American Heart Association 2005.

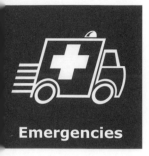
For an infant under 1 year of age

1. Position 2 fingers just below the inter-nipple line. Push down on the infant's breastbone to 1/3 to 1/2 the depth of the chest.
2. Compress **fast**, at a rate of about 100 times per minute, but **allow the chest to recoil fully after each compression.**
3. Give 2 rescue breaths for every 30 chest compressions.

For a child 1 to 8 years of age

1. **Hand position for a child of this age is different from that for an infant.** Place the heel of your hand or use two hands in the centre of the child's chest, on the inter-nipple line. Push down to 1/3 to 1/2 the depth of the chest.
2. Compress **fast**, at a rate of about 100 times per minute, but **allow the chest to recoil fully after each compression.**
3. Give 2 rescue breaths for every 30 chest compressions.
4. If two rescuers are present, take turns compressing and ventilating, switching quickly (in less than 5 seconds) every 2 minutes or so.

A to Z first aid measures

Abdominal pain and injuries

Abdominal pain is a common and usually minor symptom in children that may, occasionally, signal a more serious problem. Advise parents to pick up their child early and see a doctor if abdominal pain is severe, persistent or accompanied by any one of the following signs:

- fever,
- pale skin,
- nausea or vomiting,
- blood in stool or vomit,
- bilious (green) vomit,
- diarrhea, or
- a distended abdomen.

Suspect an abdominal injury if the child is feeling persistent pain, looks very pale and seems faint or nauseated. In that case:

1. Obtain immediate medical care.
2. Ensure the child does not drink or eat.

If you see bruising or evidence of injury on the child's back or stomach area, record this in writing and report it. If there is no explanation for these injuries and you have concerns about maltreatment, contact child welfare authorities immediately. (See Chapter 14, *Protecting Children from Maltreatment*.)

Abrasions (scrapes)

Cleaning abrasions to remove debris (dirt or other contaminants) is important to prevent infection and permanent staining or dimpling of the skin. **Wear disposable gloves when dealing with any open or bleeding wound.**

1. Rinse the abrasion with large amounts of tap water at room temperature. Using an antiseptic solution is not necessary.
2. If debris remains, gently sponge the area with damp gauze pads. Do not scrub the abrasion. If debris cannot be removed easily, advise the child's parents to arrange for further care.
3. Cover the abrasion with a sterile non-adhesive dressing.

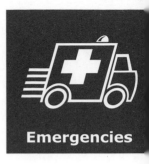

Emergencies

Anaphylaxis

Anaphylaxis is a life-threatening reaction that can follow a child's exposure to a food or substance to which he is severely allergic. It usually happens immediately but can also occur several hours later.

1. **Call 911 (or emergency services where 911 service is unavailable) if a child experiences *any* of the following signs of anaphylaxis:**
   • swelling of the mouth, lips or tongue,
   • breathing difficulty, wheezing or airway tightness,
   • hives (swollen, red skin),
   • pallor (white skin),
   • weakness, dizziness, nausea or vomiting, or
   • loss of consciousness or collapse.
2. Get the epinephrine device (e.g., EpiPen, Twinject) from its storage place.
3. Help the child lie down on the floor. It may be necessary to restrain an uncooperative child.

For EpiPen:
1. Pull out the grey safety cap.
2. Press the black-tipped end of the auto-injector against the child's upper thigh at a 90° angle (straight up), applying moderate pressure.
3. Listen for a "click" indicating that epinephrine is being injected.
4. Hold the EpiPen in place for at least 10 seconds.
5. Remove carefully, as the needle is now exposed.
6. Massage the injection site gently for 10 seconds to help the body absorb the medication.
7. Comfort the child.

For Twinject (a two-dose epinephrine device):
1. Remove the green end-caps numbered 1 and 2.
2. Place the red injector tip against the child's mid-thigh.
3. Press down firmly until the auto-injector activates.
4. Keep the Twinject in place for at least 10 seconds.
5. Remove carefully, as the needle is now exposed.
6. Massage the injection site gently for 10 seconds to help the body absorb the medication.
7. Comfort the child.

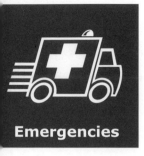

Emergencies

Administer epinephrine first.
Other medications (e.g., antihistamines, inhaled asthma medication) are **not** first-line medications when you suspect anaphylaxis. Antihistamines should be given only under medical supervision after a child has arrived at the hospital.

Don't give epinephrine through a child's snowsuit.
It's more difficult to find the injection site and maintain moderate pressure during the injection. Injecting through a single layer of clothing, including jeans, is acceptable.

Have an extra dose of epinephrine on site.
If you have to transport a child to a hospital that's more than 20 minutes away, you need to keep an extra dose of epinephrine in your first aid kit. If two adults cannot go with this child in the facility's vehicle, call an ambulance.

Any child who receives emergency epinephrine must be taken to a hospital as soon as possible.

Source: Region of Peel (Ont.) Public Health, *Keep on Track: A Health and Resource Guide for Child Care Providers in Peel*. Adapted with permission.

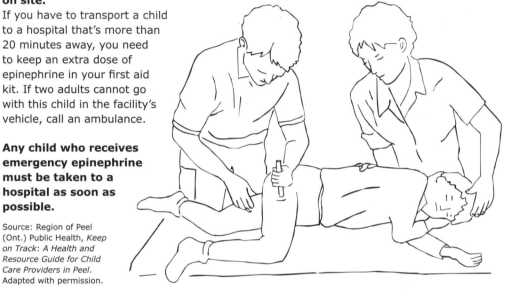

For more about anaphylaxis and allergies, see Chapter 10, *Chronic Medical Conditions*.

Asphyxiation (suffocation)

Asphyxiation occurs when a child's airway is blocked. It may be caused by choking, strangulation, smothering or near-drowning.

1. **Call 911** (or emergency services where 911 service is unavailable).
2. Move the child into fresh air.
3. **Perform CPR if the child is not breathing. (See pages 274–76.)**

Asthma

A child experiencing an asthma attack has difficulty breathing. She may experience wheezing, coughing and shortness of breath, because air is hard to expel from her lungs. You need to know how to help her use a metered-dose inhaler (MDI) and a spacer (e.g., AeroChamber), which allows more medicine to get to the lungs.

1. Remove the caps from the spacer and the MDI.
2. Shake the MDI well.

3. Insert the MDI mouthpiece into the rubber opening of the spacer, in an upright position.

4. Ask the child to breathe out as hard as she can before you place the spacer mouthpiece in her mouth. Remind her to close her lips tightly around the mouthpiece.

5. Press down on the canister, releasing one puff of medication. **Do not spray more than one puff at a time into the spacer.**

6. Help the child to breathe in and out, deeply and slowly, for 3 to 4 breaths.

7. If the child requires another puff, wait at least 30 seconds before repeating steps 4 to 6. **Remember to shake the canister well before giving the second puff.**

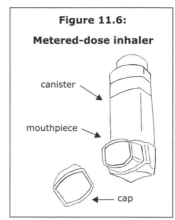

Figure 11.6:

Metered-dose inhaler

canister

mouthpiece

cap

Source: Reproduced with permission from the website of the Canadian Lung Association, www.lung.ca.

If the child's spacer comes with a **mask**, follow steps 1 to 3 and place the mask securely over her mouth and nose. Make sure there are no gaps between the mask and the child's face. Help the child to breathe in and out, deeply and slowly:

- 5 to 6 breaths if she is 18 months of age or over,
- 8 to 10 breaths if she is younger than 18 months.

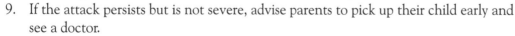

Figure 11.7:

Spacer (e.g., AeroChamber)

canister

mask

MDI

body   mouthpiece

inhaler adapter

Source: Children's Hospital of Eastern Ontario, "How to administer your child's inhaled asthma medication." Adapted with permission.

8. If the attack seems unusually severe or persistent, **call 911** (or emergency services where 911 service is unavailable).

9. If the attack persists but is not severe, advise parents to pick up their child early and see a doctor.

10. Comfort the child and reassure others.

For more about asthma, see Chapter 10, *Chronic Medical Conditions*.

Bites

Animal bites

1. Try to identify the animal and its owner, or the area where the animal may be found. Don't try to catch the animal but notify animal control officers or police as soon as possible.

2. Wearing disposable gloves, wash the wound with large amounts of tap water at room temperature.

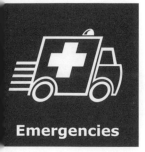
3. Advise parents to pick up their child early and see a doctor for a rabies and/or tetanus shot if needed, wound closure and/or antibiotic treatment.
4. Write your report and notify your local public health unit.

Animal attacks are rare but extremely serious. If a child is attacked by an animal, **call 911** (or emergency services where 911 service is unavailable).

Human bites

Bites occur frequently among toddlers in child care, but the vast majority cause bruising only and need little treatment. See **Bruising**, below. (If a bite breaks the skin and draws blood, see Chapter 9, *Managing Infections*, page 214.)

Snake bites

1. **Call 911** (or emergency services where 911 service is unavailable).
2. Keep the bitten body part as low (below heart level) and still as possible.
3. Do not apply ice.
4. Comfort the child and reassure others.

Bleeding

Blood loss may be visible (external) or hidden (internal). **If a wound looks serious, call 911** (or emergency services where 911 service is unavailable). Do the following until medical help arrives:

External bleeding

1. Apply firm, direct pressure on the wound with a gauze pad for 10 to 15 minutes. Wear disposable gloves.
2. If bleeding continues, apply a large pressure dressing. Maintain pressure until the bleeding stops. For serious or persistent bleeding, resist peeking under the dressing to see if the bleeding has stopped.
3. If bleeding continues and seeps through the material covering the wound, do not remove it. Simply place another cloth over the first one.
4. Once bleeding stops, place a wound dressing over the cut with firm pressure, wrapping it with adhesive tape or a piece of clean clothing. Apply a cold pack over the dressing.
5. If bleeding persists, advise parents to pick up their child early and see a doctor.

If the bleeding is severe, take steps to prevent shock:

1. Lay the child flat and immobilize the injured body part.
2. Raise his feet about 30 cm (12 in.).
3. Cover him with a coat or blanket. **Do not place the child in this position if there has been a head, neck, back or leg injury, or if the position makes him uncomfortable.**

Internal bleeding

If a child vomits blood or passes blood through the rectum or has a large and spreading bruise, **call 911** (or emergency services where 911 service is unavailable).

Bruising

Most bruises are minor and don't require medical attention. Apply cool compresses to a developing bruise for 10 to 15 minutes immediately after an injury to decrease the size of the bruise. **If the bruise continues to enlarge, call 911** (or emergency services where 911 service is unavailable).

Watch for unusual bruising (e.g., in infants who are not yet mobile), which may indicate maltreatment. If you see bruising or evidence of injury on the child's back or stomach area, record this in writing and report it. If there is no explanation for these injuries and you have concerns about maltreatment, contact child welfare authorities immediately. (See Chapter 14, *Protecting Children from Maltreatment*.)

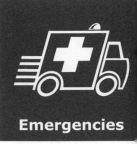

Emergencies

Burns and scalds

1. Remove child from the heat source immediately.
2. If necessary, **shout** for help. **Call 911** (or emergency services where 911 service is unavailable).
3. If clothes are on fire, smother the flames with a blanket or coat, making the child roll on the floor.

Minor burns

1. Immerse a child's burned finger or hand in cold water for 10 minutes or cover the burned area repeatedly with cold, wet cloths until the pain stops (at least 15 minutes). Change cloths often.
2. If the burn is as large as the child's hand or you see blisters, advise parents to pick up their child early and see a doctor for wound dressing and/or antibiotic treatment.
3. Do not break blisters.

ALERT

If you suspect a severe burn

Call 911 (or emergency services where 911 service is unavailable).

Do not apply water, ointment, butter, ice, medications, cream, oil, dressing or any household remedy to a severe burn.

Do not try to remove clothing that is stuck to the skin.

Severe or third-degree burns

Severe burns involve all layers of the skin and are painless because the nerves have been destroyed.

1. **Call 911** (or emergency services where 911 service is unavailable).
2. Cover the child with a clean sheet and then a blanket to keep her warm.
3. Do not apply ointment or other substances to a severe burn.
4. Do not try to remove clothing or material that seems fused with the burn.

Chemical burns

1. Remove any contaminated clothing before rinsing the child's skin with water. If the chemical product is dry (powder or crystals), brush off all you can with a clean cloth.

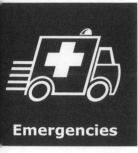

2. Rinse the area under cool, running water for 20 minutes. Avoid contact between healthy skin and used rinse water.

Cold injuries

Freezing to metal objects

If a child's tongue becomes frozen to a metal object:

1. Try to prevent the child from pulling away from the metal.
2. Try breathing hard on the area or pour warm water onto the object to warm it. Gently release the child.
3. If bleeding occurs, grasp the tongue with folded sterile gauze and apply direct pressure. Wear disposable gloves.
4. Advise parents to pick up their child early and see a doctor for treatment.

Frostbite

Frostbite is a condition in which the skin and underlying tissue are frozen. In the early stages, swelling and redness occur along with tingling, burning and numbness. As frostbite progresses, the skin becomes white, waxy and hard to the touch.

1. Move the child to a warm area and remove wet clothing. Cover him with a blanket or dry clothing.
2. Do not rub the area or apply dry heat (e.g., a heating pad).
3. Warm the affected area slowly using your own body heat or by immersing it in warm (never hot or boiling) water.
4. Offer a warm drink.
5. Advise parents to pick up their child early and see a doctor for assessment.

Hypothermia

Hypothermia is the most severe type of cold injury. Body temperature drops below normal, and the child may be drowsy, apathetic, shivering, irritable or confused, and have stiff muscles, slurred speech, fatigue, discoloured lips and/or skin that feels cold. Hypothermia becomes life-threatening when shivering stops, the child loses consciousness and/or cardiac arrest occurs.

1. **Call 911** (or emergency services where 911 service is unavailable).
2. Move the child to a warm area and remove wet clothing. Cover him with a blanket or dry clothing.
3. Use your own body heat to raise the child's body temperature slowly.
4. Do not use hot water bottles or electric blankets.

Convulsions (See Seizures, page 287.)

Croup (See Respiratory distress, pages 286–87.)

Dental emergencies

A knocked-out or broken tooth requires immediate dental care. Other dental emergencies may require medical attention.

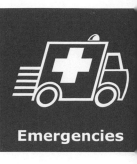

Emergencies

A knocked-out primary tooth

A primary tooth is rarely saved, but a dentist's decision to try will depend on the age of the child and how soon the tooth would fall out naturally.

1. Advise parents to pick up their child early and **see a dentist immediately**.
2. Find the tooth if possible and follow the same steps as for permanent teeth, below.

A knocked-out (or broken) permanent tooth

1. Advise parents to pick up their child early and **see a dentist immediately**.
2. Find the tooth—or tooth chip—if possible. Do not wash, rub or scrub the tooth.
3. Wearing disposable gloves, place the tooth in one of the following solutions:
   - milk. Put the milk on ice to keep it cold.
   - If the child isn't too upset and can produce saliva, ask her to spit into a small, clean container a few times and keep the tooth in the saliva. Don't ask the child to hold the tooth in her mouth, as there is a risk that she may swallow or inhale it into her lungs.
   - normal saline solution.
   - a commercial tooth preservative from the pharmacist, but only if you have this solution on hand and it is fresh.
4. Try to clean dirt or debris from the injured mouth area with warm water.
5. Place cold compresses (e.g., ice wrapped in a washcloth) on the child's face over the injured area to minimize swelling.

Toothache

1. Ask the child to swish warm water round her mouth and spit, to clean out food debris.
2. If swelling is present, place cold compresses (e.g., ice wrapped in a washcloth) on the child's face over the tooth that hurts. Do not use heat. Give acetaminophen to relieve pain.
3. Advise parents to pick up their child early and see a dentist as soon as possible.

Bitten tongue or lip

1. Wearing disposable gloves, apply direct pressure to the bleeding area with a sterile or clean cloth.
2. If there is swelling, apply cold compresses (e.g., ice wrapped in a washcloth).
3. If bleeding doesn't stop quickly or the cut is severe, advise parents to pick up their child early and **see a doctor immediately**.

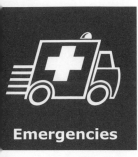

Fractured jaw

If you suspect a fractured jaw, support it with a soft pad held in place by hand—not with a bandage—and take the child to the nearest hospital emergency room. **Call 911** (or emergency services where 911 service is unavailable) if both you and another adult cannot go with him.

Drowning (near-drowning)

1. Remove the child from the water.
2. **Shout** for help. **Call 911** (or emergency services where 911 service is unavailable).
3. Don't try to remove water from the child's mouth and lungs. If the child is not moving (unresponsive), and is not breathing, **begin CPR** by opening the airway and giving 2 rescue breaths followed by 30 chest compressions. (For **CPR**, see pages 274–76.)
4. Continue to give 2 rescue breaths for every 30 chest compressions, switching with another trained person if possible, until help arrives.

Electric shock or burns

1. **Only if it is safe to do so**, disconnect electrical power.
2. Do not touch the child with your bare hands if the power is still on. To avoid injury to yourself if the power is on, keep a piece of wood, a thick dry cloth or a thick jacket between your hands and the child's body. Pull the child away from the power source.
3. **Shout** for help. **Call 911** (or emergency services where 911 service is unavailable).
4. If the child is not moving (unresponsive), and is not breathing, **begin CPR** by opening the airway and giving 2 rescue breaths followed by 30 chest compressions. (For **CPR**, see pages 274–76.)
5. Continue to give 2 rescue breaths for every 30 chest compressions, switching with another trained person if possible, until help arrives.

Eye injuries

If a strong chemical is splashed in the eye:

1. Gently rinse the eye, using tap water at room temperature, for at least 15 minutes.
2. Ask the child to keep her eye in the position that hurts least, and not to press or rub it.
3. Take her to the nearest hospital emergency room. **Call 911** (or emergency services where 911 service is unavailable) if both you and another adult cannot go with her.

If debris gets into the eye:

1. Allow natural tearing to occur for a few seconds while you ask the child to look slowly to the right and left, up and down.
2. If a particle is located under the eyelid or in the corner of the eye, remove it with the moistened corner of a small gauze pad.
3. If the child has sand in her eye, have her bend her head toward the side of the injured eye and gently rinse the eye with room-temperature tap water.

4. If debris is difficult to see or flush out, or seems stuck in the eye, take the child to the nearest hospital emergency room. **Call 911** (or emergency services where 911 service is unavailable) if both you and another adult cannot go with her.

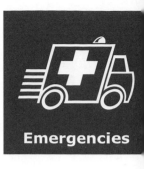

Fractures

If an injured body part is very painful, swollen or deformed, or if moving it causes the child pain, suspect a fracture. **If you suspect a neck or back injury, do not move the child.**

1. **Shout** for help. **Call 911** (or emergency services where 911 service is unavailable).
2. Have the child lie down or sit in a comfortable position and ask him to keep still.
3. Stabilize the injured part with pillows or other soft material to limit movement and reduce pain.

Head injury

The signs of a head injury usually occur immediately following an incident but may also, occasionally, develop slowly over several hours. Even if a child's skull isn't fractured, a concussion (when the brain collides against the skull during an injury and is bruised) may have occurred. The child's head might look fine, but complications can result from bleeding inside the skull.

A mild head injury may not need specific treatment. If a child begins to play or run immediately after getting a bump on the head, serious injury is unlikely. However, both you and the child's parents should monitor her closely for 24 hours after the incident.

If serious head trauma is suspected:

1. **Shout** for help. **Call 911** (or emergency services where 911 service is unavailable).
2. If the child has neck pain, is unable to move her head or feels numbness or tingling in her arms or legs, she should be kept in the position she was found in, with her head supported, until help arrives.

Low blood sugar (hypoglycemia)

A child with diabetes who is experiencing early signs of hypoglycemia might tremble, be very hungry or have blurred vision. Each child reacts differently. If you suspect a reaction, give him one of the following:

- 15 g of glucose in tablet form,
- 15 mL (1 tbsp.) or three packets of table sugar dissolved in water,
- 125-200 mL (4 to 6 oz.) of fruit juice or a regular soft drink, or
- 15 mL (1 tbsp.) of honey, jam, syrup or equivalent.

Wait 10 to 15 minutes and if there is no improvement, repeat this treatment. If the child is unable to eat or drink but is still conscious and can swallow, rub glucose gel, cake icing from a tube, jam or syrup on the inside of his cheeks or gums with your finger. Once the reaction subsides, offer the child a glass of milk or half a meat or cheese sandwich. **Don't leave the child unattended until you're sure recovery is complete.** Don't change the time of the next scheduled meal or snack.

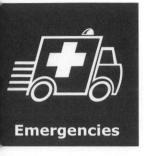

Do not give food or drink if the child is:

* unable to swallow,
* having a seizure, or
* unconscious.

1. Roll the child onto his side (see Figure 11.5, page 275), and disconnect his insulin pump.
2. **Call 911** (or emergency services where 911 service is unavailable).
3. Inject glucagon, if you have been trained to administer this shot.
4. Notify the child's parents.
5. Record the reaction in the child's daily log book.

For more about diabetes, see Chapter 10, *Chronic Medical Conditions*.

Nosebleeds

1. Wearing disposable gloves, have the child sit up and lean forward.
2. Loosen any tight clothing around her neck.
3. To stop bleeding, pinch the lower end of the nose to close the nostrils. Don't press on the bony part of the nose because this doesn't work. Apply pressure firmly for 10 to 15 minutes before checking to see if the bleeding has stopped.
4. Do not try to remove blood clots by blowing the nose after the bleeding has stopped.

Poisoning

Any non-food substance is a potential poison. If you suspect that a child has ingested something dangerous:

1. Call your local poison control centre and follow instructions or **call 911** (or emergency services where 911 service is unavailable).
2. Notify the child's parents.
3. If the child needs to go to the hospital emergency room, take a sample of what he swallowed (e.g., the container or piece of the plant).
4. **Do not make the child vomit.**

Respiratory distress (trouble breathing)

Respiratory distress can have many causes, including asthma, an allergic reaction, croup, pneumonia or an object blocking the child's airway. Severe respiratory distress is signalled by laboured or noisy breathing (wheezing), blue, greyish or very pale skin, anxiety and loss of consciousness.

1. **Shout** for help. **Call 911** (or emergency services where 911 service is unavailable).
2. Keep the child sitting upright if she is still conscious.
3. Administer medication as required for this child's underlying condition, if there is one (e.g., bronchodilator [inhaler], EpiPen or Twinject).
4. If the child is not moving (unresponsive), and is not breathing, **begin CPR** by opening the airway and giving 2 rescue breaths followed by 30 chest compressions. (For CPR, see pages 274–76.)

5. Give 2 rescue breaths for every 30 chest compressions.
6. Continue performing CPR, switching with another trained person if possible, until help arrives.

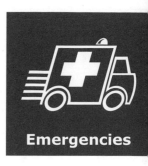

Emergencies

Seizures (convulsions)

Despite their frightening appearance—stiffening of the body, eyes rolling upward and jerking movements of the face and limbs—most seizures are not dangerous. They usually last from 30 seconds to 2 minutes.

The most common is the **febrile seizure**, which can occur at the first sign of fever in 2 to 5 per cent of children between 6 months and 5 years of age. Febrile seizures may start early in life, but they usually stop completely by the time a child is 5 years old.

1. Advise parents to pick up their child early and see a doctor as soon as possible after a febrile seizure.
2. If the seizure lasts longer than 3 minutes or the child is younger than 6 months of age, **call 911** (or emergency services where 911 service is unavailable).

Seizures are also associated with epilepsy. Children with this condition usually take daily medication to control their seizures. When an epileptic seizure occurs, the main goals are to protect the child from injury and to help with breathing if needed.

1. Lay the child on a flat surface, on his side. Do not move the child unless he is in danger or near something hazardous, and do not restrain him.
2. Wipe away vomit or saliva outside the mouth but do not put anything between the child's teeth during a seizure (including your fingers).
3. **Call 911** (or emergency services where 911 service is unavailable) if a seizure lasts longer than 5 minutes or if multiple seizures happen and the child doesn't awaken in between.
4. After the seizure stops, roll the child onto his side. (See Figure 11.5, page 275.)
5. Allow the child to sleep post-seizure and wake up gradually.

For more about epilepsy, see Chapter 10, *Chronic Medical Conditions*.

Shock

Shock happens when the body is not getting enough blood flow (oxygen). It can have many causes, including an injury with heavy bleeding, a breathing emergency or a serious infection. When a child goes into shock, her skin turns pale, then bluish-grey and is cold and clammy. Lips, earlobes and fingernails are a bluish-purple colour. For a non-Caucasian child, check the inside of the lip. Mucous membranes should be pink. The child's pulse is weak and rapid, and breathing is shallow and irregular. She may feel faint, dizzy or nauseous and gradually lose consciousness.

1. **Shout** for help. **Call 911** (or emergency services where 911 service is unavailable).
2. Give first aid appropriate to the injury (e.g., stop external bleeding).

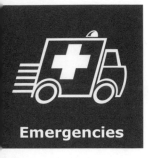
If the child is unconscious, but still breathing:

1. Lay the child on a flat surface, on her side. If she has difficulty breathing, a resting, half-seated position may help.
2. Loosen tight clothing.
3. Warm her with a blanket.
4. Moisten her lips with water if she is thirsty but don't give her anything to eat or drink.

If the child is unconscious and *not* breathing:

1. **Begin CPR** by opening the airway and giving 2 rescue breaths followed by 30 chest compressions. (For **CPR**, see pages 274–76.)
2. Give 2 rescue breaths for every 30 chest compressions.
3. Continue performing CPR, switching with another trained person if possible, until help arrives.

Stings
Bees, wasps and hornets

If the child is known to be allergic to stinging insects:

1. Give epinephrine (e.g., EpiPen or Twinject) **immediately** (see pages 277–78).
2. **Call 911** (or emergency services where 911 service is unavailable) after giving the epinephrine.
3. Call the child's parents.

If the child is not known to be allergic to stinging insects:

1. Remove the stinger by scraping gently with a straight-edged object (e.g., a credit card or blunt table knife). Do not use tweezers to pull out the stinger, because the squeezing action can produce more venom.
2. Wash the sting site with large amounts of tap water at room temperature.
3. Place a cold compress (e.g., ice wrapped in a washcloth) on the sting for 10 minutes, then off for 10 minutes. Repeat this process.
4. **Call 911 (or emergency services where 911 service is unavailable) if a child experiences *any* of the following signs of anaphylaxis:**
   • swelling of the mouth, lips or tongue,
   • breathing difficulty, wheezing or airway tightness,
   • hives (swollen, red skin),
   • pallor (white skin),
   • weakness, dizziness, nausea or vomiting, or
   • loss of consciousness or collapse.
5. Give epinephrine (e.g., EpiPen or Twinject) **immediately** (see pages 277-78).
6. Call the child's parents.

For more about allergies and anaphylaxis, see Chapter 10, *Chronic Medical Conditions*.

Ticks

1. Use tweezers to grasp the tick as close to the skin surface as possible.
2. Pull gently but firmly, using an even, steady pressure. Do not jerk or twist, and do not squeeze, crush or puncture the body of the tick, which may contain infectious germs.
3. After removing the tick, wash the skin with water and soap. If the tick's mouth parts are lodged in a child's skin, leave them alone. They will work out of the skin without treatment.

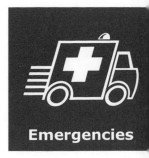

Emergencies

Procedures in the event of sudden collapse

If a child appears to have stopped breathing:

1. **Shout** for help. **Call 911** (or emergency services where 911 service is unavailable).
2. **Begin CPR** by opening the child's airway and giving 2 rescue breaths followed by 30 chest compressions. (For **CPR**, see pages 274–76.)
3. Give 2 rescue breaths for every 30 chest compressions.
4. Continue performing CPR, switching with another trained person if possible, until medical help arrives.
5. Collect the child's emergency record to take with you to the hospital.
6. Contact the child's parents immediately. Ask them to meet you at the hospital or ask police to contact the parents and help them get to the hospital.

When you reach the hospital

Give medical staff all the information you can about the child's schedule that day, his last feeding or meal, allergies (if any) and any medical problems or recent injuries.

The investigation

If there is a death, police and other authorities will begin their investigation within an hour or two after it is confirmed. This investigation may include staff interviews and site photographs. Do not remove items or alter the scene where the child's collapse occurred. Investigators may remove items as evidence. In the event of a SIDS death, for example, investigators may remove an infant's last feeding bottle, bedding and diapers.

If a death occurs at your child care centre, the director is responsible for completing a signed and dated account of the child's activities during the day, making a note of the presence and function of all staff who attended the child during the day. Staff should also prepare their own reports (dated and signed) of contact with the child. These records are to be written as soon after the death as possible, preferably the same day. Child care practitioners in a home care setting must also write a report, with the same details and time frame.

Same-day follow-up

Contact your provincial/territorial child welfare office to report a child's death. The office will investigate and prepare an independent report. Contact the facility's insurance

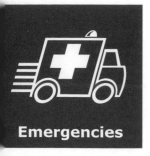
agent, who will probably conduct an independent investigation as well. In the event of media calls, do not disclose any details about the incident, or the names or contact information of the family involved. Direct all official and personal inquiries to the centre director or administrator. Contact parents of other children in the same program to inform them of the death and arrange for early pick-up. Follow provincial/territorial privacy guidelines about the release of personal health information when informing others of the death.

The centre director must speak individually with all staff, try to assess their need for immediate psychological assistance, provide them with a number to call for help, and offer to phone a relative or friend to take them home.

Always ready

Being prepared for emergencies is essential for ensuring the safety of children in your care. Training in first aid and CPR is only a first, though vital, step. Keeping your skills current and practicing drills for emergencies are important too. An early and effective response can spell the difference between a minor crisis and a true emergency, and that difference rests in your capable hands.

Selected resources

Emergency preparedness

Manitoba Child Care Association. 1998. *Crisis Response Manual for Child Care Facilities*. Book, disks. Winnipeg, Man.: MCCA. www.mccahouse.org

National Association of Child Care Resource and Referral Agencies (U.S.). Disaster planning. www.naccrra.org/disaster

National Child Care Information and Technical Assistance Center (U.S.). 2007. Emergency preparedness for child care programs. www.nccic.org

Public Safety Canada. Is your family prepared? www.getprepared.ca

Emergency procedures

American Heart Association. 2006. *Heartsaver CPR Student Workbook*. Book and CD-ROM. www.americanheart.org

Canadian Paediatric Society (Paediatric Emergency Medicine Section). 2007. Paediatric basic and advanced life support guidelines: An update. *Paediatrics & Child Health*, 12(3), July/August), 495–497.

Canadian Red Cross. 2006. Child Care First Aid & CPR Manual. Ottawa, Ont.: Canadian Red Cross. www.redcross.ca

Les publications du Québec. 2002. *Guide to First Aid for Children in an Educational Childcare Setting*. Sainte-Foy, Quebec: Les publications du Québec.

Manitoba Child Care Association. 1998. Crisis Response Manual for Child Care Facilities. Book, disks. Winnipeg, Man.: MCCA. www.mcahouse.org

St. John Ambulance. First Aid for Emergencies: Infants and Children (poster #9900).

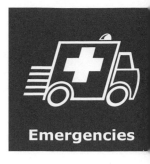

Emergencies

Websites

Allergy/Asthma Information Association. www.aaia.ca

Allergy Safe Communities. www.allergysafecommunities.ca

Anaphylaxis Canada. www.gosafe.ca

Canadian Association of Poison Control Centres. www.capcc.ca

Canadian Lung Association. www.lung.ca

Canadian Medic Alert Foundation. www.medicalert.ca

Canadian Red Cross. www.redcross.ca

Children's Asthma Education Centre. www.asthma-education.com

Children's Hospital of Eastern Ontario. Childhood asthma. www.cheo.on.ca

Heart and Stroke Foundation of Canada. www.heartandstroke.ca

St. John Ambulance. www.sja.ca

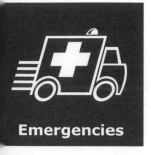

Emergencies

Appendix 11.1: Sample consent form for emergency care and transportation

Name of child: _____

Date: _____

If, at any time, due to such circumstances as an injury or sudden illness, medical treatment is necessary, I authorize the child care staff to take whatever emergency measures they deem necessary for the protection of my child while in their care.

I understand that this may involve contacting a doctor, interpreting and carrying out his or her instructions, and transporting my child to a hospital or doctor's office, including the possible use of an ambulance.

If possible, the hospital will be _____

or the doctor contacted will be (include doctor's name and address) _____

_____ .

I understand that this may be done prior to contacting me, and that any expense incurred for such treatment, including ambulance fees, is my responsibility.

Parent's signature _____

Centre director's or child care operator's signature_____

12

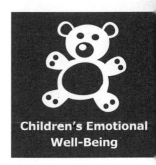

Children's Emotional Well-Being

Children's Emotional Well-Being

Child care practitioners play an essential role in nurturing emotional well-being by developing a warm and caring relationship with each child in their care. They do this by providing caring routines, being supportive of each child's unique personality and temperament, and offering appropriate guidance for behaviour. Learning to meet children's emotional needs requires an understanding of their emotional development. It also takes practice and experience in applying the basic principles of child guidance, a process that encourages children to develop self-confidence, respect for others and an ability to cope with their daily lives.

Understanding emotional development

From infancy, children move through stages of emotional and social development, just as they develop physically and psychologically. The foundation for positive social relationships is a secure relationship with a parent. Babies engage their parents in play; then as toddlers, they learn to play alongside and later **with** other children.

Attachment

Attachment begins as the connection of understanding between an infant and the most significant people in his life—his parents. As parents respond to their baby's first cues of hunger or distress, they signal to their child that he can trust them to meet these needs.

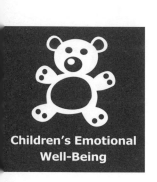

Children's Emotional Well-Being

This first attachment, which is crucial to a child's development, almost always unfolds quite naturally. A mother responds to her crying infant, offering whatever she feels her baby needs—feeding, a diaper change, cuddling. The infant settles, gazes into his mother's eyes, signalling that he has what he needs. As parents become better at reading their infant's non-verbal signals and respond in a predictable and consistent manner, the infant experiences less stress. He learns that his parents are dependable and always there. This positive relationship is called **attachment**. Secure attachment provides strong protection against stress and is critical to a baby's long-term emotional health. Responding quickly to a baby's cries is the best way to offer security and should not be misconstrued as "spoiling." Babies cannot be spoiled.

From an early age, children can develop secure attachments to more than one significant adult without jeopardizing the primary attachment to parents. As a child care practitioner learns to understand a child's needs and responds appropriately, promptly and with emotional warmth, attachment between her and a child grows. In large centres with many children and several staff, it is important for each child to establish a secure attachment with at least one adult. A high staff-to-child ratio makes this easier to achieve.

Personality and temperament

All children have a unique personality that will influence how they respond to events and people in their world. They also have a unique temperament, an inherent style of behaviour that parents will recognize very early on and come to understand and appreciate more fully over time. A child's activity level, mood, distractibility, intensity of response, and tolerance for (or frustration with) change are all part of temperament. For example, some babies are easygoing, while others are more demanding and may have intense reactions. Both the child-rearing environment and how well parents and child care practitioners can accommodate a child's temperament will significantly affect a child's behaviour and emotional development.

It is important to consider personality and temperament when interacting with a child. One easygoing 6-month-old might react positively to being held by someone new, whereas a baby who is slower to adapt may find this situation stressful and become upset. Some babies have very predictable sleep rhythms, while others won't easily adopt a schedule. One toddler might sleep restfully in a bright, noisy room, while another needs a dark, quiet environment. The arrival of a new caregiver might be welcomed enthusiastically by one child, but cause another to become anxious and upset. You can help parents by reinforcing how differences like these are normal variations in temperament.

Separation

Between 6 and 12 months of age, babies become aware of and begin to experiment with separateness from the significant adults in their lives. A baby who has started to crawl might move off a little way for a brief time, only to scoot back quickly. She begins to enjoy a game of "peek-a-boo," which also teaches her that an adult is still there even when she can't be seen.

At about 8 months, babies begin to exhibit separation anxiety, where they can't bear to be away from a parent, usually their mother. They may also show fear in the presence of a stranger. This stage of development slowly resolves as children gain understanding of time and of the fact that their parents will return to them. However, separation may continue to be stressful for some children (and parents) throughout toddlerhood and beyond.

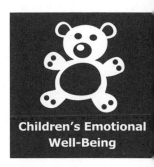

Children's Emotional Well-Being

Autonomy

A sense of autonomy is a component of personality that child care practitioners can foster whenever they encourage babies or toddlers to act independently. Overcoming each new challenge gives a child a sense of success and encourages her to attempt the next developmental step. For example, during tummy time, when a baby reaches for a toy and succeeds in grasping it, she will look for approval. You need to be there to provide encouragement and approval as often as possible. With a good understanding of how each child is developing, child care practitioners can offer experiences that challenge without frustrating. They can be sensitive to situations where a child needs help or encouragement to complete a task independently.

Emotion regulation

Children's ability to identify and appropriately express negative and positive emotions develops gradually as they interact with family members, child care providers and, eventually, peers. Books, TV and video games can also influence how children express their emotions.

Child care practitioners can help guide children to express their feelings in healthy ways. Naming and talking about emotions will help children develop language to describe their feelings. For example, when a toddler cries and resists leaving the park, the caregiver can say: "You're angry that it's time to go home. It's okay to be angry, but we have to go. We'll come back tomorrow." You can also help preschoolers to connect feelings with experiences by encouraging them to talk without imposing your own views: "How do you feel about Tommy taking the truck?"

REMEMBER

You act as a role model when you take responsibility for your own anger or other negative feelings and express them in direct and non-aggressive ways. Telling children that they are too big to cry or that they are making a fuss over "nothing" won't help. Saying "I understand just how you feel. Let's try to work this out together" is a better opening at stressful moments.

Helping children make the emotional transition to child care

Regardless of a child's age, the first time he enters child care is often upsetting for both him and his parents. You can help families make the transition positive by coaching parents and comforting the child.

The child and his parents should visit the child care centre or home setting to familiarize themselves with the surroundings, staff, activities and the other children. It may be helpful to schedule these visits during various points in the daily routine—such as snack time, lunchtime, nap time and so on. If ratios and schedules permit, you might arrange a visit with the parents and child in their own home to become better acquainted. Sharing a photo album of program facilities and activities with a family before enrolment is another way to make the transition easier for both parents and child.

Make the transition gradual

Help families ease into full-time child care by encouraging parents to attend with their child for short periods over the first few days.

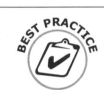

Shortened visits during their first few days in the program give children more time to adjust to being in child care and allow them to learn by experience that parents will return.

- Greet children and parents by name when they arrive. Whenever possible, the same staff member should meet the child on arrival. Welcome each child cheerfully, saying something like: "I'm so glad to see you here today. Your friends are waiting for you at the art table, and they're glad to see you too."
- When parents do leave, encourage them to say goodbye rather than slipping out, even when their child is very young. Suggest that they make their goodbye short and upbeat, and that they link their return to an activity—"I'll be back after your nap"—rather than the time of day, which a young child won't understand.
- Offer a child extra physical reassurance during the first few days. Hold him on your lap, hold hands or offer a hug when his parents leave.
- Talk to children, even the very young, about feelings. You might say: "You're sad that it's time for Mom to go to work. She'll be back to pick you up later. It's okay to be sad."
- Plan an interim activity that children enjoy for the time immediately after parents have left. Go feed the fish together or listen to some music.
- Encourage children to bring a favourite toy or blanket for comfort and a sense of continuity with home. Suggest to parents that they bring in photos of family and pets.
- Help children get used to their new environment by showing them their cubby, the washroom and activity areas. Avoid overloading them with too many rules and routines at once. Allow them to observe the daily routine and take part in activities

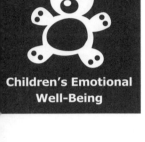

Children's Emotional Well-Being

only when they're ready. Give them some opportunities to explore activity areas on their own and to handle unfamiliar objects and toys.

- Plan group activities that help a new child learn the names of other children. These activities can involve music, stories or cooperative games. Allow the new child to start out as an observer and to join in when he wants.
- Encourage children to borrow a book or toy to take home and bring back the next time to help them understand that they will be returning.
- Talk with parents daily about their child's progress in making the transition and invite them to give you their own observations.
- Consider writing about the child's day in a daily log book for parents. You can highlight how their child is fitting in, his stages of development and his interests.

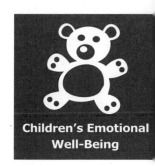

Children's Emotional Well-Being

Encourage attachment

- Assign one child care practitioner to each child.
- Be alert to situations where children are upset because they are frightened, sad or physically hurt. Offer warm physical reassurance.
- If a child asks about her parents, reassure her that they are thinking about her. Provide opportunities to talk about her parents by engaging her in a conversation about what they might be doing.
- Offer lots of hugs and reassuring words so children feel safe and cared for in their new environment.

Creating emotional attachment and security through daily care

The emotional well-being of babies and toddlers depends on having responsive and warm relationships with the adults who care for them. These relationships are enhanced by comforting, consistent and predictable routines. Each interaction between you and a child in your care—feeding, diapering, preparing for nap time, play or socializing—contributes to the strength of the practitioner–child relationship and to the child's emotional well-being. Comfortable, regular routines provide children with the attention, conversation, security and closeness needed for building warm, trusting and stable relationships. Work with parents to set routines for eating and sleeping, adapting them to accommodate children's ongoing development, as well as their routines at home. For example, you may need to schedule nap or feeding times to coordinate with parents' evening schedules.

Baby and toddler feeding

Responding appropriately to hunger cues as a child reaches each new stage of development is a key component of quality child care. While a baby is bottle-feeding, respond emotionally to her need for intimacy and security by holding her close, chatting and looking into her eyes. (See Chapter 3, *Nutrition*, for a full discussion on feeding children in your care.)

Diaper changes and dressing

Diaper changes and dressing offer natural opportunities in a child's routine care for one-on-one interaction through eye contact, smiling, talking, singing and playing games. These games might include playing "peek-a-boo," identifying body parts or learning the names of articles of clothing. These interactions enhance the connection between child and caregiver, build and strengthen mutual trust, and are good opportunities for language development. As children grow, they can participate more actively or independently in each routine. Children who learn to help during diaper changes—by lifting their legs, for example—are more likely to be willing participants.

Toilet learning

When it comes to toilet learning, each child is different. While some are ready to start as early as 18 months, most will start between the ages of 2 and 4 years. Being aware of signs that a child is ready to toilet learn, following his cues so that he doesn't feel rushed, and being patient will ensure a positive learning experience.

Signs of readiness to toilet learn

A child:

- shows an interest in toileting (watches others, likes books about the potty),
- can walk to the potty (or adapted toilet seat),
- is steady and balanced when sitting on the seat,
- can stay dry in diapers for several hours in a row,
- has regular and predictable bowel movements,
- can follow one or two simple instructions ("Time to go pee," "Let's wash our hands"),
- may let you know when he needs to go,
- wants to please, or
- is eager to be more independent.

Never rush a child to toilet learn. It can be frustrating for everyone.

When a child shows signs of readiness, it's time to discuss the toileting routine with parents and decide on words to use when asking their child to use the toilet. Consistency is important. Using common words, such as pee and poo, will help the child be understood. Take a relaxed and patient approach to toilet learning, offering lots of encouragement and praise when children are successful and responding to "accidents" by simply and calmly helping children to change their clothing without criticism. Toileting accidents are common for some children until about the age of 5. A child should never be forced to use the toilet—this can lead to a power struggle and more problems in the future.

Toilet learning is easier when:

- it begins in spring or summer, when children have fewer layers of clothing to remove.
- children are dressed in loose pull-down pants rather than overalls, which are more difficult to take off and put back on again.
- your facility has child-sized toilets or an adult toilet modified for children's use with steps, a footstool or a toilet seat adapter. Children feel more secure and stable when their feet can touch the floor. Toilets are also easier to clean than potty chairs.

Children's Emotional Well-Being

Sleep and napping

The routines of settling a baby or child down for sleep can reinforce feelings of security and comfort. As with feeding, it is important to attend to a child's cues for sleep readiness and respond appropriately. Establish a quiet routine to signal nap time. This can be as simple as a diaper change or a trip to the bathroom, a story or a quiet song, a cuddle and tucking in with a favourite toy or blanket, then dimming the lights.

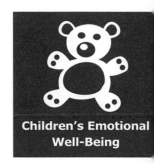

Children's Emotional Well-Being

How much sleep do children need?

Every child is different. Some sleep a lot and others much less. This chart is a general guide to the amount of sleep children need over a 24-hour period, including nighttime sleep and naps.

Newborns (birth to 6 months)	16 hours (3 to 4 hours at a time)
Older babies (6 months to 1 year)	14 hours
Toddlers (1 to 3 years)	10–13 hours
Preschoolers (3 to 5 years)	10–12 hours

A consistent, predictable routine helps a child develop regular sleep habits and makes it easier for him to relax into sleep. However, sleep habits change frequently, so routines will need adjusting too. For an infant under 6 months, follow a soothing bedtime routine and lay him on his back in his crib to sleep. If the baby doesn't settle (and you're sure that he is tired), you might pat him gently to encourage sleep. If he continues to cry, pick him up for a cuddle and help him relax. Ask parents how they handle sleep issues at home and try to adapt your system to be consistent with theirs. It's important to respond quickly to a crying baby. A quick response reinforces feelings of security and trust and will probably lead to less crying later on.

Babies over 6 months are learning to self-soothe, to fall asleep on their own or to get back to sleep when they wake up. Follow the child's sleep cues (eye rubbing, yawning) and put him down for a nap only when he is ready. Get in the habit of laying the child down for a nap while he is still awake but sleepy, so that he drifts off to sleep on his own. Discuss with parents how to respond to crying at nap time. One suggestion is to attend to the child, patting him gently without picking him up, then leave the room and return to pat and soothe for short periods as needed. Always listen to the tone of a child's cry—if it sounds urgent, check right away. A consistent response to crying by both parents and caregivers helps children develop good sleep habits.

Communicating

Long before they say their first words, babies actively communicate with the significant adults in their lives. As early as 6 months, a baby may look at a toy and then at you, to signal that she wants it. Pay close attention to a child's attempts to communicate and respond appropriately. Pick up the toy, pass it to her and talk about it: "Here's your teddy. I think he'd like a hug." By responding with emotional warmth to a child's attempts at communication, by offering appropriate words for this interaction, sometimes adding new words and concepts, you help develop language. This interactive process of responding and amplifying continues as children begin to use words and develop spoken language.

Playing

Playing comes naturally to children—it's how they learn. When children feel emotionally connected to caregivers, they are more open to playing with them. The easy interaction of finger games and tickles, for example, is an early form of play that helps build emotional connection.

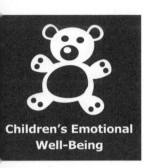

Children's Emotional Well-Being

A child care practitioner supports "play learning" by being available to share in play if children want her to. As children embark on independent play, you can support this by being nearby while they explore, offering help when there is a difficulty, and allowing them to take the lead in directing play. Follow a child's lead by playing face to face, imitating sounds and actions, commenting on what's happening and taking turns.

The relationship that children develop with you during play will deepen their sense of trust and of themselves as separate and distinct persons. By expressing approval or delight in children as they play, you nurture their sense of autonomy, as well as building self-esteem, self-confidence and self-control.

Follow the natural activity patterns of children in your care. For toddlers and preschoolers, play tends to be spontaneous and intermittent, so introducing short activities, staying "in the moment" and allowing children to stop, change or adapt play will add to the fun. Children enjoy play more when you pay attention and sometimes join in.

Helping children with their fears

Fears are a normal part of children's development. They are usually temporary and fade as children mature emotionally.

- Between the ages of 6 and 8 months, babies are interested in new faces but sometimes fear strangers or show anxiety when held by them. Even a familiar person with a new haircut or wearing glasses for the first time may seem frightening. Babies are also afraid of falling and of loud noises.
- Toddlers often fear things that make a loud noise, such as the vacuum cleaner or a flushing toilet. They may also be afraid of the dark while falling asleep. Many toddlers are scared of costumed characters, such as Santa Claus or clowns.
- Preschoolers may continue to exhibit some toddler fears, such as fear of the dark, while overcoming others, such as fear of loud noises. Preschoolers have a rich imagination and are able to ask "What if…?," which may lead to new fears, perhaps of imaginary creatures (e.g., ghosts) or of experiencing something that they've heard in a story or seen on TV.
- Children can also develop fears from their own experience or because an adult has demonstrated a fear. For example, they might be afraid of dogs, spiders or snakes.

How to deal with fears and anxieties

While children often show fear in situations that adults know are harmless, their feelings need to be acknowledged as real. Child care practitioners can help children manage and overcome fear by responding in a calm, empathetic way.

- Acknowledge that a child is afraid and offer your support, but let her know that you don't share her fear.
- Give the child the opportunity to talk about a fear, and listen with understanding. Assure her that you'll stay close while, at the same time, letting her know you're confident that she can handle her fear.
- Teach the child to take slow deep breaths to reduce feelings of stress. Give hugs and hold hands to help her feel more secure.
- Don't overreact to a new fear. Children who play together may sometimes "borrow" one another's fears or mimic a friend's frightened reaction.
- Don't force a child to confront her fear. For example, if a child is afraid of dogs, don't force her to pet one. Let her take her time and encourage her to stay close to you.
- Offer age-appropriate play opportunities to process a fear. Drawing a picture of what she's afraid of can give a child a sense of control over her feelings.
- Encourage role-playing to help children resolve fears. A child might use stuffed animals or toys to act out a situation that makes her fearful.
- Read stories where overcoming fear is a theme.
- Prepare children for experiences that they might find frightening by letting them know what will happen. Sometimes they can work out their response through role-play.
- Keep your own fears in check.

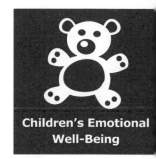

Children's Emotional Well-Being

Helping children learn social skills

By giving lots of feedback about social interactions and by modelling appropriate behaviours, child care practitioners help children make friends and interact with others in positive ways. Here are some specific ways to encourage healthy social interactions:

- Teach children how to approach others in a friendly way. Show them how to say "Hi" when meeting, and how to ask another child to play.
- Model a pleasant demeanour—a smile, a friendly look and voice, eye contact—and encourage children to share their smile with others.
- Show children how to listen by remaining still and looking at the person who is speaking. Demonstrate good listening skills by being attentive when children speak.
- Suggest that a new child approach one particular child or a group of children with whom she's likely to

REMEMBER

You reinforce sharing and other good behaviours by noticing and commenting on them. When children share, help or cooperate, research shows they are more likely to do it again if you acknowledge their actions. Say "It was kind of you to share with Kathy," and "Thank you for waiting your turn." Other children will be more likely to copy good behaviours that are reinforced in this way.

be comfortable. Join the group and encourage everyone to meet and greet. Once children are playing together, withdraw discreetly.

- Encourage children to practice social interaction in pretend play with other children and with dolls.
- Help children share when they are developmentally ready. While toddlers aren't yet ready, by age 5 most children will share toys with encouragement. Ways to help children share include:
  - ➤ having more than one of a popular toy item,
  - ➤ providing "extras" of desirable craft items that children can pass to one another,
  - ➤ playing games that involve taking turns or passing an object,
  - ➤ playing games that encourage sharing special friends (e.g., dancing, changing partners on cue), and
  - ➤ modelling, by offering to share things yourself.

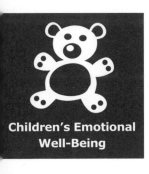

Children's Emotional Well-Being

Encouraging healthy sexual development

Children begin to explore their own bodies, including the genital area, during infancy. They become aware of gender differences between the ages of 2 and 3, when they begin referring to other children as boys or girls. Child care practitioners play an important role in promoting healthy sexual development by responding appropriately to early sexual behaviour, providing developmentally appropriate sexual information, and encouraging and modelling gender equality. Being sensitive to the cultural norms around sexuality for the families of children in your care is important too.

- Respond to children's sexual behaviour calmly. Expect children to be curious and want to explore each other's bodies in the preschool years. Treat this behaviour casually. If children engage in more overt sexual play, stop it in a neutral manner, being careful not to make them feel shame. Ignore the occasional use of inappropriate words and correct children gently only if they persist.
- Ignore masturbation in babies and young toddlers. Once a child is age 2 or 3, teach him that masturbation is acceptable only in a private place like his bedroom at home.
- Listen carefully to questions about sexuality. Ask the child what he thinks, before offering an answer. Offer sexual information in a matter-of-fact way. Use the proper names for genitals, rather than nicknames. Answer questions with simple, accurate explanations. A child will likely ask more questions if he is not satisfied with the answer or needs more information. Reading an age-appropriate book together may help children to understand sexual development.
- Encourage gender equality by treating boys and girls in the same way. Don't discourage natural curiosity about gender differences.
- Monitor children's toys and books and eliminate any that suggest or encourage overt sexual stereotyping. Use gender-inclusive language.
- Encourage boys and girls to engage in all types of play. Ensure that children don't exclude others from play because of gender.

The philosophy of child guidance

Child guidance is positive discipline that teaches children appropriate behaviour, as opposed to punishing them for inappropriate behaviour. This approach to discipline respects the dignity of children as developing human beings and sees them as capable—with help—of problem-solving and self-control.

Accept children as autonomous individuals, regardless of how they behave, and guide them as they learn about self-control and problem-solving. Respecting children's personal identity, feelings and developmental stage involves showing that you:

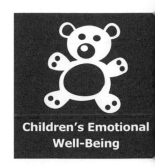

Children's Emotional Well-Being

- value every child's family,
- care about a child's feelings and thoughts,
- encourage ideas and contributions from children,
- are honest with children,
- listen actively to what a child is communicating, and
- understand a child's stage of development and gauge your own expectations for behaviour appropriately.

Understanding the influence of environment on behaviour

Children's environment, and the responses of adults around them, have a significant impact on behaviour. By adjusting this environment, you can help children change their behaviour. Aspects of the environment that affect a child's behaviour include:

- *Physical space.* Spaces that are calm, comfortable and organized promote positive behaviour. Whenever possible, create separate activity areas for quiet times, active movement and messy activities.
- *Materials.* Choose age-appropriate materials and circulate toys to create a stimulating environment for play. Label materials and their coordinating storage units to ease clean-up routines and to prevent materials from getting mixed up.
- *Schedule.* A daily schedule that unfolds in a series of familiar, comforting routines, allowing for structured and unstructured play as well as quiet and active play, promotes positive behaviour. The schedule should provide you with enough time to simply enjoy the company of children in your care.
- *Group size.* A high staff-to-child ratio helps ensure optimal participation and learning. When a group gets too large, there is too much activity and noise, and not enough personal or one-on-one interaction. (See staff-to-child ratios, pages 4–5.)
- *Peer behaviour.* How children treat each other affects their behaviour. Be alert to teasing and bullying.
- *TV and other media.* Minimize or eliminate TV viewing in your program and discourage access to computer games. While high quality children's programming may promote positive social behaviour, violent programming and games are known to increase children's feelings of insecurity, dull their ability to empathize and increase aggressive behaviour. **Encourage parents to limit and monitor their child's "screen time."**

Assessing and modifying behaviour

To help children change unacceptable behaviour, you first need to understand why it is happening. Observe carefully, noting factors that might trigger or explain the negative behaviour. Ask other staff members and a child's parents for their observations and opinions about what events ("antecedents") preceded the behaviour. Keeping a simple log of antecedents, behaviours and consequences ("the ABCs") can help you identify patterns and make links between what is happening in the child's world and behaviour.

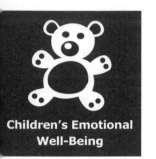

TABLE 12.1

Sample log entry, with prompts

Date/time	Antecedents *What's going on? Where? Who is present? Any other environmental notes?*	Behaviours *What did the child do? How many times? For how long? To whom?*	Consequences *What happened as a result? What did others/caregivers do? How many times/for how long? How did the child respond? If a command was given at the start, did the child comply?*	Review *In retrospect, what went wrong? If behaviour is repeated, what would I do differently?*
Monday 8 a.m.	Sally in high chair. I (child care provider) was feeding her oatmeal. She'd had most of the bowl and half her milk.	Sally threw her bowl on the floor and laughed.	I told her "No" firmly, and she cried until I cuddled her.	My strategy may have backfired when Sally got a lot of attention for her behaviour. An alternative approach, such as ignoring the event and simply removing Sally from the high chair, might be considered next time.
Right after		She threw the spoon and cup at my head.		

Source: Robert E. O'Neill et al., *Functional assessment and program development for problem behaviour.* Adapted with permission.

Once you've identified a pattern, work with parents to make a plan to modify their child's behaviour. Together you may decide that a child who is having more frequent tantrums isn't getting enough sleep and try for an earlier bedtime. A child who is whining more than usual may need more one-on-one attention with her child care practitioner.

Implement a plan and continue to record the child's behaviour, watching for signs of improvement. If there is no change, revisit the plan and ensure that everyone is taking the same steps and following through with consequences. If there is a persistent inappropriate behaviour that puts a child at risk of hurting herself or other children, you can ask parents to consult a doctor for additional guidance or a psychological referral.

Practicing preventive guidance techniques

Offer praise and show affection

Offer praise and show affection to children on an ongoing basis, not just when they are seeking attention. Guard against interacting with a child only when it's necessary to alter behaviour. Make sure most of your interactions with any child are positive ones.

When children demonstrate self-control, provide positive reinforcement. Verbally praise a child by using an "I" message to recognize the specific behaviour: for example, "I like the way you helped Curtis clean up the blocks." Use positive reinforcement to recognize effort, not just results or accomplishments.

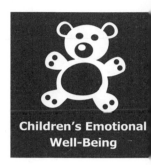

Children's Emotional Well-Being

If a child often demonstrates attention-seeking behaviour, provide attention more often when she behaves appropriately. A child who is cuddled, spoken to and made to feel important throughout the day will be less likely to demand attention by disrupting other activities.

Know what to ignore

Ignore annoying but harmless behaviours such as whining. Actively discouraging these behaviours tends to draw attention to them, reinforcing them as "attention-getters," and often increases their frequency. While ignoring these behaviours takes time (and patience), it's worth pursuing. A child will be surprised when an adult ignores a behaviour that used to win attention and, initially at least, the inappropriate behaviour may even increase. However, if you consistently ignore the behaviour, it may eventually subside.

Plan transitions

Moving from one activity to another or stopping an enjoyable activity to initiate a less enjoyable one, such as tidying up or breaking for a diaper change, can be frustrating or confusing for children. These are times when they are more likely to display inappropriate behaviour. Minimize the possibility of outbursts by developing a routine for transitions that helps children recognize and deal with what is coming next. The routine should involve giving children regular notice of any new activity. Keep both the notice and its timing age-appropriate. For example, give a toddler a few minutes' warning, saying: "Time to change your diaper soon." Give older children regular 15-minute, 5-minute and 1-minute warnings of a change in activity. Offer regular reminders of an upcoming activity. For example, in the morning, let children know about an outing after lunch. Help children understand time by using a visual clock. Set the clock to show that there are 15 minutes left until clean-up time, then 5 minutes, then 1 minute.

Make transition times pleasant with songs or games that encourage children to move easily from one activity to the next. Whenever possible, prepare the next activity ahead of time to avoid having children wait.

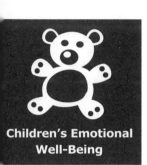

Offer choices

Providing limited and realistic choices encourages children to think independently. For example, you might ask a child whether he would like banana or strawberry yogurt, or whether he prefers to wear his blue or green socks.

Accept mistakes

All children make mistakes and need every opportunity to learn from them. When a child makes a mistake, be neutral and give her some time to find her own solution. When a natural and age-appropriate solution presents itself, such as wiping up a spill, help the child do it. Younger children who are unable to come up with their own solutions may need you to suggest a few options.

Use "I" messages

"I" messages are personal statements about how undesirable behaviour affects the child care practitioner. "I" messages help the child see the effects of behaviour, such as: "When you throw sand, I'm afraid it will go in my eyes." Choose "I" messages that are appropriate for the child's level of understanding.

Act as a role model

Children learn through imitation. When dealing with co-workers and children, demonstrate the qualities you hope to encourage—respect, generosity, cooperation, kindness and helpfulness.

Set limits

Let children know your expectations and rules for acceptable behaviour. Knowing these limits in advance helps children develop self-control. An appropriate limit is one that a child can understand and follow most of the time. The most necessary limits are those that prevent children from hurting themselves or others, or from damaging property. Remind children regularly about rules and limits. They may forget, particularly when they are busy, excited or concentrating on another activity. As a child develops, rules and limits will need to be reviewed and revised.

A good limit:

- is developmentally appropriate,
- helps a child achieve self-control,
- protects children's health and safety,
- is explained using simple language,
- is enforced firmly, respectfully and kindly.

Guidance interventions

When children do act out, using intervention techniques can help them return to appropriate behaviour.

Redirect

Redirection—when inappropriate behaviour is diverted to an appropriate activity—is the most developmentally appropriate and effective guidance technique for toddlers. It is also a helpful strategy for older children. A toddler climbing on a table can be redirected to a climbing apparatus instead. The redirection should be accompanied by words that teach the child what it is you want her to do rather than what you don't want her to do: "The climber is the best place for you to climb. Let's see you go up."

Encourage problem-solving

Invite children to help find a solution to their inappropriate behaviour. Children who are involved in solving a problem are more likely to implement the solution. For example, if two children are arguing over a toy, invite them to discuss the fairest way to take turns. When children are encouraged to offer solutions, it develops a sense of responsibility for their own actions as well as for the needs of others. Use a specific and consistent problem-solving approach with clear and easy steps that caregivers **and** children can understand and apply.

Use logical consequences

When a child behaves inappropriately and redirection is unsuccessful, apply clear consequences for the action. For example, a child who is drawing on a wall should be directed to use paper, while you explain that you want him to draw on that instead. If he draws on the wall again, repeat the explanation and take away the crayons as a consequence. When an obvious consequence doesn't present itself, apply a "response cost," where the inappropriate behaviour costs the child the loss of a privilege. For young children this "cost" must be immediate. For example, a child who is playing too roughly can be made to play separately from other children for a short time.

Give time-outs

During a time-out, a child is physically separated from the child care practitioner and the other children. A time-out should take place in a safe, quiet corner or chair, away from others and without distractions. Briefly explain the reason for the time-out—"No hitting"—and send the child to the designated spot. If he refuses, take him by the hand or carry him. During the time-out, ignore the child, even if he shouts or apologizes. When the time-out is over, clear the air by offering a new activity. Don't lecture the child about the behaviour. Time-outs should last 1 minute for every year of the child's age, to a maximum of 5 minutes. Never suggest or make a child feel as if a time-out means that you love or care for him any less.

Restrain and hold

When a child becomes so upset and out of control that she's at risk of hurting herself or others and all other discipline strategies have proved unsuccessful, a child care practitioner should hold the child, using just enough strength to restrain her. This must be done carefully, both to avoid hurting the child and to prevent the child from hurting herself. Once the child settles down, apply a time-out or logical consequence.

At no time should a child be spanked, shaken, or subjected to any form of physical punishment or verbal abuse while in your care.

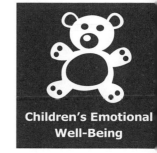

Children's Emotional Well-Being

Handling typical discipline issues

Tantrums

Tantrums are a normal part of child development. These outbursts are caused by intense negative emotions that the child hasn't yet the ability or self-control to express in other ways. You can prevent some tantrums by:

- paying attention to good behaviour,
- reducing obvious triggers, such as allowing a child to become hungry or overtired,
- inviting the child to express himself in another way: "How do you feel?" or "I can see that you're angry. How can I help?"

Tantrums can often be avoided or shortened by intervening before a child loses complete control. Speak in a calm voice, acknowledge the child's frustration and help him work out his problem appropriately.

When a tantrum does occur, ignore the behaviour so that a child is not rewarded for his outburst by your attention. Observe him discreetly from a distance to ensure he stays safe. If a child is thrashing about, ensure his immediate environment is safe by moving furniture, toys or other children out of the way. Refusing to pay attention until the tantrum stops can be difficult, but it will help the child regain control. Once the tantrum is over, offer a drink of water or a face wash and redirect him to a new activity. If the tantrum occurred because he didn't want to comply with a direction, try to regain the child's compliance by gently repeating what you're asking him to do.

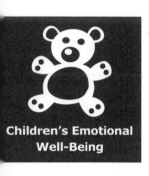

Children's Emotional Well-Being

When a child is out of control

When nothing works and a child loses control, give her space to collect herself.

- Stand between her and the rest of the world—but at a safe distance. Don't try to move her unless she is in danger of hurting herself or others.
- Don't confront her. To keep her from feeling trapped, stand sideways, compose your face and don't look her in the eye.
- Don't speak. She isn't ready to listen yet.
- When she's calmer, speak with her quietly. Help her to name her feelings ("You were pretty angry") and to distinguish between feelings and actions ("It's okay to feel angry, but it's not okay to throw chairs"). Let her know that you love her, and help her to think about how she can solve the problem next time.

Source: Canadian Child Care Federation, "Tips for parenting children with challenging behaviour." Adapted with permission.

Interrupting, name-calling, shouting

When a child interrupts, tell her: "It's your turn to listen now and my turn to talk. Later we can trade." Tell a child who is name-calling: "She likes to be called by her name, which is Mary." Tell a child who is shouting: "Please use your quiet voice. It helps me listen better" or "Loud voices are for outside; quiet voices are for inside."

Unacceptable language

Ignore the occasional unacceptable word. If swearing persists, tell the child that the use of such words is not allowed and offer some alternatives. Apply a time-out or the loss of a privilege if swearing continues.

Storytelling and lying

As a child's imagination develops, making up stories is entirely normal and healthy. Don't discipline a child or make him feel guilty for telling stories, but do let him know the difference between his version of events and reality. You might say: "Cars can't really fly. But it would be very cool if they could." When a child makes up a story to avoid taking responsibility for a mistake, explain the reality, encourage him to tell the truth and offer an opportunity to make amends: "I think you spilled the juice, not the dog. It's always best to tell the truth. Let's get a cloth and you can clean it up."

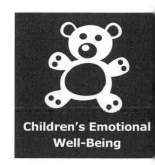

Children's Emotional Well-Being

Destructiveness

When a child is damaging an object, first redirect her or show her how to use the object properly. For example, show how to turn pages of a book gently, without tearing them. If the destructive behaviour persists, take away the object or remove the child from the area. Reinforce the importance of respecting property.

Rough play

In acting out fantasies or pretending to be "superheroes," children can play roughly with each other. Allow the play, while carefully monitoring behaviour to ensure no one is getting hurt. Set limits so that children know what is expected of them when they are playing. You might say: "When you play Batman, capture the bad guys by tagging them. Don't pull on anyone."

Aggression

Aggression is a behaviour that injures a person or object, and in children it usually takes one of two forms. A child might use physical aggression such as hitting and kicking to get back an object that has been taken away, such as a toy. This is more common in very young children. Sometimes you can prevent this form of aggressive behaviour by having more than one of the favourite toys on hand. Older children may show more intentional physical aggression, where they hurt another child to get even or to express anger. Hostile aggression can also be psychological, such as not playing with a certain child, telling others not to play with her, or teasing. These behaviours are forms of bullying that should not be ignored.

When aggression occurs, deal with it immediately. If necessary, interrupt physical fighting and separate the children. If a child is hurt, comfort him first. Ignore the aggressor (if it's clear who that was). Only once a child is consoled should you give your attention to the aggressor. Firmly restate the rules: "No hitting" or "No scratching." Show clear disapproval with a face-to-face conversation with the child at eye level. It is important to acknowledge the feelings that led to a child's aggression: "I know you are mad at Susie because she took your book, but I won't let you hit her. Let's see how you can ask her to give it back." Finally, if this doesn't work, impose a consequence, such as a time-out or the loss of a privilege.

Aggressive behaviour can be minimized by providing lots of opportunities for physical play to help release pent-up energy and diffuse stressful encounters, while setting clear and consistent limits on behaviour ("No hitting allowed"). Encourage children to share, take turns and express their feelings.

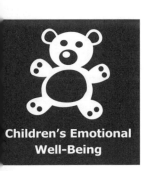

Children's Emotional Well-Being

Connecting with parents

When child care practitioners and parents work together to meet the needs of children, their positive relationship contributes to the emotional well-being of all concerned. You can, in practice, provide emotional support to a whole family. This can range from having a friendly and supportive conversation when parents drop off and pick up their children, to helping connect a family with a community agency. Children sense the cooperation between parents and caregivers and feel more secure as a result.

Actively respect the ethnic and linguistic backgrounds, cultural values and traditions of families connected with your program. You can foster cultural understanding among families in the child care community in small ways: by adding ethnic foods to the menu, inviting parents and children to tell their stories, or celebrating their holidays.

In all dealings with families, a high standard of confidentiality is essential for building trust. Every program should have a written confidentiality policy that outlines when and how any information about children or families may be disclosed to a third party and stipulates the need for parental consent. If a parent's first language is not spoken by any of the child care staff, it may be necessary to have an interpreter present at the time of enrolment to explain when parents can give or withhold their consent in a child care setting. All staff, including those who do not work directly with children, need to understand and follow the facility's confidentiality policy.

The heart of caregiving

Child care practitioners play an essential role in the emotional lives of children in their care by developing nurturing and loving relationships with them, responding to them individually in age-appropriate ways and offering guidance for behaviour. Day-to-day interactions are opportunities to model and enhance language and social skills while building each child's sense of security and self-esteem. Encouraging children to be inquisitive about their environment, and expressive and caring in their interactions with others, is at the heart of caregiving.

Selected resources

The Canadian Paediatric Society's website for parents and caregivers, Caring for Kids, has information on topics described in this chapter. Parent notes can be downloaded at www.caringforkids.cps.ca, reproduced, and shared with families. The following brochures are also available:

————. 2008. Colic and crying.

————. 2008. Guiding your child with positive discipline.

————. 2008. Healthy sleep for your baby and child.

————. 2008. Toilet learning.

————. 2008. When your child misbehaves: Tips for positive discipline.

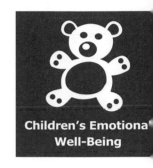

Children's Emotional Well-Being

General

Canadian Child Care Federation. 2008. *Supporting our children's social well-being: It's a team effort*. Ottawa, Ont.: CCCF. Online resource kit includes articles, resource sheets and workshops on building practitioner–family partnerships in support of children's social well-being. Covers specific topics such as behaviour guidance, communication, self-esteem, resiliency and cultural identity. www.cccf fcsge.ca

————, Canadian Institute of Child Health. 2001. *Nourish, nurture, neurodevelopment: Neurodevelopmental research; Implications for excellent caregiver practices*. Learning kit. Ottawa, Ont.: CCCF/CICH. www.cccf-fcsge.ca

Canadian Mental Health Association and Hincks-Dellcrest Treatment Centre. 2004. *Handle with Care: Strategies for promoting the mental health of young children in community-based child care*. Booklet. Ottawa, Ont.: CMHA. www.cmha.ca

Centre of Excellence in Early Childhood Development. Includes bulletins and online encyclopedia on several topics related to the social and emotional development of young children, including attachment and aggression. www.excellence-earlychildhood.ca

Centre of Knowledge on Healthy Child Development, Offord Centre for Child Studies. www.knowledge.offordcentre.com

Fearn, Terrellyn. 2006. *A sense of belonging: Supporting healthy child development in Aboriginal families*. Toronto, Ont.: Best Start Resource Centre. Produced in collaboration with Spirit Moon Consulting, Waabinong Head Start, Ontario Federation of Indian Friendship Centres, Ontario Native Women's Association, Pauktuutit Inuit Women of Canada, Ontario Native Women's Association, Union of Ontario Indians, Métis Nation of Ontario and Nishnawbe-Aski Nation. www.beststart.org

George Brown College, Centre for Early Childhood Development and Hincks-Dellcrest Institute. *Ideas: Emotional well-being in child care*. Published in the spring and fall issues (various years) of *Interaction* magazine. Past issues available at www.cccf-fcsge.ca

Invest in Kids. Comfort, Play and Teach: A Positive Approach to Parenting. Tip sheets for parents on topics such as challenging behaviour and self-esteem. www.investinkids.ca

Jewish Family Services of the Baron de Hirsch Institute. 2004. *Family front and centre: A support resource promoting healthy child development*. Five booklets addressing attachment, attention, anxiety, aggression and self-esteem. www.familyfrontandcentre.com

Region of Peel (Ont.) Public Health. Great beginnings: Build your child's brain, build your child's future. 2006. Learning kit. www.peelregion.ca

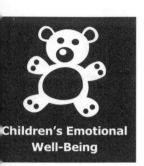

Children's Emotional Well-Being

Attachment and separation

Canadian Child Care Federation. 2001. Coping with separation anxiety. Resource sheet #41. www.cccf-fcsge.ca

Goldberg, Susan. 2004-2005. Attachment. Feature series (6 parts). www.aboutkidshealth.ca

Hospital for Sick Children, Infant Mental Health Promotion. A simple gift. Videos or DVDs, with guides for parents/caregivers or professionals. Toronto, Ont.: Hospital for Sick Children.www.sickkids.ca/imp

———. 1998. Comforting your baby.

———. 2001. Helping young children cope with emotions.

———. 2005. Ending the cycle of hurt.

Manitoba Child Care Association. 1997. Let babies be babies: Caring for infants and toddlers with love and respect. Set of 6 DVDs. Winnipeg, Man.: MCCA.

Nichols, Alison. 2001. Right from the start: An attachment-based course for parents of infants under 2 years; Leader manual. Infant-Parent Program, Hamilton Health Sciences and McMaster University, Hamilton. www.communityed.ca

Public Health Agency of Canada. 2003. First connections... make all the difference: Resource kit on infant attachment. www.phac-aspc.gc.ca

St. Joseph's Women's Health Centre. 2004. Attachment across cultures. Toolkit and website. www.attachmentacrosscultures.org

Behaviour and behaviour management

Canadian Child Care Federation. www.cccf-fcsge.ca

———. 2000. Tips for parenting children with challenging behaviour. Resource sheet #48.

———. 2001. Fear and loathing: A guide to bullying behaviour. Resource sheet #56.

———. 2001. Resolving conflicts, promoting peace. Resource sheet #51.

Child Development Resource Connection, Peel. *Setting the stage for successful behaviour: The teamwork approach to challenging behaviour*. Manual and video. Also available in French, Punjabi, Cantonese, Polish and Spanish. www.cdrcp.com

Faber, Adele and Elaine Mazlish. 2nd ed., 1999. *How to Talk So Kids Will Listen and Listen So Kids Will Talk*. New York, NY: Avon Books.

Gordon, Mary. 2006. Roots of Empathy: Changing the world child by child. Toronto, Ont.: Thomas Allen and Son. See also a program designed for early childhood settings entitled Seeds of Empathy, at www.seedsofempathy.org

Kaiser, Barbara and Judy Sklar Rasminsky. 1999. *Meeting the Challenge: Effective Strategies for Challenging Behaviours in Early Childhood Environments*. Ottawa, Ont.: Canadian Child Care Federation. www.cccf-fcsge.ca

———, *Meeting the challenge: An Aboriginal perspective* (CD-ROM), and *Meeting the challenge online* (an e-learning program).

Kurcinka, Mary Sheedy. 2nd ed., 2006. *Raising Your Spirited Child: A Guide for Parents Whose Child is More Intense, Sensitive, Perceptive, Persistent, Energetic*. New York, NY: HarperCollins.

Phelan, Thomas. 3rd ed., 2004. *1-2-3 Magic: Effective Discipline for Children 2–12*. Glen Ellyn, IL: ParentMagic.

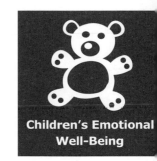

Children's Emotional Well-Being

Connecting with parents

Kaiser, Barbara and Judy Sklar Rasminsky. 1999. *Partners in Quality: Relationships*. Ottawa, Ont.: Canadian Child Care Federation. www.cccf-fcsge.ca

Wilson, Lynn. 2005. *Partnerships: Families and Communities in Canadian Early Education*. Toronto, Ont.: George Brown College.

Self-esteem

Canadian Child Care Federation. 1989. 98 ways to say "very good." Resource sheet #5. www.cccf-fcsge.ca

Pearson, Jennifer and Darlene Kordich Hall. 2006. *Reaching IN… Reaching OUT Resiliency Guidebook: "Bounce back" Thinking Skills for Children and Adults*. www.reachinginreachingout.ca

Sexual development

Region of Peel (Ont.) Public Health. 2004. *Keep on track: A health and resource guide for child care providers in Peel*. Section 9: Health and safety, mind and body, pages 9-6 to 9-10. www.region.peel.on.ca/health/keep-on-track/pdfs/entiremanual.pdf

Society of Obstetricians and Gynaecologists of Canada. Sexuality and child development. www.sexualityandu.ca

International organizations

National Center for Clinical Infant Programs (U.S.). Zero to Three. www.zerotothree.org

Parenting and Family Support Centre (University of Queensland, Australia). Triple P: Positive Parenting Program. www.pfsc.uq.edu.au

Raising Children Network (the Australian parenting website). www.raisingchildren.net.au

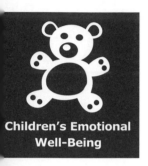

Children's Emotional Well-Being

chapter

13

Including Children with Special Needs

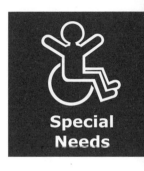

Special Needs

I ncluding children with special needs is an increasingly important aspect of quality early learning and child care. Promoting inclusion may require additional training, resource allocation and adjustments to programming, but it is well worth the effort and acknowledges that children with special needs have a right to quality child care. Including children with special needs provides them with opportunities to build independence and participate in the wider community. Inclusion also benefits other "typically developing" children (that is, those without special needs) within the child care facility by making them more aware, sensitive and compassionate. Many programs now have policies and strategies in place for including children with special needs.

What are special needs?

Children with special needs have disabilities, delays or disorders in their physical, social, intellectual, communicative, emotional and/or behavioural development. About 10 per cent of children have special needs that require some kind of additional support and/or consultation and staff training to ensure that they can fully participate in community-based child care programs. Special (also called exceptional) health care means care beyond that typically provided by child care practitioners, and for which they will require additional information, training and support.

A system known as the International Classification of Functioning, Disability and Health (ICF), developed by the World Health Organization, is providing a new context for thought and practice in the field of childhood disability. This system encourages an approach to care that puts more emphasis on children's function ("activity") and social engagement ("participation") than on their impairment.

Children may enter a child care program having one clearly defined diagnosis with identified needs (e.g., children with cerebral palsy or Down syndrome are usually diagnosed early), or their needs may emerge only after enrolment, as with language delay. In either scenario, the observations and involvement of child care staff can help clarify a child's needs, establish appropriate supports and monitor progress.

Children with and without special needs usually come together in a child care facility in one of two ways: a community-based child care facility may broaden its services to include children with special needs; or a program designed specifically for children with special needs may broaden its services to include children without special needs. The latter is sometimes called reverse integration rather than inclusion. Although both types of facility exist in Canada, inclusive community-based programs are more prevalent.

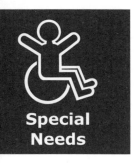

Special Needs

Creating an inclusive child care facility

Making inclusion work involves a few essential steps. Creating an inclusive child care facility begins with building trusting relationships among parents, staff and community support personnel, all of whom need time and opportunities to share their views, concerns and requirements. This sharing promotes a culture of inclusion, which is crucial to success.

Inclusion may be as specific as accommodating one child who uses crutches in a home setting, or as broad as reconfiguring a centre designed specifically for children who are hearing impaired to include other children. How inclusion is accomplished depends on the type of need as well as the intensity of the condition. For example, children with cerebral palsy vary widely in their abilities. In all cases, achieving inclusion for an individual child requires four basic steps:

1.   A needs assessment
2.   An inventory of the child's skills, abilities and supports
3.   An inclusion support plan
4.   Ongoing training, support and additional staffing, as needed

At the end of this chapter, you'll find selected resources to help you assess your program's readiness for inclusion and develop inclusion support and individual care plans.

1. Needs assessment

In collaboration with a child's parents, treating physician and community support personnel—the individuals who make up the child's existing "circle of care"—you should identify what the child needs from your program to reach certain personal developmental goals. This assessment will include physical, cognitive, emotional and social dimensions and will highlight the areas where additional supports may be necessary. You'll also be taking stock of potential environmental or equipment needs that can optimize the child's active participation in the program.

2. Inventory of skills, abilities and supports

Taking this inventory determines what resources are already available, within both the facility and the community, to meet a child's special needs. For example, a centre may be designed (or retrofitted) with ramps and wider doorways to accommodate wheelchairs, or a staff member may have experience feeding children who have difficulty swallowing. A local agency may offer individualized support for children with autism spectrum disorders within the child care setting.

The types and levels of staff support will depend on both the needs of the child and the centre's experience and training. **Types** of staff support include consultative support only, part-time extra staffing or full-time extra staffing. **Levels** of staff support indicate the duration of external support—frequency of consultative visits and the time periods for which extra staff will be provided. An experienced staff may require less support than a group with more limited experience.

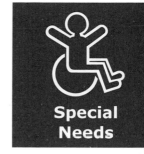

Special Needs

3. Inclusion support plan

An individualized inclusion support plan (which, depending on location in Canada, is variously known as an Individual Program Plan [IPP], an Individual Family Service Plan [IFSP], an Individual Education Plan [IEP] or a Routine-based Plan [RBP]) must be developed for all children with special needs. This plan should be:

- created for the individual child,
- used for planning and programming, and
- regularly monitored for usefulness and updated when required.

Some plans will be more detailed than others, depending upon the child's needs and the centre's capacities. Each one should be updated annually or every 6 months, as required.

Many children with special health care needs do not require additional developmental supports. When they do, their inclusion support plan identifies specific developmental, functional or social goals to work toward in the child care program. These might include:

- building relationships and interpersonal skills,
- improving communication,
- developing gross (large) and fine motor skills,
- helping with self-care, and
- learning (e.g., activities, sense of self, life skills). See Appendices 13.2–13.3, pages 350–51, for forms to help with routine-based planning.

The inclusion support plan identifies how a child's health and/or non-medical needs are to be met and stipulates what additional supports must be provided. The types and levels of training needed by staff who enrol this child depend on four main factors:

- The child's health and/or non-medical issues and their intensity,
- The staff's experience in working with children with special needs,
- The overall quality of the centre, and
- The inclusion capacity of the centre.

Consultation with a health care provider or an expert in behaviour management might be a first step in your inclusion support plan. Many preschoolers with special needs are involved in stimulation/early intervention programs that help children fulfill their potential and meet specific developmental goals. These programs provide both functional support (e.g., communication, social, academic, behavioural and daily living skills) and a team of professionals who may design an individualized program to be implemented at home and in child care.

The inclusion support plan should also specify which resources are available to achieve necessary supports (e.g., which government, community or other funding resources will help cover additional costs). The centre should budget for additional costs associated with the inclusion of a child with special needs, such as staffing issues, insurance, equipment and supplies, and facility modifications. Most provinces and territories provide some support to centres that include children with special needs, in the form of funding, consultation, training, and equipment and/or accommodation grants.

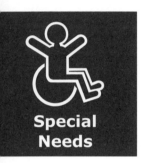

Special Needs

4. Ongoing training, support and additional staffing, as needed

Staff in centres that enrol children with special needs require training in specific strategies for dealing with conditions and needs, as well as training related to inclusion strategies in general. Many agencies and provinces offer this type of in-service training. As well, an increasing number of early childhood education students are graduating with higher levels of experience and confidence in working with children with special needs.

REMEMBER

An important measure of the overall quality of any program is its capacity to make modifications and adjustments to ensure the success of every child. What often matters most is how open the staff are to making changes and learning how to accommodate children with special needs.

Training for child care staff should include four stages:

1. Orientation
2. Condition-specific background training
3. Child-specific skill development
4. Skill maintenance

While the need for appropriate training is clear, arranging it is not always straightforward and may be difficult in some communities. Staff training is generally a collaborative effort, involving families, health professionals, consultants and child care staff.

Appropriate assessment, training, evaluation, monitoring and skill maintenance training by health professionals are essential prerequisites for enrolling a child with special health care or other needs.

Developing an individual health care plan for each child with special needs

While about 10 per cent of children have some kind of special need, only about 1 per cent require special health care. In addition to the inclusion support plan, an individual health care plan must be developed before these children enter a program. Often drafted by a nurse, a treating physician or a centre director in collaboration with parents, other child care staff and professionals involved in a child's circle of care, this plan is developed to address health needs specifically. It contains information about the child's medical history, current status, and the kind of care she will need while attending the program. These "how-tos" of specialized health care often include:

Completing a child's circle of care might pose challenges, but child care staff need to know precisely what tasks they are responsible for and how to perform special health care procedures when required.

- medication to be given, with dosage, schedule and possible side effects,
- medical equipment or supplies that are needed on site,
- dietary needs or restrictions,
- warning signs and symptoms to watch for, and
- emergency procedures and actions that may be needed.

The individual health care plan also details the specific adaptations to space or programming needed to accommodate a particular child, any activity restrictions or precautions, and the roles and responsibilities of staff in daily programming.

The individual health care plan is a legal document that must be approved and signed before enrolment by the health care provider, the child's parents and the program director. It stipulates a schedule for review, risks inherent in the child's attendance, and parents' acknowledgement of these risks along with their consent to the implementation of the individual care plan. (For more about health care plans and sample condition-specific forms, see Chapter 10, *Chronic Medical Conditions*.)

Implementing an appropriate individual care plan for a child with more complex needs might mean coordinating with one or more community rehabilitation centres. Child care providers often participate in yearly reviews and in helping the child achieve specific developmental or functional goals set out in these plans. Additional support staff, extra training and a reduced child-to-staff ratio may also be required to respond effectively to the child's special needs. Finally, it is important to have special health care services (e.g., nursing) in place before the child is enrolled to avoid last-minute scrambles, which can be stressful for parents and staff and disruptive for programming.

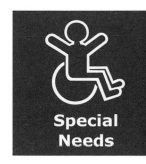

Special Needs

Supporting parents of children with special needs

The parents of a child with special needs may face everyday challenges that are not experienced by parents of other children. They often provide more physical care to their child for longer periods, and are more likely to encounter medical emergencies. They may be providing specialized care from home, or dealing with exceptional behavioural issues, sleep disorders or more frequent illnesses. While all parents advocate for their children within the medical and educational systems, parents of children with special needs often act as "case manager" and service seeker as well. Raising a child with special needs requires a degree of energy and focus that can strain relationships between spouses and among family members. Parents may find it difficult or impossible to juggle paid work and family responsibilities. Their family income and professional/vocational identity may suffer because of these additional challenges.

Whenever possible, plan meetings and appointments with parents of children with special needs at times convenient for them, and be flexible about scheduling. Encourage them to bring along a trusted relative and/or advisor. Parents may wish to act as care coordinators for their child, making sure services such as speech or language therapy, physiotherapy and medical care are in place. **Be supportive of whatever choices parents make to coordinate services for their child.**

For all children, "family-centred" care means that parents are primarily responsible for determining their child's developmental goals, while care providers collaborate and communicate openly with them. Starting child care may be the first time that a child with special needs hasn't been in the care of a parent or primary caregiver since birth, making this transition an anxious time for parents. Contact with child care staff can help alleviate their anxiety. The child care experience provides all parents with new insight into their child's personality and abilities.

Supporting other children and their parents

Open communication with all families involved in your child care program is an important aspect of inclusion. Administrative issues, such as how to notify and prepare parents of other children for integration, should be handled well before inclusion becomes policy. Revising parent orientation information, including children with special needs in program photos and holding public tours of a new or retrofitted facility are examples of how to make the space feel truly inclusive.

All staff, children and their parents should be aware that certain expectations and rules may apply to some children and not others, depending on their needs. For example, a child

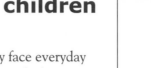

You provide vital "life support" to the parents of children with special needs by collaborating closely with them about all aspects of their child's care, being sensitive to their feelings and acknowledging the special issues and extra workload they must deal with every day. Just speaking with you about their child's development and behaviour provides information, reassurance and a sense of shared experience that can be especially empowering for these families.

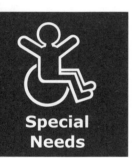

Special Needs

with a disability might require help with dressing or eating, while others are expected to do these tasks independently. When a child with special needs requires extra attention or is treated differently, other children in the program, or their parents, may need help to understand why. Usually, both parents and peers become more empathetic and patient as they grow to understand that people with different needs sometimes require special accommodation, especially as they learn that their own needs receive the same respect.

Children's questions about a perceived difference or special need should always be answered honestly and at their developmental level. You can also use picture books or photos to help children understand special needs.

Tapping into community supports

A child with special needs often requires additional care from the community, and health professionals and other resource staff may be just as involved as the child care program. Depending on the level of need and availability, a child may also receive specialized support from any number of professionals in a multidisciplinary team, including:

A child's circle of care, however big or small, can be a rich source of information, insight, approaches and resources for your child care program.

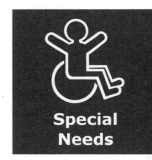

Special Needs

- physicians,
- public health and other nurses,
- physiotherapists,
- occupational therapists,
- speech and language specialists,
- early childhood consultants,
- resource teachers,
- staff at rehabilitation or specialized training centres,
- social workers,
- psychologists and behavioural specialists,
- recreation therapists.

Community supports may also be available to child care facilities promoting inclusion. These may include a provincial/territorial child care office, with access to assistance and funding for inclusion, or local community or religious organizations.

The benefits of inclusion

Like their peers, children with special needs in child care benefit from opportunities to realize their full potential. In many respects, their program won't differ from programming for other children. Their interests and preferences should be considered and engaged in the same ways and at the same times as those of their peers. Having separate activities for children with special needs is seldom necessary and may even hinder the process of inclusion. (See Appendix 13.2 for a template to help you adapt/record daily routines.)

The same principles for guiding behaviour apply to all children, so be sure to discuss a child's behaviour and progress with his parents often. You should agree about and use consistent behaviour management strategies, both at home and in child care. It is always important to be aware of and sensitive to children's emotional or psychological needs, especially those of a child with special needs, who may occasionally feel heightened frustration or have difficulty in social situations.

Inclusion strategies for children with specific needs

This section describes some common needs of and inclusion strategies for children with specific conditions. These basic adaptations are only a starting point, and should be expanded, modified and refined for each child in your care.

Attention deficit hyperactivity disorder

Attention deficit hyperactivity disorder (ADHD) is a condition that makes it difficult for a child to pay attention, sit still and exercise self-control. All children may exhibit these behaviours, particularly when excited or under stress. However, children with ADHD are consistently inattentive, impulsive and/or hyperactive, in ways inappropriate to their age and stage of development. These behaviours impair their ability to function. ADHD occurs in approximately 5 out of 100 children and is three times more common in boys than in girls. Children can sometimes be diagnosed with this disorder by 4 years of age. An observant child care practitioner who is charting a child's behaviour can help identify some of the symptoms of this condition.

While the exact cause of ADHD is unknown, a genetic component has been identified and may be linked to an imbalance of certain chemicals in the brain. A child's environment can either aggravate ADHD or help reduce its symptoms.

Treatment

In the preschool period, treatment for ADHD is mainly behavioural. While medication is less frequently used in this age group, it may be prescribed before the age of 6 if a child's behaviour impedes his developmental progress. ADHD medication acts on that part of the nervous system responsible for concentration and helps children focus on the task or activity at hand.

Observe children on medication for any changes in behaviour and possible side effects, and report back to parents. Side effects of the commonly used medications for ADHD can include:

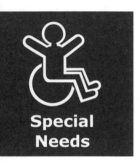

Special Needs

> **BEST PRACTICE**
>
> If you have questions about the safety of a particular game or activity for any child with special needs, seek information and approval from that child's treating physician before making it part of your program.

- decreased appetite, especially for lunch,
- mood changes (especially as medication wears off),
- difficulty sleeping (especially at nap time; nighttime sleep difficulties can also occur, but often improve over time),
- being too quiet. Careful adjustment of the dosage by the child's treating physician should resolve this.

Dietary restrictions to control ADHD have not been proven effective. Studies have shown that children do not become "hyper" because of sugar intake. While adults may note increased activity levels in children after they've eaten a sugary treat, this is probably caused by excitement surrounding the treat (such as having cake at a birthday party). Another possible explanation is "observer bias"—adults making the observation really believe that sugar is the cause of the behaviour.

Caring for a child with ADHD

With appropriate supports, a child with ADHD can be effectively included in a child care setting. The following basic adaptations provide more outlets for high activity and extra help with focusing and concentration.

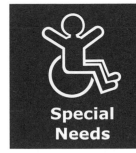

Special Needs

Child's behaviour or limitation	Strategy
Seems not to listen to instructions	Give directions in small, manageable steps that can be accomplished as separate tasks. Check to make sure child has understood before moving on to next step.
Doesn't finish projects	Structure short activities that emphasize starting, doing and finishing, to help teach focus.
Has trouble concentrating, even on a chosen task	Provide more and longer opportunities for large motor play in an open play setting.
Flits frequently from one activity to another	Have fewer toys available to choose from at one time.
Is easily distracted	Make changes to the environment to decrease noise, visual distractions.
Appears disorganized, loses things	Provide child with personal checklists.
Has difficulty sitting still	Provide frequent breaks and opportunities to move.
Fidgets	Provide child with a specified "fidget" toy that is not distracting to the rest of the group.

Charting good behaviour and providing regular positive reinforcement are important everyday strategies, just as they are with other children. In fact, most of these strategies would also apply to other conditions, such as autism, behavioural or developmental disorders, and fetal alcohol spectrum disorder.

Autism spectrum disorders

Autism spectrum disorders (ASDs) include a range of neurologically-based developmental disorders affecting communication, social understanding, behaviour and play. "Spectrum" refers to the continuum of intensity or "shades" of disability. Children with an ASD have difficulty communicating and interacting, but show significant individual differences in the number of symptoms, their intensity, age of onset and levels of functioning.

There are five ASDs, all categorized under the medical diagnosis of pervasive developmental disorder:

- Rett's syndrome,
- childhood disintegrative disorder,
- Asperger's syndrome,
- autistic disorder (also called autism), and
- pervasive developmental disorder not otherwise specified.

The term "ASD" is commonly used because the differences between these disorders are often unclear.

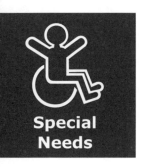

Special Needs

Children with an ASD vary widely in their intelligence, behaviours and abilities. Some don't speak at all; others use language that is highly repetitive or have trouble with back-and-forth conversation. Children with better language skills may focus on a small number of topics and have difficulty with receptive language (understanding what is said to them) and expressing abstract ideas. Children with an ASD may play repetitively, have few interests and have limited social skills. Stereotypical behaviours include rocking, hand flapping, resisting changes in the daily routine and difficulty with transitions. These children have trouble processing incoming sensory information and may exhibit unusual sensitivities (e.g., bothered by loud noises, lights, or certain textures in clothes and food). Children with an ASD are often dyspraxic, a disorder affecting motor activity development. Children with dyspraxia might experience difficulty with:

- eye movement,
- handling eating utensils, drinking from a cup or buttoning clothing,
- activities such as walking, skipping or jumping,
- speech.

ASDs are present in about 1 of every 166 children and are four times more likely to occur in boys than in girls. The signs are commonly present before a child turns 3 years of age.

The causes of ASDs include genetic factors, so the condition tends to run in some families. ASDs are not caused by psychological factors, but a child's environment can either aggravate the disorder or help reduce the symptoms. **There is no evidence that immunizations contribute in any way to the development of ASDs.**

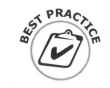

BEST PRACTICE

Child care practitioners often find that modifications to the environment and curriculum for a child with an ASD also benefit other children in their program.

Treatment

Children with an ASD are treated using educational approaches, such as tailoring instructions to their developmental level, using repetition, presenting information in a variety of ways and settings to help children generalize, and involving as many senses as possible in learning. Treatment interventions designed by a multidisciplinary team of professionals benefit from a child care practitioner's input if a child is enrolled in a program. Children with an ASD often need to be taught skills directly that other children learn through casual observation. Treatment by therapists trained in applied behavioural analysis (ABA) is proving particularly effective in improving language and cognition. ABA assesses of a child's responses and designs ways to motivate him within a developmental skills training program. Behaviour management strategies are also a major component of treatment. (For more about behaviour management, see Chapter 12, *Children's Emotional Well-Being*.) In some cases, medication can help reduce aggressive, difficult or hyperactive behaviours in children with an ASD.

Caring for a child with an ASD

With appropriate supports, a child with an ASD can usually be effectively included in a child care setting.

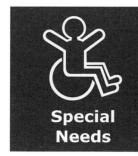

Special Needs

Child's behaviour or limitation	Strategy
Has difficulty coping with change and transitions	Adhere to a consistent and predictable daily routine.
Has trouble understanding what is being said	Give information or guidance visually, using gestures or pictures, as well as verbally.
Exhibits repetitive behaviours, such as rocking, hand flapping	Discourage separate, self-stimulatory activities.
Is socially withdrawn	Involve child in group learning activities for as long and as often as possible. Encourage positive interaction among peers.
Has difficulty speaking	Encourage communication using gestures and pictures as well as speech.
Exhibits inappropriate/disruptive behaviours	Have at least one trained, experienced staff member to deal with difficult behaviours, initiate individual interventions and guide other staff.
Is hypersensitive to certain stimuli (e.g., loud noise, bright light)	Make changes to the environment/activities to reduce sensory overload. Implement a sensory "diet"—a planned and scheduled activity program designed to meet child's specific sensory needs, thereby achieving and maintaining optimal levels of alertness and performance.

Inclusive child care settings and group activities that promote communication and appropriate social skills are known to contribute to best outcomes for children with an ASD. Let parents know when a child isn't responding to your intervention attempts, so that they can discuss alternative strategies with their treatment team or physician.

Behavioural disorders

Children with a behavioural disorder or emotional disturbance can exhibit one or more of the following characteristics:

- hyperactivity (short attention span, impulsiveness),
- non-compliance with rules or requests,
- excessive reactions to being frustrated, such as inappropriate crying, tantrums and other poor coping skills,
- aggression and/or self-hurting behaviour, and
- withdrawal, not initiating interaction with others, retreating from social interaction, excessive fear or anxiety.

While many children exhibit some of these behaviours occasionally, a child with a behavioural disorder will behave inappropriately often, more intensely and for prolonged periods, a sign that she is not coping with her peers or her environment.

There are many causes of behavioural disorders, including heredity, brain abnormalities and family dysfunctions. Recent research suggests that the number of preschoolers with a behavioural disorder is increasing.

Treatment

Children with a behavioural disorder are treated using educational approaches and interventions designed by a multidisciplinary team of professionals, which should include a child care practitioner if a child is enrolled in a program. Behaviour management strategies are a major part of this treatment. In some cases, medication can help reduce aggressive, difficult or hyperactive behaviours. Let parents know when a child isn't responding to your intervention attempts, so that they can discuss alternative strategies with their treatment team or physician.

Caring for a child with a behavioural disorder

With appropriate supports, many children with severe behavioural disorders can be successfully included in a community-based child care program. However, children with these disorders often require additional staff support to make this possible.

Child's behaviour or limitation	Strategy
Does not comply well with routines or requests	Give directions in small, manageable steps that can be accomplished as separate tasks. Check to make sure child has complied before moving on to next step.
	Give frequent verbal reinforcement for compliance.

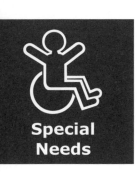

Special Needs

Has a short attention span, is impulsive	Structure short activities that emphasize starting, doing and finishing, to help teach focus. When child seems overexcited, slow activities down, speak softly and slowly, ask questions.
	Provide more and longer opportunities for large motor play in an open play setting.
	Provide frequent breaks and opportunities to move.
Shows excessive frustration (yelling, inappropriate crying, tantrums)	Apply basic behaviour management techniques consistently (prepare child for transitions, give timely reminders, reinforcement, rewards, redirection, time-outs).
Flits frequently from one activity to another	Have fewer toys available to choose from at one time.
Is easily distracted	Make changes to the environment to decrease noise, visual distractions.
Is aggressive (pushing, hitting, biting)	Intervene immediately, comfort hurt child first, restate the rules ("no hitting"). Speak seriously, face to face, acknowledge possible reasons for aggression. Apply time-out or loss of privilege consistently.
Is socially withdrawn	Involve child in group learning activities for as long and as often as possible. Encourage positive interaction among peers.
Shows excessive fear or anxiety	Encourage child to speak about fears and anxieties and reassure while encouraging coping strategies.
Exhibits inappropriate/disruptive behaviours	Have at least one trained, experienced staff member to deal with difficult behaviours, initiate individual interventions and guide other staff.

Adaptations to programming depend on the child's level of ability and specific needs. Various specialized training programs for staff are available.

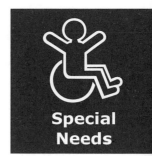

Special Needs

Cerebral palsy

Cerebral palsy is a condition that affects movement and muscle coordination and is caused by an abnormality in the child's developing brain. It affects approximately 3 out of 1,000 children. Abnormal development of or injury to the brain at any time from early pregnancy to the age of 2 years can result in cerebral palsy. The condition is non-progressive—that is, it doesn't get worse with time, although its impact may be greater as a child matures. There is a wide range of functional disabilities associated with this condition, and there are several types of cerebral palsy. Each child presents differently—from a slightly awkward walk or difficulty with hand control to a lack of muscle control throughout the body affecting all movement and speech. Depending on which areas of the brain are affected, a child may experience:

- muscle tightness or spasms (or the contrary, low muscle tone or floppiness),
- involuntary movements,
- difficulty with large motor skills (e.g., walking, running),

- difficulty with fine motor skills (e.g., writing),
- difficulty with perception.

Issues with feeding, breathing, bladder and bowel control, and pressure sores may arise, as well as orthopedic complications. Some children with cerebral palsy may also have seizures, learning disabilities or developmental delay. Some will have functional limitations, such as difficulties with dressing, toileting, eating, playing and pre-academic skills (e.g., drawing, cutting).

The degree of physical disability that a child with cerebral palsy experiences is not an indication of intelligence level.

Treatment

Treatment is tailored to improving a child's physical functions and is focused on increasing functional independence and participation with the least amount of stress or strain on a child's body. Exercises to maintain and build strength, control and range of motion and to prevent muscle contractures are the main treatment. Current medical treatments include botulinum toxin ("Botox") injections, muscle relaxant medications, surgery (tendon release or lengthening) and neurosurgery (on spinal nerve roots, to reduce spasticity).

Some children with cerebral palsy use assistive devices such as splints, braces, crutches, walkers or wheelchairs to increase mobility, or supportive seating, and may learn to use technologies such as a communication board or interactive computer programs. You may need to learn child-specific tasks, such as:

- feeding and positioning a child for optimal comfort and safety,
- using adaptive equipment,
- using assistive technologies, such as communication devices.

Depending on individual need, children with cerebral palsy may also receive regular physical, occupational, and speech and/or language therapy.

Caring for a child with cerebral palsy

With appropriate supports, a child with cerebral palsy can be effectively included in a child care setting. Staff training in both cerebral palsy and child-specific tasks such as positioning and feeding is required, and collaborating closely with the child's parents, treating physician and therapists will reveal other ways to provide program support.

Child's behaviour or limitation	Strategy
Experiences spasticity or involuntary body movement	Provide a special chair that offers additional support and a standing frame to allow child to participate actively in a standing position.
	Use a splint to help place child's hand in a functional position when holding a marker or eating utensil.
	Hold child in a flexed position during transfers to reduce spasticity.

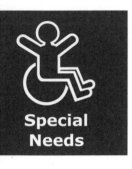

Special Needs

Has limited large motor skills	Arrange environment and remove obstacles for optimal access and mobility (e.g., for wheelchairs).
Has limited fine motor skills	Use adapted tools and materials (e.g., special scissors with "spring" to assist with opening and closing, a slanted board to prevent paper from sliding around when colouring).
	Use supportive strategies for feeding, dressing and play that are child-specific (e.g., using a curved spoon for feeding, dressing the weaker hand first, using pictures to model play).
	Adapt learning activity (e.g., alphabet) to allow child to point to a letter instead of writing it. Pre-cut and paste parts of a craft project so that child can complete the activity and feel successful.

Depending on the child's needs, additional long-term staffing support may be required.

Developmental delay

Children may show a delay in one or more important areas (e.g., speech or cognitive abilities or fine and large motor activity). If all are affected, the condition is described as global developmental delay. Each child with delayed development has a unique profile of abilities and needs, and may be affected mildly, moderately or severely. Although diagnosis comes later, most developmental disabilities are present from birth. A cause isn't always evident. Appendix 13.1 outlines the ages at which most children reach certain developmental milestones. If a child in your program hasn't developed one skill by a certain age, it doesn't necessarily indicate a problem. But if observing a child day to day leads you to check "No" for more than one item at or below his age, advise parents to consult their physician.

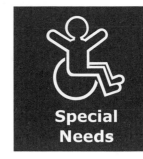

Special Needs

Treatment

A child with a developmental delay may need an individualized program of treatment. Special educational approaches and interventions designed by a multidisciplinary team, including a child care practitioner if the child is enrolled in a program, can be a major part of intervention. Behaviour management techniques that help reduce anxiety and hyperarousal may also be beneficial. Oral motor difficulties and speech delay can be addressed through speech and language therapy, oral motor therapy and occupational therapy. In some cases, medication can help reduce associated aggressive, difficult or hyperactive behaviours. Let parents know when a child isn't responding to your intervention attempts, so that they can discuss alternative strategies with their treatment team or physician.

> **"MATCH" any program activity to a child's abilities:**
>
> - **M**odify the task to accommodate the child.
> - **A**lter expectations.
> - **T**each in adaptive ways to suit the child's abilities.
> - **C**hange the environment for optimal access, participation and enjoyment.
> - **H**elp by understanding the nature of the child's disability.

Caring for a child with a developmental delay

With appropriate supports, a child with a developmental delay can be effectively included in a child care setting.

Child's behaviour or limitation	Strategy
Has trouble understanding what is being said	Give directions in small, manageable steps that can be accomplished as separate tasks. Check to make sure child has understood before moving on to next step.
	Give information or guidance visually, using gestures or pictures, as well as verbally.
Has difficulty with large motor skills	Arrange environment and remove obstacles for optimal access and mobility.
Has difficulty sitting unsupported	Provide good support for sitting to allow child to use hands more freely.
Has difficulty with fine motor skills	Adapt activities, play schedules and toy options to child's abilities rather than to age.
	Adapt learning activity (e.g., alphabet) to allow child to point to a letter instead of writing it. Pre-cut and paste parts of a craft project so that child can complete the activity and feel successful.
Has difficulty speaking	Encourage communication using gestures and pictures as well as speech.
Has difficulty accomplishing tasks	Structure short activities with graduated challenges. Encourage practice and celebrate improvement.
Flits frequently from one activity to another	Have fewer toys available to choose from at one time.
Has difficulty sitting still	Provide frequent breaks and opportunities to move.
Fidgets	Provide child with a specified "fidget" toy that is not distracting to the rest of the group.

Encourage children with a developmental delay to participate in activities with other children their age by making games, schedules and toy options flexible enough so that all children can feel successful.

Down syndrome

Down syndrome is caused by a chromosomal anomaly, or difference, called trisomy 21. All children with Down syndrome have a developmental disability, although the degree can vary from very mild to severe. In preschool years, some children show only mild delays in their cognitive development. Hypotonia, where the child's basic muscle tone is lower than normal, is often present and can cause delayed head control and delays with sitting and walking. Tasks involving fine motor skills, such as playing with smaller toys (e.g., large

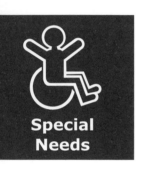

Special Needs

beads, Lego), holding a crayon or cutting, may be difficult as well. Many children with Down syndrome are prone to respiratory tract infections and ear infections caused by a build-up of fluid in the middle ear. This can lead to a hearing loss that requires medical or surgical care. Children with Down syndrome often require eyeglasses and may experience other associated medical problems that need to be monitored by a physician.

Many children with Down syndrome are very social and an easy fit in a group setting. They may show oppositional behaviour, often have difficulty communicating, and usually experience functional delays (e.g., learning to dress, eat and use the toilet independently more slowly than other children).

Treatment

Children with Down syndrome can benefit from educational approaches and interventions designed by a multidisciplinary team of professionals, including all involved child care practitioners.

Caring for a child with Down syndrome

With appropriate supports, a child with Down syndrome can be effectively included in a child care setting.

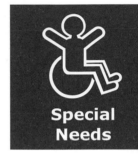

Special Needs

Child's behaviour or limitation	Strategy
Has difficulty with expressive language (the manner of speech)	Use sign language, a communication board or pictograms, or other special communication strategies or devices recommended by child's speech and language pathologist.
	Involve other children in learning sign language.
Has difficulty with fine motor skills	Adapt activities, play schedules and toy options to child's abilities rather than to age.
	Provide a range of materials (e.g., puzzles ranging from 4-piece insets to 24-piece jigsaws and helper scissors for crafts as well as regular school scissors).
Has difficulty sitting unsupported	Provide good support for sitting to allow child to use hands more freely.
Has atlantoaxial instability (a condition where vertebrae at the top of the spine are looser than normal)	Restrict child diagnosed with atlantoaxial instability from activities with forceful bending of the neck (e.g., somersaults), or activities where there is a risk of falling on his head (e.g., indoor/outdoor climbers).
Has difficulty accomplishing tasks	Structure short activities with graduated challenges. Encourage practice and celebrate improvement.

Encourage children with Down syndrome to participate in activities with other children their age by making games, schedules and toy options flexible enough so that all children can feel successful. If you have questions about the safety of a particular game or activity for a child with Down syndrome, seek information and approval from that child's treating physician before making it part of your program.

Fetal alcohol spectrum disorder

Fetal alcohol spectrum disorder (FASD) refers to a set of disabilities associated with maternal alcohol consumption during pregnancy. Characteristics of FASD include:

- restricted growth,
- neurological abnormalities, developmental delays, behavioural and learning disabilities, and skull and brain malformations,
- characteristic facial features, including smaller eye openings, a thin upper lip, flattened cheek bones and flattening out of the groove between the upper lip and nose.

The word "spectrum" refers to a continuum of effects: from physical (alcohol-related birth defects or ARBD) to neurological (alcohol-related neurodevelopmental defects or ARND). The term "FASD" is commonly used because the differences between these two disorders are often unclear.

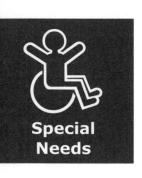

Special Needs

Toddlers and preschoolers affected by FASD may be:

- hyperactive,
- unable to follow simple instructions,
- much too friendly, even with strangers,
- developmentally delayed.

Psychological characteristics may include slow thinking and auditory processing, difficulty remembering and generalizing, concrete/literal thinking, poor judgment and difficulty linking cause and effect, persistent repetitive behaviours, difficulty with change and transitions, impulsivity, distractibility, and difficulty sorting (regulating) sensory input or stimuli.

The exact prevalence of FASD is unknown, but studies suggest it may run as high as 9 in 1,000 births.

Treatment

Children with FASD show significant individual differences in the number and severity of their symptoms, and in their levels of functioning. Treatment involves using educational approaches and interventions designed by a multidisciplinary team of professionals that should include a member of the child care staff if the child is enrolled in a program. Behaviour management strategies are often a major part of this treatment. The earlier that FASD-associated problems are recognized, the sooner effective management can begin.

Caring for a child with FASD

With appropriate supports (including anticipatory guidance—i.e., guiding behaviour before a problem arises), a child affected by FASD can usually be effectively included in a child care setting. Additional staff may be needed to support a child with FASD if he has severely disruptive behaviour.

Child's behaviour or limitation	Strategy
Has difficulty coping with change and transitions	Adhere to a consistent and predictable daily routine.
	Use a visual schedule and lots of advance notice to help with transitions.
Has trouble understanding what is being said	Establish clear and simple rules and be prepared to repeat them every day, using the same words.
	Give directions in small, manageable steps that can be accomplished as separate tasks. Check to make sure child has understood before moving on to next step. Praise her as she masters any new step and be encouraging even when things don't go well.
	Speak softly and gently.
	Find extra opportunities for child to make choices or decisions for herself.
	Give information or guidance visually, in different contexts or situations. Be concrete: Use gestures or pictures as well as speaking.
Is hypersensitive to certain stimuli (e.g., loud noise, bright light)	Make changes to the environment/activities to reduce sensory overload.
	Provide an area that is cozy and quiet, with a dimmer light level, to help calm an overstimulated child.
	Implement a sensory "diet"—a planned and scheduled activity program designed to meet child's specific sensory needs.
	Keep physical contact during dressing or other tasks exceptionally gentle.
Doesn't finish projects	Structure short activities that emphasize starting, doing and finishing, to help teach focus.
Has trouble concentrating, even on a chosen task	Provide more and longer opportunities for large motor play in an open play setting.
Flits frequently from one activity to another	Have fewer toys available to choose from at one time.
Is easily distracted	Make changes to the environment to decrease noise, visual distractions.
Has difficulty sitting still	Provide frequent breaks and opportunities to move.

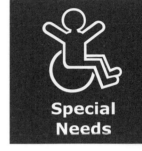

Special Needs

Collaborating closely with the child's parents, treating physician and therapists, and providing regular written reports on behaviour and learning patterns will contribute to best outcomes for children with FASD. Let parents know when a child isn't responding to your intervention attempts, so that they can discuss alternative strategies with their treatment team or physician.

Hearing disorders

The first two years of a child's life are critical for language development, and the most important early sign of possible hearing loss is an absence of or a delay/difficulty in developing language. If children have difficulty hearing, their speech and language will also be affected. Sound is measured by its intensity (loudness) and its frequency (pitch). A hearing impairment can involve intensity and frequency and be in one or both ears. Hearing loss can be slight, mild, moderate, severe or profound, based on how well a child can hear the intensities or frequencies associated with speech.

Children can experience various hearing disorders. **Conductive hearing loss** occurs when sound is prevented from moving freely along the ear canal, through the eardrum and the bones of the middle ear, to the inner ear. Ear infections, excessive earwax or malformations of the ear can cause conductive hearing loss. This loss is often temporary and may be treated medically, surgically or with hearing aids. **Sensorineural hearing loss** is the result of a problem with the inner ear or auditory nerve. This loss is usually permanent and can't be improved by medical or surgical treatment. However, hearing aids or a cochlear implant—a tiny receiver implanted in the bony part behind the ear and connected to a microphone—can help alleviate the effects of a neurosensory loss. A **mixed hearing loss** refers to a combination of conductive and sensorineural loss.

The impact of hearing loss depends on whether it affects both ears and when it develops. Children who experience hearing loss after they have developed good speech and language skills will not have the same difficulties as children affected from birth. It is estimated that 2 to 3 infants per 1,000 have at least a mild hearing impairment. A child care practitioner may be the first person to detect an anomaly or delay in the development of language skills.

Table 13.1 outlines the ages at which most children reach certain speech, language and hearing milestones. If a child in your program hasn't developed one skill by a certain age, it doesn't necessarily indicate a problem. But if observing a child day to day leads you to check "No" for most items at or below his age, advise parents to consult their physician.

Behavioural implications for a child experiencing hearing loss may include:

- a tendency to isolate himself in a group setting and be upset or distant during large group activities where there is a lot of noise,
- being unresponsive to instructions,
- an inability to focus on auditory activities (stories, music, circle time), or
- avoiding games and toys with an auditory component.

Children with hearing loss may tire more quickly than others from the strain of listening and watching for long periods of time. They can experience difficulties with balance, which might delay learning to walk.

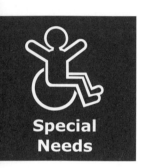

Special Needs

TABLE 13.1

Speech, language and hearing milestones

Birth to 3 months		
Does the child:	**Yes**	**No**
make cooing sounds?		
have different cries for different needs?		
smile at you?		
startle at loud sounds?		
soothe/calm at a familiar voice?		
3 to 6 months		
Does the child:	**Yes**	**No**
babble and make different sounds?		
make sounds back when you talk?		
enjoy games like peek-a-boo?		
turn his eyes toward a sound source?		
respond to music or toys that make noise?		
6 to 12 months		
Does the child:	**Yes**	**No**
wave hi/bye?		
respond to her name?		
let you know what she wants using sounds, and actions like pointing?		
localize correctly to sound by turning her head toward the sound?		
pay attention when spoken to?		
12 to 18 months		
Does the child:	**Yes**	**No**
use common words and start to put words together?		
enjoy listening to storybooks?		
begin to follow simple directions (e.g., "Point to your nose")?		
point to body parts or pictures in a book when asked?		
look at your face when talking to you?		
18 to 24 months		
Does the child:	**Yes**	**No**
understand more words than she can say?		
say two words together (e.g., "More juice")?		
ask simple questions (e.g., "What's that?")?		
take turns in a conversation?		
2 to 3 years		
Does the child:	**Yes**	**No**
use sentences of three or more words most of the time?		
understand different concepts (e.g., in-on; up-down)?		
follow two-part directions (e.g., "Take the book and put it on the table")?		
answer simple questions (e.g., "Where is the car?")?		
participate in short conversations?		

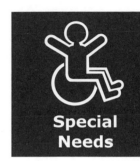

Special Needs

3 to 4 years		
Does the child:	**Yes**	**No**
tell a short story or talk about daily activities?		
talk in sentences with adult-like grammar?		
generally speak clearly so people understand her?		
hear you when you call from another room?		
listen to TV at the same volume as others?		
answer a variety of questions?		

4 to 5 years		
Does the child:	**Yes**	**No**
pronounce most speech sounds correctly?		
participate in and understand conversations even in the presence of background noise?		
recognize familiar signs (e.g., stop sign)?		
make up rhymes?		
hear and understand most of what is said at home and school?		
listen to and retell a story and ask and answer questions about a story?		

Source: Canadian Association of Speech/Language Pathologists and Audiologists. 2006. "Speech, language and hearing milestones: Prevent, protect, act." Adapted with permission.

Table 13.2 describes the degrees of hearing loss and specific educational and medical supports.

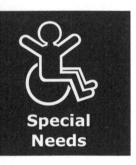

Special Needs

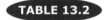

TABLE 13.2

Degrees of hearing loss and specific supports

Degree of hearing loss	Implications/Recommendations
Normal hearing -10 to +15 dB HL [decibels hearing loss]	Child should detect all speech.
Borderline 16 to 25 dB HL	Child may have difficulty hearing faint speech. Requires seating close to the child care practitioner.
Mild loss 26 to 40 dB HL	Child may miss from 25 to 40 per cent of speech if not wearing hearing aids. Requires hearing aids, seating close to the child care practitioner.
Moderate loss 41 to 55 dB HL	Child has difficulty understanding speech and likely has speech problems. Requires hearing aids, speech therapy, seating close to the child care practitioner and an FM system.
Moderate to severe loss 56 to 70 dB HL	Without hearing aids, child may miss 100 per cent of speech. Language is delayed and child care practitioners have trouble understanding him. Child has the same requirements as for moderate loss.
Severe loss 71 to 90 dB HL	Without hearing aids, child may hear loud voices about 30 cm (1 ft.) from his ear. Child has speech problems and the same requirements as for moderate loss.
Profound loss 91 dB HL	Child is likely aware of only vibrations when not wearing hearing aids. Speech and language don't develop spontaneously. In addition to the requirements for moderate loss, child may be a candidate for a cochlear implant and a structured therapy program. Some children may require a special education program.

Treatment

Because the age of diagnosis has a direct impact on the development of communication skills and future academic achievement in children with permanent hearing loss, universal newborn hearing screening is an essential strategy to improve long-term outcomes. Provincial or regional newborn hearing screening programs already exist in many provinces and are at different stages of development in others. Screening means an accurate and complete audiological assessment can be done for otherwise healthy children by 3 to 6 months of age.

In most children, the cause of a conductive hearing loss is an ear infection. (See Chapter 9, *Managing Infections*.) Recurrent or chronic ear infections may be relieved using ventilation tubes. Inserted by an ear, nose and throat surgeon, tubes equalize pressure in the middle ear and allow the area to ventilate. Some cases of conductive hearing loss are due to a malformation of bones in the middle ear. If this cannot be surgically corrected, the child may be fitted with hearing aids.

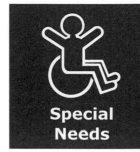

REMEMBER

Children wearing ventilation tubes in their ears usually require no special care, but be sure to ask parents whether their child's doctor placed limits on bathing or swimming.

Special Needs

Sensorineural hearing loss results from damage to the inner ear or auditory nerve. If loss is considered permanent, hearing aids can be prescribed for infants as young as 3 months old, usually for both ears. For young children with only mild sensorineural hearing loss, the decision to fit with hearing aids is made on a case-by-case basis. Even children with profound loss usually have some residual hearing that can be amplified with a hearing aid. A cochlear implant should ideally be surgically inserted by 1 year of age in children with profound hearing loss, increasing their access to auditory information. Children diagnosed after the age of 2 are more likely to have life-long deficits in language, speech and literacy.

The use of sign language as a form of communication is becoming much less common. Today, most children with a permanent hearing loss learn to communicate using oral language because of technological advances such as the cochlear implant. FM units are often used in group situations—the child care practitioner wears a microphone and the child wears a receiver adapted to his amplification devices. The child hears the speaker's voice while the impact of noise is minimized.

Children with a hearing loss benefit from special education services, including:

- speech, language and auditory training,
- amplification systems (e.g., personal hearing aids, cochlear implants, FM systems),
- sign language and lip-reading instruction, and
- a Picture Exchange Communication System (PECS), also known as a communication board or pictograms, which teaches children to use picture cards to make their wishes clear.

Preschool children who have been fitted with a hearing aid or cochlear implant need to be followed in a structured parent-centred therapy program. These services are usually provided by local hospitals or school boards.

Caring for a child with a hearing disorder

With appropriate supports, a child with a hearing disorder can be effectively included in a child care setting.

Child's behaviour or limitation	Strategy
Has trouble understanding what is being said	Seat child face to face with the child care practitioner during group activities.
	Give information or guidance visually, using gestures or pictures, as well as verbally.
	Use an FM system when child is in a group situation.
	Ensure that child care practitioners don't cover their mouths when speaking (e.g., during meals).
Is hypersensitive to certain stimuli (e.g., loud noise, bright light)	Make changes to the environment/activities to reduce sensory overload: Matted rooms reduce noise, felt pads (or even slit tennis balls) on chair and table legs eliminate scraping noises.
	Provide an area that is cozy and quiet, with lower light, for child to retire to if she feels worn out.
Is inattentive	Find other ways to make contact: Tap child on the shoulder, flick a light on and off or tap a desk so child feels a vibration.
Has tendency to withdraw	Offer extra visual support (e.g., gestures, pictures) to children in group activities. Keep play groups small, to minimize noise, distraction or the sense of being "left out."
	Involve other children in learning sign language, if applicable.
	Encourage other children to act as "social coaches."

Children with hearing loss pick up a lot of information with their eyes that other children get from listening. Paying extra attention to visual materials, lighting (e.g., ensuring a child isn't facing the window, which can be hard on the eyes) and noise levels will ease stress and help with concentration. Respect for personal spaces (e.g., a cubby) and "labelling" items in the child care environment visually, with pictures that illustrate their importance or use, will help make children with hearing loss feel they are part of the group.

Staff training on how hearing loss affects communication is essential. Where applicable, staff training in sign language and other communication aids will enrich the program. Depending on the child's needs, additional staff may be required, especially during playground activities, while crossing roads and during field trips.

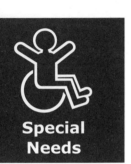

Special Needs

Speech and language difficulties

While most preschoolers are too young to be diagnosed with a specific language disorder, there may be early signs that a child is having trouble with one or both areas of language development:

- receptive language, defined as what is understood when being talked to, or
- expressive language, defined as the manner of speaking.

Repeating or hesitating on the first syllable of words is common and considered normal until a child is over 4 years of age. In addition to the signs identified in Table 13.1, the following may—but don't necessarily—indicate an emerging language disorder:

- Difficulty with **pragmatics** or the social use of language may mean the child has difficulty knowing how to use speech and non-verbal language to get along with others.
- **Dysphasia** means a child has trouble finding the words or grammar to communicate.
- **Dyspraxia** means a child has serious difficulty making sounds and coordinating the motor movements of the mouth.
- **Phonological** difficulty means a child has trouble pronouncing the sequence of sounds that form words. Speech is difficult to understand.
- Difficulty with **articulation** means a child has trouble pronouncing very specific sounds, such as *th, s, f.*
- **Stuttering** means a child involuntarily repeats the first consonants of words.

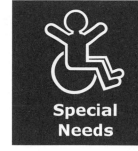

Special Needs

True stuttering, which occurs in about 1 per cent of children (and more often in boys than in girls), is different from normal developmental stuttering and speech difficulties, which occur in about 90 per cent of children between the ages of 18 months and 5 years. As children develop language, they often repeat words or phrases, mispronounce words, leave out words or sounds and speak some words that are difficult to recognize. Normal developmental stuttering and speech problems usually improve over 2 to 3 months.

Speech and language difficulties may be associated with other conditions, such as hearing loss, neurological disorders, brain injury, developmental disabilities or a specific physical impairment (e.g., cleft lip or palate). Lack of social stimulation may also be a factor, adding to a child's feelings of frustration and social isolation. Often, however, the cause is unknown. Most children with language disorders are born with them. The problem is usually detected when the child is around 18 months to 2 years of age. Language delay is the most common developmental problem identified in the preschool period.

Treatment

Children experiencing speech and language difficulties are treated by speech and language therapists. If a child has a serious difficulty with expressive language, a therapist may introduce her to another communication method—an augmentative (enhancing) communication system. One of the most popular systems is the Picture Exchange Communication System (PECS), which teaches children to use picture cards to make their wishes clear.

Caring for a child with speech and language difficulties

With appropriate supports, a child with speech and language difficulties can be effectively included in a child care setting.

Child's behaviour or limitation	Strategy
Has difficulty speaking	Give many opportunities to interact verbally during the day, particularly in situations that prompt child to make a request, make a choice or otherwise communicate her wishes. These opportunities can be spontaneous during activities or structured as part of child's day.
	Give child lots of time to get thoughts expressed. Don't verbally rush her and discourage others from speaking for her. This is especially important for stuttering.
	Use pictures both to reinforce your verbal instructions (receptive language) and to assist child to express herself.
Has difficulties with the social use of language (pragmatics)	Organize play so that other children in a small group may act as language models. Child care practitioners can help to facilitate communication between child and other children in the group.
Is reluctant to speak	Respond consistently to child's non-verbal behaviour, which is an important form of communication.

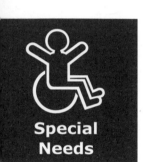

Special Needs

Teaming up with speech and language professionals and training programs will help child care practitioners provide optimal support to children who have difficulty speaking. If signs of difficulty persist, recommend that parents take their child to a specialist for assessment. Although many speech/language programs have long waiting lists, some offer parent workshops for use-at-home strategies while children are waiting for treatment.

Vision disorders

There is a wide range of vision disorders. Normal vision is defined as 20/20. A child with a vision disorder may be described as being partially sighted or having low vision (defined as vision between 20/60 and 20/190), as legally blind (defined as less than 20/200 vision) or as totally blind.

Vision problems are common and can be present at birth or can develop over time. It is important to pick up vision problems as early as possible. A physician should examine any child over 3 months of age whose eyes cross, even intermittently. Persistent eye turn in a newborn or a child of any age should be promptly assessed by a physician. Vision loss can be caused by various eye disorders as well as infections, congenital disorders and injury. The effect of visual problems on a child's development depends on the severity and type of loss, the age at which the vision loss occurs and whether other disorders are involved. Children with neurological or developmental disorders are at higher risk for vision disorders.

Child care practitioners play an important role in detecting vision disorders in infants and toddlers and alerting parents. Signs of a vision disorder include:

- delayed social smiling,
- floppiness or head tilting,
- delay in reaching for objects, in passing an object from hand to hand or in looking at hands,
- excessive blinking, squinting or eye rubbing,
- startling easily,
- seeking out sunlight or other bright light,
- peering closely at objects, or bringing them unusually close to the face,
- showing little or no interest in age-appropriate visual material, or in activities taking place across the room,
- wandering eye movements.

Almost all children who are visually impaired have some degree of vision, so the impairment may not be recognized immediately.

Treatment

Children with vision disorders receive treatment from specially trained vision therapists, as well as their physician and ophthalmologist. A child may be fitted with glasses or contact lenses, or have one eye patched to strengthen the vision in the other eye. The Canadian National Institute for the Blind offers resources to parents and child care practitioners.

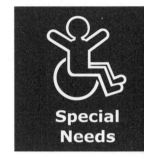

Special Needs

Caring for a child with a vision disorder

With appropriate supports, a child with a vision disorder can be effectively included in a child care setting.

Child's behaviour or limitation	Strategy
Has difficulty seeing objects or activity	Use bright lights, toys and clothing in strong and contrasting colours, or fluorescent paint to create a highly visual environment and encourage child to exercise partial sight.
	Highlight an object with a flashlight or other light source to help child concentrate on it.
Has tendency to withdraw	Plan games and activities where child can participate fully.
	Keep play groups small, to minimize noise, distraction or the sense of being "left out."
	Provide motivation and a sense of direction during play. This helps with development and can be achieved verbally or by using other sensory cues. A child with a visual impairment will reach for a noisy toy just as a typically developing child will reach for a brightly coloured one.

Has difficulty with orientation	Adjust environment for optimal participation and access.
	Keep centre layout and furnishing simple, stable and consistent, and always help child get oriented in new surroundings.
Appears uninterested	Always supplement visual cues or instructions with verbal ones.
	Make lots of "audio-tactile links": Bring any new object close to child's eyes (10 to 15 cm [4 to 6 ins.] away), tell child its name and encourage handling. Introduce just one object at a time.
	Describe concepts and things visually, in ways child can appreciate. A farm is "a big place where food grows and there are lots of animals."

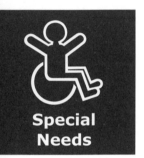

Special Needs

Rights and benefits of inclusion

Inclusion is a right, not a privilege. Children with special needs have the right to attend the same child care programs as other, typically developing children. While the process of including children with special needs usually begins with personal efforts on a small scale, over time it can have a profound impact on the overall quality of life in any community. Inclusion benefits everyone in child care, where each child can be recognized, accommodated and celebrated in an accepting environment.

Selected resources

General

American Academy of Pediatrics, American Public Health Association, National Resource Center for Health and Safety in Child Care. 2nd ed., 2002. *Children with Special Needs: Applicable Standards from* Caring for Our Children; *Guidelines for Out-of-Home Child Care*. Elk Grove, IL: American Academy of Pediatrics. See Appendix T for a list of adaptive equipment for physical/occupational therapy and physical activities.

Baker, Bruce L., Alan J. Brightman and Jan B. Bacher. 4th ed., 2004. *Steps to Independence: Teaching Everyday Skills to Children with Special Needs*. Baltimore, MD: Brookes Publishing.

Canadian Child Care Federation. www.cccf-fcsge.ca

———. 2001. Communicating with a child who has special needs. Resource sheet #38.

———. 2001. Early identification for children with special needs. Resource sheet #56.

Carr, Anne. 1997. Play and relationships: Programming for inclusion. www.cfc-efc.ca

Gould, Patti and Joyce Sullivan. 1999. *The Inclusive Early Childhood Classroom: Easy Ways to Adapt Learning Centres for All Children*. Beltsville, MD: Gryphon House.

Hemmeter, Mary L. et al. 2005. *Division for Early Childhood (DEC) Recommended Practices Workbook: Improving (DEC) Practices of Young Children with Special Needs and their Families*. Missoula, MT: Division for Early Childhood Education.

Irwin, Sharon Hope. 2005. *Inclusion Voices: Canadian Child Care Directors Talk about Including Children with Special Needs*. Wreck Cove, N.S.: Breton Books, or www.specialinkcanada.org

————, Donna S. Lero and Kathleen Brophy. 2004. *Inclusion: The Next Generation in Child Care in Canada*. Wreck Cove, N.S.: Breton Books, or www.specialinkcanada.org

Norton, Trudy. 1997. Special health care for child care settings: Minimize the risks. www.cfc-efc.ca/docs/cccf

Patchen, Ginger. 1997. Physical challenges in child care: Let the children lead. www.cfc-efc.ca/docs/cccf

Sandall, Susan R. and Ilene S. Schwartz. 2002. *Building Blocks for Teaching Preschoolers with Special Needs*. Baltimore, MD: Brookes Publishing.

See also Selected resources for Chapter 2, *Healthy Activities*

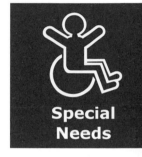

Special Needs

Inclusion preparedness and supports

City of Toronto Children's Services. 2007. *Inclusion: Policy development guidelines for early learning and care programs*. www.toronto.ca/children

Early Childhood Environment Rating Scale-Revised (ECERS-R). www.fpg.unc.edu/~ecers

Gerlach, Alison. 2007. *Steps in the right direction: Connecting and collaborating in early intervention therapy with Aboriginal families and communities in British Columbia*. B.C. Aboriginal Child Care Society. www.acc-society.bc.ca

————, and Deanne Zeidler. 2004. *A Guide for Culturally-Focused Early Intervention Therapy Programs for Aboriginal Children and Families in British Columbia*. Vancouver, B.C.: B.C. Aboriginal Child Care Society. www.acc-society.bc.ca

Irwin, Sharon Hope. 2005. SpeciaLink Inclusion *Child Care Inclusion Profile* and *SpeciaLink Child Care Inclusion Principles*. www.specialinkcanada.org

Littlechild, Shelly. 2006. *Community assessment toolkit*. www.scdp.bc.ca

Smith, Monique Gray. 2006. *Aboriginal supported child development handbook*. www.scdp.bc.ca

SpeciaLink. 2005. How to measure inclusion quality in child care: A SpeciaLink training video for the inclusion scales. DVD. www.specialinkcanada.org

Supported Child Care, Province of British Columbia. 2004. *Support guide* and *Support guide user handbook*. www.scdp.bc.ca

Attention deficit hyperactivity disorder

Canadian Paediatric Society. 2002. Medical treatment for attention deficit hyperactivity disorder. www.caringforkids.cps.ca

———. 2003. Alternative treatments for attention deficit hyperactivity disorder. www.caringforkids.cps.ca

Children and Adults with Attention Deficit/Hyperactivity Disorder (CHADD). www.chadd.org

Learning Disabilities Association of Canada. www.ldac-taac.ca

Learning Disabilities Association of Quebec. www.aqeta.qc.ca

National Institute of Mental Health (U.S.). www.nimh.nih.gov

Autism spectrum disorders

Autism Canada Foundation. www.autismcanada.org

Autism Society Canada. www.autismsocietycanada.ca

Canadian Paediatric Society. 2004. Early intervention for children with autism. www.cps.ca

———. 2007. Autistic spectrum disorder: No causal relationship with vaccines. www.cps.ca

Centers for Disease Control and Prevention (U.S.), Autism Information Centre. www.cdc.gov/ncbddd/autism

Health Canada. 2008. Diseases and conditions: Autism. www.hc-sc.gc.ca

Mount St. Vincent University. 2004. *Supporting children with autism in child care settings: Final report*. www.msvu.ca. See also the Resource reference list (books, videos and websites) at this site.

SpeciaLink. 2007. The mainstream is the right stream: On the road to mainstream daycare. VHS/DVD. See "Autism in the mainstream: A treatment approach." www.specialinkcanada.org

Behavioural disorders

Canadian Child Care Federation. 2001. *Tips for parenting children with challenging behaviour*. Resource sheet #48. www.cccf-fcsge.ca

———. 2005. DVD. Meeting the challenge: An Aboriginal perspective.

Irwin, Sharon Hope, ed. 1999. *Challenging the Challenging Behaviours: A Sourcebook Based on the SpeciaLink Institute on Challenging Behaviours in Child Care*. Wreck Cove, N.S.: Breton Books, or www.specialinkcanada.org

Kaiser, Barbara and Judy Sklar Rasminsky. 1999. *Meeting the challenge: Effective strategies for challenging behaviours in early childhood environments*. Ottawa, Ont.: Canadian Child Care Federation. www.cccf-fcsge.ca

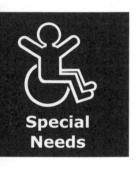

Special Needs

Positive Parenting Program (Triple P). www.pfsc.uq.edu.au

See also Selected resources for Chapter 12, *Children's Emotional Well-Being*

Cerebral palsy

American Academy for Cerebral Palsy and Developmental Medicine. www.aacpdm.org

Bloorview Kids Rehab. 2007. Community resources: Cerebral palsy guidebook. www.bloorview.ca

Geralis, Elaine, ed. 2nd ed., 1998. *Children with Cerebral Palsy: A Parent's Guide*. Bethesda, MD: Woodbine House.

Rosenbaum, Peter. Cerebral palsy: What parents and doctors want to know. *British Medical Journal*, 326 (May 2003): 970–974.

SpeciaLink. 2007. The mainstream is the right stream: On the road to mainstream daycare. VHS/DVD. See "Shawn and his mainstream parents." www.specialinkcanada.org

Developmental delay

Division for Early Childhood of the Council for Exceptional Children. www.dec-sped.org

Early Intervention Canada. McGill University and Yaldei Developmental Centre. www.earlyinterventioncanada.com

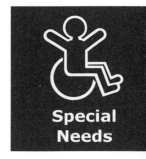

Special Needs

Down syndrome

Canadian Down Syndrome Society. www.cdss.ca

Down Syndrome: Health Issues. www.ds-health.com

Down Syndrome Research Foundation. www.dsrf.org

National Association for Down Syndrome (U.S.). www.nads.org

Fetal alcohol spectrum disorder

Canadian Centre on Substance Abuse. FASD Information Service. www.ccsa.ca

Canadian Child Care Federation. 2001. Caring for children with fetal alcohol syndrome. Resource sheet #70. www.cccf-fcsge.ca

Canadian Paediatric Society. 2002. Fetal alcohol spectrum disorder: What you should know about drinking during pregnancy. www.caringforkids.cps.ca

Centre for Excellence in Early Childhood Development. www.excellence-earlychildhood.ca

First Nations of Quebec and Labrador Health and Social Services. FAS information kit: Our children, our future; Put an end to FAS/FAE. www.cssspnql.com.

Motherisk. www.motherisk.org

Ontario Federation of Indian Friendship Centres. 2005. *FASD toolkit for Aboriginal families.* Aboriginal Children's Circle of Early Learning. www.accel-capea.ca

Public Health Agency of Canada. 2008. Fetal alcohol spectrum disorder. www.phac.aspc.gc.ca

VON Canada. 2005. *Let's Talk FASD: Parent driven strategies in caring for children with FASD.* Ottawa, Ont.: VON Canada. www.von.ca/FASD

Hearing disorders

Canadian Academy of Audiology. www.canadianaudiology.ca

Canadian Association of the Deaf. www.cad.ca

Canadian Child Care Federation. 2001. Ear infections, hearing loss and children. Resource sheet #27. www.cccf-fcsge.ca

Carver, Roger. 2001. *Deaf Childcare in Canada: A Deaf-friendly Vision for the 21st Century.* Ottawa, Ont.: Canadian Association of the Deaf. www.cad.ca

Hearing Foundation of Canada. www.hearingfoundation.ca

Speech and language difficulties

American Speech and Hearing Association, Child speech and language. www.asha.org

Canadian Association of Speech/Language Pathologists and Audiologists. www.caslpa.ca

————. 2000. Pre-school speech and language development. Fact sheet.

————. 2000. Hearing health in children. Fact sheet.

Canadian Language and Literacy Research Network. www.cllrnet.ca

Childhood Apraxia of Speech Association of North America. www.apraxia-kids.org

Vision disorders

Canadian National Institute for the Blind. www.cnib.ca

SpeciaLink. 2007. The mainstream is the right stream: On the road to mainstream daycare. VHS/DVD. See "James: Blind and in the mainstream." www.specialinkcanada.org

Websites

Active Living Alliance for Canadians with a Disability. www.ala.ca

American Academy of Pediatrics. www.aap.org

Bloorview Kids Rehab. www.bloorview.ca

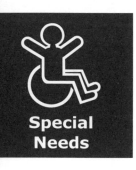

Special Needs

Brookes Publishing. www.brookespublishing.com

Canadian Association of Community Living. www.cacl.ca

CanChild Centre for Childhood Disability Research. www-fhs.mcmaster.ca/canchild

Centers for Disease Control and Prevention (U.S.). www.cdc.gov

Centre for Excellence in Early Childhood Development. www.excellence-earlychildhood.ca

Centres of Excellence for Children's Well-Being: Children and Adolescents with Special Needs. www.coespecialneeds.ca

Child Care Plus: The Center on Inclusion in Early Childhood. www.ccplus.org

Learning Disabilities Association of Canada. www.ldac-taac.ca

Learning Disabilities Association of Quebec. www.aqeta.qc.ca

National Institute of Neurological Disorders and Stroke. www.ninds.nih.gov

SpeciaLink: The National Centre for Child Care Inclusion. www.specialinkcanada.org

Supported Child Development Program (B.C.). www.scdp.bc.ca

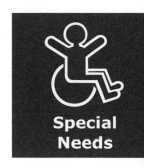

Special Needs

Appendix 13.1: Developmental milestones

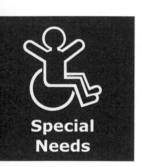

Special Needs

Age	Large motor skills	Fine motor skills	Psychosocial (interactive) skills	Cognitive skills
At the end of 3 months, most infants can...	roll from front to back control head and neck movement when sitting raise their head and chest when lying on their stomach stretch out and kick their legs when lying on their stomach or back push down with their legs when feet are on a firm surface	bring their hands together open and shut their hands bring their hands to their mouth take swipes at a dangling object	smile responsively and spontaneously be expressive and communicate with their face and body imitate some body movements and facial expressions	watch faces intently follow moving objects recognize familiar objects and people
At the end of 8 months, most babies can...	roll both ways (front to back, back to front) sit unsupported support their whole weight on their legs control their upper body and arms	grasp and shake a hand toy transfer an object from hand to hand use their hands to explore an object	reach for a familiar person smile at their image in a mirror respond to expressions of emotion from other people imitate speech sounds	track a moving object, and find one that is partially hidden explore with hands and mouth struggle to get objects that are out of reach look from one object to another watch a falling object
At 12 to 14 months, most babies can...	reach a sitting position without help crawl on hands and knees, or scoot around on their behinds get from a sitting to a crawling or prone (on their stomach) position pull up to stand cruise, holding onto furniture stand momentarily without support walk holding an adult's hand, and maybe take two or three steps without support start to climb stairs with help	finger-feed using the pincer grasp (thumb and forefinger) put objects into a container (and take them out again) release objects voluntarily poke with an index finger push a toy begin to drink from a cup scribble with a crayon begin to use a spoon	be shy or anxious with strangers imitate during play show a preference for certain people and toys test parental response to actions and behaviour extend an arm or leg to help when being dressed take off socks come when called (i.e., respond to their name) say "mama" or "dada" and at least one other word with meaning indicate a need without crying stop an action if you say "no"	explore objects in different ways (shaking, banging, throwing, dropping) recognize the names of familiar objects respond to music begin to explore cause and effect

Age	Large motor skills	Fine motor skills	Psychosocial (interactive) skills	Cognitive skills
At 18 months, most babies can...	climb into chairs walk without help climb stairs one at a time with help	build a three-block tower use a spoon well turn a few board-book pages at a time turn over a container to pour out the contents drink easily from a cup	follow a simple instruction remove some clothing on their own point to a named body part point to familiar objects when asked help with simple tasks	use objects as tools fit related objects together
At 24 months, most toddlers can...	pull a toy while walking carry a large toy or several toys while walking begin to run kick or throw a ball climb into and get down from chairs without help walk up and down stairs with help	build a tower of four blocks or more complete a simple shape-matching puzzle turn board-book pages easily, one at a time	imitate the behaviour of adults and older children get excited about being with other children engage in parallel play with other children show increasing independence show defiant behaviour	begin "make-believe" play
At 3 years, most toddlers can...	walk up and down stairs, alternating feet (one foot per stair) run easily jump in place throw a ball overhand	make up-and-down, side-to-side and circular lines with a pencil or crayon build a tower of more than six blocks hold a pencil in writing position screw and unscrew jar lids or big nuts and bolts string big beads work latches and hooks snip with children's scissors	show spontaneous affection for familiar playmates begin to take turns understand the concept of "mine" vs. "someone else's" object to changes in routine ask a lot of questions anticipate daily activities put toys away ask for help know their full name	match an object in their hand or the room to a picture in a book expand make believe play to animals, dolls and people sort easily by shape and colour complete a puzzle with three or four pieces understand the difference between "one" and "two" name body parts and colours
At 4 years, most preschoolers can...	hop and stand on one foot for up to four seconds kick a ball forward catch a bounced ball	draw a person with two to four body parts use children's scissors draw circles and squares twiddle thumbs do a finger-to-thumb sequence (e.g., Itsy-bitsy spider)	look forward to new experiences cooperate with other children play "Mom" or "Dad" be very inventive dress and undress imagine monsters negotiate solutions to conflicts	understand counting follow a three-part instruction recall parts of a story make up and tell simple stories understand "same" and "different" engage in rich fantasy play know their address

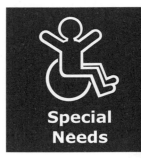

Special Needs

Appendix 13.2: Routine-based programming suggestions

Insert facility letterhead here

Child's name: _____

Date initiated: _____

Review schedule: _____

Dates revised: _____

Italics indicate latest additions or modifications to the routine-based plan

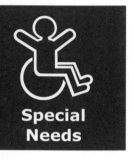

Special Needs

Routine (with time of day)	Goal	Suggested activities
Arrival		
Free play		
Directed activity		
Circle time		
Snack		
Hygiene routine		
Outdoor play		
Puzzle or story		
Hygiene routine		
Lunch		
Rest time / Walk / Quiet / Free time		
Free play		
Departure		
Developed by:		

Appendix 13.3: Action planning form

Focus area: _____

Team members:_____

_____

_____

Purpose:_____

_____

_____

Practices to be addressed	Action steps to be taken	Timelines and persons responsible	Resources and supports needed	Indicators of success	Status/Date completed

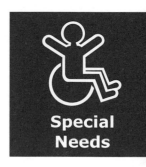

Special Needs

Practices to be addressed	Action steps to be taken	Timelines and persons responsible	Resources and supports needed	Indicators of success	Status/Date completed

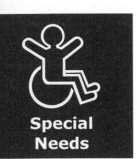

Special Needs

Date: _____ Present: _____

Notes: _____

_____

_____

Date: _____ Present: _____

Notes: _____

_____

_____

Date: _____ Present: _____

Notes: _____

_____

_____

Source: Hemmeter, Mary L. et al. 2005. *Division for Early Childhood (DEC) Recommended Practices Workbook: Improving Practices of Young Children with Special Needs and their Families*. Missoula, MT:*Division for Early Childhood Education.

14

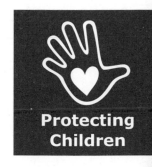

Protecting Children from Maltreatment

Most child care practitioners will encounter child maltreatment during their working lives. Almost 4 per cent of all children in Canada are assessed by child welfare authorities. Maltreatment is substantiated in almost half those cases, which include all forms of child abuse and child neglect. Many more children and youth likely suffer maltreatment without ever coming to the attention of child welfare authorities. In an Ontario population survey of adults, almost one-third of all men and women reported being physically and/or sexually abused as children. The most common types of child maltreatment are neglect, physical abuse and exposure to domestic violence.

Child maltreatment occurs within all socio-economic and cultural groups. In all provinces and territories, it is a legal responsibility to report cases of suspected abuse and neglect to child welfare authorities. All child care practitioners must be trained to recognize and deal with suspected cases of maltreatment. This chapter outlines how to recognize possible maltreatment, what to do if you have concerns, how to create a child care environment free from abuse and how to help families that may be at risk.

Reporting suspected child maltreatment is the first step to helping both the child and his family. This is a crucial step in the important work of protecting children from immediate and long-term physical and emotional damage that can result from maltreatment. Simply making a phone call to child welfare services may protect a child or his siblings from further maltreatment—and perhaps even prevent more serious harm. You may help to break a pattern of maltreatment—such as repetitive head injury—by reporting, and also help parents get the support they need if they are having difficulties with parenting.

Your legal responsibility is to **report** any suspicion or concern that a child is, or is at risk of, being abused or neglected. It is **not** your responsibility to investigate or substantiate the maltreatment, or to identify an offender. This is the role of child welfare services and the police.

Child care practitioners are in a unique position to recognize subtle changes in a child's physical and emotional health or behaviour. You have an ongoing relationship with that child and regular opportunities to observe a family interacting over a period of time. You may be more sensitive to warning signs than family, friends or neighbours. You may also be seen as a "safe" confidant for a child wishing to disclose maltreatment, as well as for parents who have concerns or questions about life at home that they are reluctant to share with others.

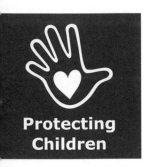

Protecting Children

Types of maltreatment

Neglect

Neglect is the omission of care resulting in harm—or risk of harm—to a child. It may also include the failure to provide parenting appropriate for a child's physical, emotional and psychological health and development. Neglect is the parent/caregiver's failure to provide any one or a combination of the following:

- physical necessities, such as food, appropriate nutrition, weather-appropriate clothing and shelter,
- a safe environment, and supervision appropriate to the child's age and/or development,
- medical care,
- affection, emotional support and nurturing,
- developmentally appropriate stimulation,
- protection from harm, or
- regular schooling.

Although neglect may occur as an isolated incident or under particular circumstances, it is often seen as a chronic pattern. For example, you may notice that:

- a child's failure to thrive seems to be caused by noticeably poor physical, dental or mental health.
- parents don't seem willing to seek medical attention.
- clothing seems consistently inadequate.

- patterns of injury suggest lack of supervision.
- there is a routine lack of personal hygiene and proper food.

Neglect may also result in progressively worsening delays in development, especially in babies and toddlers. Language delay, attachment problems, a negative view of self and others, social withdrawal or isolation during free play, avoidance of social interactions, and confusion in interpreting the emotions of others can all be early signs of neglect. A child who is neglected might also be consistently aggressive, uncooperative or behave out of keeping with her age and developmental stage. Remember that all of this observed behaviour and development may be due to an underlying condition or have an explanation other than neglect. By themselves, such signs would not be reason enough to report to child welfare authorities, but they should prompt you to watch for other possible signs.

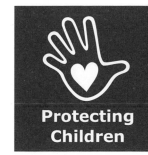

Physical abuse

Physical abuse can occur just once, or repeatedly. Physical abuse is the use of force against a child in a way that causes injury or the risk of injury. This type of abuse includes hitting, slapping, shaking, pushing, choking, biting, burning, kicking, pulling, or using a weapon or an object to assault a child. Using force to restrain a child in a painful or harmful way, such as holding a child under water or requiring him to assume a painful position (e.g., forced kneeling on a painful surface), is also physical abuse. Physical abuse is **not**:

- the use of protective restraints intended to protect the child from pain or harm to himself or others (rather than to punish).
- the use of defensive measures to protect oneself or a child in danger from harm (rather than to correct behaviour).

Signs of physical abuse appear in many different ways. Any bruise on a very young child that does not have an adequate explanation is concerning and may warrant a report to child welfare services. Other bruises to be concerned about include those that have the shape of recognizable objects or appear on fleshy areas of the child's body, such as the buttocks and thighs. Multiple or patterned bruises are highly suspicious. Don't confuse bruising with dermal melanosis (Mongolian spot), a blue-grey pigmentation often found on the back or buttocks of healthy, darker-skinned infants at birth. (See Appendix 14.1, page 364, for questionable bruise sites.)

ALERT

Bruises are rarely seen on babies who are not yet cruising—especially on babies younger than 9 months of age.

Also of concern are burns that have no reasonable explanation and significant burns that did not receive medical attention. Pay attention to injuries such as:

- any fracture in a child who is not yet walking,
- abnormal use of a limb (e.g., limping, or not using an arm normally) without a reasonable explanation and/or without seeking medical attention, and
- unexplained injuries to unusual parts of the body (e.g., the face—other than the forehead—genitalia, backs of the arms and legs, and abdomen).

In infants, toddlers and preschoolers, injuries to the head and brain are particularly serious and difficult to recognize. They can manifest first with signs such as vomiting, unexplained irritability or lethargy, trouble breathing, persistent crying, and limpness or seizures.

Emotional abuse

Emotional abuse damages a child's sense of self. Emotionally abusive behaviour can be acts or omissions that put children at risk of developing serious cognitive, emotional or psychological problems. Emotional abuse may include exploitation, intimidation, social isolation, verbal threats, or unreasonable demands or comments that "put down" or demean a child. Exposing children to family violence is also considered emotional abuse, and is reportable to child welfare services.

Sexual abuse and exploitation

Sexual abuse includes any activity with a child, by an adult, for sexual purposes. Any sexual behaviours or acts that are for the pleasure of an adult by a minor are considered abusive. Minors cannot legally consent to sexual relations with adults or those in a position of authority. Sexually abusive behaviour includes fondling, subjecting or exposing a child to sexual gestures, asking a child to touch or allow sexual touching, exposing genitals, viewing pornographic materials, exhibitionism, and involving a child in pornography, prostitution or intercourse.

Exposure to domestic violence

The link between spousal assault and child maltreatment

A violent environment always places children at risk, both in their present lives and for the future. Experiencing abuse as a child increases not only the risk of being revictimized as an adult—accepting violence as normal in adult relationships—but also the likelihood of becoming an abuser. For many families, spousal assault and child maltreatment overlap. When one parent (most often the mother) is being abused, the probability that children will also be hurt increases greatly. Boys who witness abuse of their mother are more likely to abuse their partners in adolescence and adulthood. Girls who witness abuse are more likely to accept abusive relationships as adults.

REMEMBER

Witnessing the abuse of a parent is child maltreatment. It is very painful for a child to see or hear a parent being abused. The experience has a lasting effect on a child's behaviour, physical and mental health, and ability to socialize with others and to perform in school.

The link between physical punishment and child maltreatment

Physical punishment is an action by an adult or caregiver that inflicts physical discomfort or pain with the intention of changing a child's behaviour.

Research shows that physical punishment:

- cannot be distinguished from abuse in terms of degree of force, parental intent or extent of injury,

- does not improve long-term behaviour or compliance in children, and
- can have lasting negative consequences for children.

Some forms of physical punishment, such as slapping or spanking a child under 2 years of age, using objects (e.g., a belt or ruler) to punish, or delivering any slap or blow to a child's head, are criminal offences.

Unfortunately, the use of physical discipline is common, with 50 to 85 per cent of Canadian parents reporting spanking or slapping their children. At the same time, more than three-quarters of parents in Canada recognize that physical punishment is harmful, unnecessary and ineffective. Nearly all parents feel they need more information and education on child discipline.

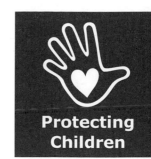

Protecting Children

The most common risk factors for physical punishment are:

- parental approval of physical punishment as an effective method of discipline. The more strongly a parent approves of its use, the more frequent and harsher the physical punishment tends to be.
- parental anger in response to conflict with a child.
- parental experience of physical punishment as a child.
- parental interpretation of their child's misbehaviour as either intentional or serious (i.e., as defiance instead of normal behaviour for the child's age or developmental stage).

The use of physical punishment places children at risk of abuse, mental health problems, antisocial behaviour, poor relationships with parents, confusion about personal rights (both their own and those of others), and an increased tolerance of violence.

Child care practitioners can support families by demonstrating and promoting non-physical approaches to guiding children's behaviour. You are uniquely qualified to suggest resources to parents so they can learn more about developmentally appropriate behaviours, effective discipline and how to manage difficult behaviours.

REMEMBER

You can "set the tone" for families and the community by explicitly and unequivocally discouraging the use of physical punishment.

The child care practitioner's responsibility

Children must be cared for in a safe environment, free from risk of abuse or neglect. Child welfare laws in Canada require that all cases of suspected child abuse or neglect be reported to appropriate child welfare authorities, which in most cases is the local Children's Aid Society. **In some provinces, the law also requires that concerns about children *at risk* of abuse or neglect be reported to child welfare authorities.** These authorities are charged with investigating the situation and determining whether a child is in need of protection.

While all citizens have a duty to report suspected cases of child maltreatment, mandatory reporting laws place a special responsibility on professionals, such as child care practitioners, who work closely with children and are especially aware of those who may be in need of protection. Child care practitioners who fail to report suspected abuse or neglect can be charged with and convicted of failure to report. Anyone making a report of suspected child maltreatment to child welfare services is protected under the law from civil liability, as long as the report has been made in good faith (i.e., without bad intent).

If you suspect a child has suffered—or is at risk of suffering—abuse or neglect, take the steps set out in Figure 14.1.

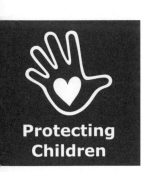

Protecting Children

How to document suspected maltreatment

Recording information about possible abuse should be done accurately, promptly and in detail, in a journal or other permanent record kept at the facility (e.g., an attendance record). Your documentation may be used in an investigation or court proceedings. Make notes as soon as possible of any observations that raise your suspicion of maltreatment. These notes should include a description of what was seen, heard or said. For instance, document the size and shape of any bruise or other injury. If a child discloses information in conversation, write down the exact words the child used. Do not include any speculation or opinion about your observations—simply describe what you saw or heard. The date and time of events must also be documented. It's also good practice to record any calls or discussions with child welfare authorities.

Each time you record information, sign and date the entry. If something comes to mind later, that information should be added, and then signed and dated. **Do not** rewrite or change original notes. Any mistakes or additions should be added, initialled and dated.

How to support a child who discloses abuse or neglect

When a child chooses an adult to disclose information about being abused or neglected, it is because he perceives that adult as an important person in his life who can be trusted to help. The confiding child needs to be supported and helped to feel safe. Children may disclose maltreatment purposefully (by telling you), accidentally (e.g., in conversation about something else), with gentle prompting, or simply by showing behavioural signs of maltreatment (e.g., sexually explicit play). It is very common for children to later deny or recant their statements, even when there has been maltreatment. Children do this for many reasons. They may fear the consequences for themselves or for the person who maltreated them. They may have been threatened or sworn to secrecy. They may feel pressured to recant or value loyalty to family above telling the truth. Often, children may believe they are to blame, may feel concerned about not being believed, or may not realize that what has been done to them is abusive. Finally, disclosure can be traumatic.

The following tips will help you handle a disclosure more sensitively:

- Take the child to a quiet place, where you can speak privately.

FIGURE 14.1

What to do if you suspect maltreatment

Seek medical attention if necessary. If a child is in immediate danger, call 911 (or emergency services where 911 service is unavailable).

- Resolve any urgent medical issues.

Record the incident in writing.

- Use the child's own words.
- Keep this record up-to-date.
- Don't rewrite or change original notes; just add anything you think of later to the report.
- Be sure to date and initial each entry.

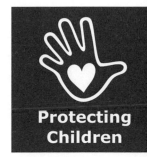

Protecting Children

Report concerns to child welfare authorities **immediately**. Remember:

- Child care practitioners are required by law to report their concerns directly to authorities themselves and not through another party, such as a supervisor.
- You should notify authorities of any new and/or ongoing concerns, even if you know they have been previously reported.
- If you're unsure of whether your concerns warrant a report, call the child welfare authorities and ask for advice.
- It is the child welfare worker's responsibility to decide whether concerns warrant further investigation.
- Do not delay in reporting concerns in order to collect more information. Report with whatever information you have at the time.

Be prepared to provide as much information as possible, including:

- the child's name, address and present location (e.g., home, child care or shelter),
- the reasons for your own concern and what first raised your suspicions,
- the details of an injury (if any) or encounter (e.g., the what, when, where) that concern you,
- the names and address of the parents and siblings of the child (and who the child is living with, if not her family),
- the child's special needs, if any, and
- child care drop-off and pick-up times and designated contacts.

Identify yourself. While any person can report anonymously, giving your name and professional position lends greater credibility to any report. Remember:

- It's difficult for child welfare services to explain to families why and how concerns have arisen when the report is made anonymously.
- If keeping your name confidential is important, discuss your reasons and concerns with child welfare services. In most circumstances, child protection authorities will respect the confidentiality of the person reporting. In Quebec, they must ensure the confidentiality of the person reporting.

- Ask open, non-leading questions (e.g., "What happened?"). Gently encourage the child to give you only enough information to evaluate your own concerns as to whether or not she has suffered abuse or neglect. Whether she needs protection is up to the child protection authorities.
- Remain calm, so as not to upset the child.
- Don't express any anger or criticism.
- Reassure the child that you believe what she has told you, that telling you was the right thing to do, and that whatever happened is not her fault.
- Let the child know that you are going to talk to someone who can help. Don't promise to keep what she has told you a secret.
- If the child expresses fears about what will happen to the person who may have abused her, explain that you don't know but that you will find out what happens next.
- Return the child to her regular activities, if appropriate.

REMEMBER

You don't need to gather the facts: that is the role of the child welfare worker. Well-intended but inappropriate questioning may interfere with the subsequent child welfare investigation.

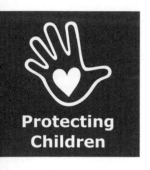

Protecting Children

Children who are unable to communicate or who rely more on adults for their care because of disability are more vulnerable to abuse and neglect. These children may not be able to disclose maltreatment. Being alert to physical signs or changes in their behaviour or mood is especially important.

Preventing child maltreatment

Because child care practitioners have ongoing and close relationships with children and their families, they play a particularly important role in preventing child maltreatment by:

- providing emotional support to families, and
- sharing and modelling best practices in caring for children.

Working in partnership with parents in a non-judgmental way, you can build a trusting relationship with families. Within that relationship, offer information on parenting issues, such as appropriate discipline, community programs or parenting classes, and family resource centres. You may be among the first to recognize when a family is falling into crisis and be able to offer links to community supports such as shelters, social workers or crisis lines.

In day-to-day interactions with children, you can be a model for individual parents and help to set a high standard for child care within your community. It's important to speak openly with parents about their frustrations with child rearing and help them identify difficult behaviours (and how to deal with them) at different developmental stages. (For more on basic guidance strategies, see Chapter 12, *Children's Emotional Well-Being*.) Certain groups of children are at higher risk of maltreatment: those with behavioural problems, a physical disability, chronic illness or a developmental delay. Children with special needs are particularly vulnerable because they are even less likely than their peers to recognize or disclose abusive behaviour.

Suspected or confirmed child maltreatment committed by a child care practitioner must be reported to child welfare authorities in the same way as for a family member or other possible abuser. You can minimize the risk of maltreatment occurring while a child is in your care—and protect yourself from allegations of maltreatment—by taking a few basic precautions.

Screen all prospective staff and volunteers for a history of maltreating children, including running a police check. Having a screening policy in place is less likely to identify someone who might harm a child than to deter unsuitable applicants, who in effect screen themselves out.

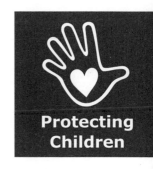

Protecting Children

- Do not leave a child alone with someone visiting the facility or the parent of another child.
- Always notify parents immediately if their child sustains an injury or experiences a traumatic event in the child care setting.
- Have a buddy system that pairs new staff members with experienced staff.
- Make parents feel welcome when they visit your facility at any time, especially if their appearance is unscheduled.
- Encourage parents to network among themselves and to share family experiences with child care staff.
- Just as you should report any suspicions you have about abuse or neglect, be open to receiving any parent's concerns. Advise them of their right and responsibility to report these concerns.

Follow common-sense practices for avoiding misunderstandings that might lead to false accusations of sexual abuse. These include:

- exercising good judgment about the kind of language to use with children (e.g., never using any words that could have a sexual connotation),
- avoiding play or care in secluded areas and keeping co-workers and parents informed of activities when you are alone with a child,
- confining touch to a child's head, back and shoulders when offering comfort, affection or reassurance,
- being sensitive to how a child feels about being touched and asking permission if you're not sure,
- learning to intervene and redirect children appropriately when they are engaged in masturbation or sexual play, and
- using correct terminology for all body parts and encouraging children in your care to do the same.

Always follow appropriate behaviour management techniques and never use corporal/physical punishment for a child. If an interaction with a child becomes unmanageable, request the help of another staff person or, if you are working alone, call the child's parents. The more you know about normal child development and behaviour techniques for different ages, the better equipped you'll be to handle difficult behaviours without parents or co-workers misunderstanding.

While child maltreatment in Canada remains all too common, child care practitioners play a crucial part in seeking help for families at risk. Observation, reporting, modelling appropriate child guidance techniques, and sharing knowledge and experience with parents in need of help are all positive steps toward protecting children in your care.

Selected resources

Resources for child care practitioners

Alberta Children's Services. 2005. *Responding to child abuse: A handbook.* www.solgen.gov.ab.ca

Baker, Linda L., Peter J. Jaffe and Kathy J. Moore. 2001. *Understanding the effects of domestic violence: A trainer's manual for early childhood educators.* London, Ont.: Centre for Children and Families in the Justice System. www.lfcc.on.ca

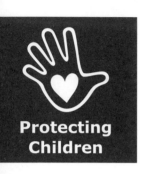

Protecting Children

――――. 2001. *Understanding the effects of domestic violence: A handbook for early childhood educators.* London, Ont.: Centre for Children and Families in the Justice System. www.lfcc.on.ca

Canadian Child Care Federation. www.cccf-fcsge.ca

――――. 2006. Hitting doesn't work. Resource sheet #82.

――――. 2005. Connecting with your community health partners: Child welfare workers. Resource sheet #74.

――――. 2001. Protecting children: Helpful rules to keep young people safe. Resource sheet #13.

――――. 2001. Respecting children's rights at home. Resource sheet #64.

――――. 2001. Tips for parenting children with challenging behaviour. Resource sheet #48.

Manitoba Family Services and Housing. 2003. *Child protection and child abuse manual: A protocol for early childhood educators.* www.pacca.mb.ca

National Center on Shaken Baby Syndrome (U.S.). 2002. *A Guide for Child Care Providers.* Ogden, UT: NCSBS. www.dontshake.com

Public Health Agency of Canada, National Clearinghouse on Family Violence. www.phac-aspc.gc.ca/ncfv-cnivf

――――. 2006. *A "what to do" guide for professionals who work with children.*

――――. 2001. *A booklet for service providers who work with immigrant families: On issues relating to child discipline, child abuse and child neglect.*

Region of Peel (Ont.) Public Health. 2004. *Keep on track: A health and resource guide for child care providers in Peel.* Children and families needing special help section: Child abuse. www.region.peel.on.ca/health/keep-on-track/pdfs/entiremanual.pdf

Saskatchewan Early Childhood Association. 2007. *A Guide to the Prevention and Detection of Child Abuse.* Regina, Sask.: SECA. www.skearlychildhoodassociation.ca

Resources for families

Alberta Children's Services. 2006. *Child abuse: Children exposed to family violence.* www.child.gov.ab.ca

Canadian Paediatric Society. www.caringforkids.cps.ca

———. 2008. Guiding your child with positive discipline.

———. 2008. When you child misbehaves: Tips for positive discipline.

———. 2002. Never shake a baby. Brochure and parent note.

Department of Justice, Family Violence Initiative. 2007. Child Abuse Fact Sheet. www.canada.justice.ca

Durrant, Joan and Ron Ensom. 2004. Physical punishment of children. Centre of Excellence for Children's Well-Being, Child Welfare. Information sheet #7E. www.cecw-cepb.ca

Health Canada. 2004. What's wrong with spanking? Tip sheet and brochure formats. www.phac-aspc.gc.ca

———. Child abuse prevention resources: Developed through the family violence initiative (April 1991 – March 1996). www.phac-aspc.gc.ca

Public Legal Education and Information Service of New Brunswick. 2007. Spanking and disciplining children: What you should know about Section 43 of the *Criminal Code*. www.legal-info-legale.nb.ca

Trocmé, Nico et al. 2004. Physical abuse of children in the context of punishment. Centre of Excellence for Children's Well-Being, Child Welfare. Information sheet #8E. www.cecw-cepb.ca

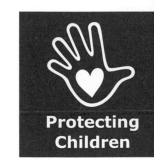

Protecting Children

Websites

Aboriginal Children's Circle of Early Learning. www.accel-capea.ca

Canadian Child Care Federation. www.cccf-fcsge.ca

Centre for Children and Families in the Justice System. www.lfcc.on.ca

Centre of Excellence for Children's Well-Being. www.cecw-cepb.ca

Child Welfare League of Canada. www.cwlc.ca

Department of Justice Canada. www.justice.gc.ca

National Center on Shaken Baby Syndrome. www.dontshake.org

National Resource Center on Child Abuse and Neglect (NRCCAN). www.casanet.org/library/abuse/nrccan.htm

Ontario Association of Children's Aid Societies. www.oacas.org

Prevent SBS (Shaken Baby Syndrome) British Columbia. www.dontshake.ca

Public Health Agency of Canada. Family Violence Initiative/National Clearinghouse on Family Violence. www.phac-aspc.gc.ca

Appendix 14.1

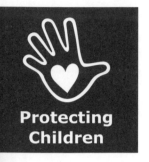

Common sites for bruises

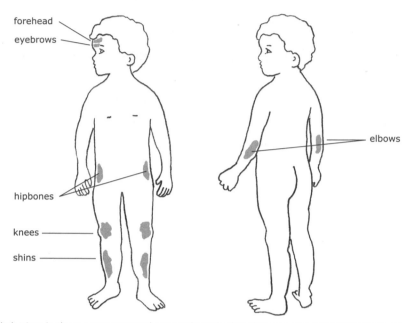

forehead
eyebrows
hipbones
knees
shins
elbows

While bruises in these areas commonly occur through play, they can also occur through abuse.

Questionable sites for bruises

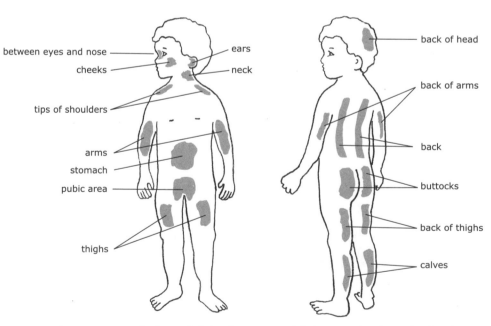

between eyes and nose
cheeks
tips of shoulders
arms
stomach
pubic area
thighs
ears
neck
back of head
back of arms
back
buttocks
back of thighs
calves

Also suspicious are bruises on infants who are not mobile (younger than 9 months of age), and bruises that have a recognizable shape or pattern.

chapter

15

Caregivers' Physical Health

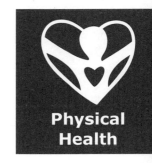

Physical Health

I n any profession, how workers feel during a typical day influences the quality of
their work. In child care, a job that requires a high level of activity and interaction,
there is a particularly strong relationship between feeling good, working well and
providing quality care. This chapter is a general overview of work-related physical
health issues affecting child care practitioners, while Chapter 16 deals with social and
emotional issues.

The most common physical injuries for child care practitioners involve the musculoskeletal
system, especially the lower back, and are the result of muscle sprains and strains. Exposure
to infections, as well as environmental exposures (e.g., to chemicals, mould and noise), can
also lead to medical problems. In the regulated sector, standards are in place to protect the
physical health and safety of children and the people caring for them. While standards vary
among jurisdictions and between child care centres and home settings, one thing is clear:
workplace health in child care is a responsibility shared by regulators, management and
child care practitioners themselves.

The physical environment

The location and layout of a child care setting are important indicators of quality care and can directly affect the well-being of children and caregivers. Facility design can make it easier or more difficult to move through a program day (e.g., whether the outdoor play space is on site or involves a walk), to interact with families (e.g., a designated space for quiet conversation, a meeting or administration) or to have some "down time" (e.g., a staff room). Further, the design of a child care facility can have a direct impact on child–staff interaction, job satisfaction and staff turnover. Other important aspects of the physical environment include the type of space allocated for child care (e.g., whether it is purpose-built or adapted), the amount of space per child, how well the space is organized, furnished and equipped, the availability of natural light and views to the outdoors, and the size and accessibility of an outdoor play area. While all provinces and territories regulate physical space for child care, specifications vary widely in scope and detail by jurisdiction.

Promoting physical well-being in child care

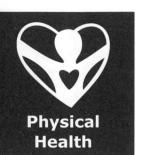

Physical Health

Maintaining a physically healthy workplace involves conducting regular safety checks, adjusting routines to balance physically intense work with quiet times, and ensuring that staff members seek timely medical advice for symptoms of illness. And while these tasks are necessary and beneficial, promoting workplace health goes further—it involves attention to ergonomics, which means adapting a workplace for the optimum benefit of workers, as well as for the work to be done. Ergonomics draws on the biophysical sciences (e.g., physiology, kinesiology and biomechanics), as well as psychology and sociology, to improve the design of workplaces and work processes. In a best-practice scenario, a facility should be designed, organized, equipped and furnished specifically for child care, and to meet the specific needs of the children and staff in attendance.

Increasingly, maintaining a healthy workplace means being aware of environmental hazards and avoiding items or substances that are potentially harmful to human health. The precautionary principle—that is, always erring on the side of caution—already shapes decisions about play equipment, indoor and outdoor surfaces, plastic products and cleaning supplies in both child care centres and home settings. Air quality is also important. If child care practitioners experience frequent headaches, fatigue, or eye, nose or throat irritations, a certified indoor air quality inspector should examine the premises for the presence of particulate matter (often caused by construction), mould spores, formaldehyde (often associated with off-gassing from furniture or carpeting) or radon gas, which occurs naturally but can accumulate in higher than healthy levels in some locations. Regular cleaning and facility maintenance eliminate dust and mould. Commercial air fresheners should be avoided. Natural light—and proper lighting in areas where windows are lacking—and manageable noise levels are other important determinants of workplace health.

Because routine cleaning is an essential daily task, child care practitioners may use household cleaning products several times a day. These products are toxic if ingested and can cause an allergic or other reaction if they are inhaled or come into contact with the skin or eyes. Safe handling (e.g., wearing household rubber gloves, never combining chemical cleaners) and storage (e.g., in original containers, out of the sight and reach of children) minimize the risk of chemical exposure. Information about the safe use of hazardous materials is available through Health Canada's Workplace Hazardous Materials Information

System (www.hc-sc.gc.ca) in the form of material safety data sheets, worker education programs and product labelling.

Physical injuries

Caring for children is physically intensive work. Consider that:

- The combined actions of bending, lifting, kneeling, standing, stretching, pushing and pulling—all required for basic set-up, interactions with children and cleaning duties—have been estimated to take up 20 to 30 per cent of a child care practitioner's normal working day.
- Child care practitioners typically sit several times a day for extended periods (10 to 20 minutes) without back support, on child-sized chairs or on the floor for play activities.
- Bending to make eye contact while speaking or listening to children happens in 2- to 3-minute increments throughout the working day.
- Bending down or lifting children to aid and comfort, dress or change clothing and diapers throughout the day takes about 3 to 5 minutes each time.
- Child care practitioners walk and stand for 3 to 4 hours a day, while leading and conducting learning activities both indoors and out.
- Lifting or assisting children on outings who cannot walk by themselves because they are hurt, tired or upset can happen on average twice a week for 15 minutes per incident.

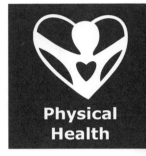

Physical Health

The physical effort required from child care practitioners on a typical day far exceeds the requirements of many professions. Injuries, particularly back injuries and muscle strains and sprains, are very common.

Fortunately, the risk of injury can be reduced by maintaining physical fitness, taking basic preventive measures and adapting behaviours whenever possible. Here's what you need to know to prevent and treat the most common physical injuries in a child care setting.

Back pain

Back pain may be the result of muscle strain or may involve injury or herniation of the spinal discs that separate vertebrae. Muscle strain is characterized by pain and stiffness; disc injury usually involves back pain radiating to a leg, or back pain with numbness or weakness of the legs or feet. For strain, a physiotherapist or registered massage therapist may recommend relaxation and gentle back exercises. For persistent pain or if a disc injury is suspected, you should consult a doctor.

Child care situations that can contribute to back injury

- lifting children, toys or equipment incorrectly,
- working at inappropriate heights (i.e., child-sized tables and chairs),
- lifting children into and out of cribs,
- sitting on the floor with an unsupported back,
- reaching above shoulder height to obtain supplies,
- lifting children on and off diaper-changing tables,
- using awkward positions and forceful motions when opening windows, and
- carrying bags of diapers or garbage to the dumpster and throwing them in.

Source: Canadian Child Care Federation. 2002. "Back Injury and Stress," *Interaction* 16(3). Adapted with permission.

Not all back pain is preventable, but there are effective ways to reduce the risk of injury and to manage pain when it does occur. Here are some suggestions:

- Change your posture, even slightly, every few minutes to help relieve pressure. This is easy to do in child care, where movement is fairly constant.
- Make time for regular physical activity—especially exercise that strengthens abdominal/core muscles—to build strength, support the back and help prevent muscle strain.
- Stretch regularly and gently to increase flexibility and help correct posture.
- Use proper lifting techniques:
  - ➤ Stand as close as possible to the object you are lifting.
  - ➤ Keep your feet about hip-width apart, with one foot slightly behind the other. This position helps with stability and reduces the likelihood of twisting or concentrating weight on one side of your body.
  - ➤ Bend your knees, but don't sit on your heels, which makes getting up more difficult.
  - ➤ Keep your arms as straight as possible when lifting an object (as opposed to a child), to prevent shoulder and back strain.
  - ➤ Look ahead before straightening your knees, to avoid turning at the waist.

See Figure 15.1 for examples of proper lifting techniques.

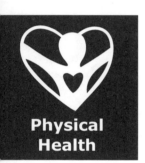

---

10 ways to protect your back on the job

1. Hold a child close to your body and avoid twisting motions. Lower the crib side before lifting a child out. If it is appropriate and safe, encourage toddlers to climb up or down stairs—with your help—rather than carrying them.
2. Have some full-sized furniture as well as child-sized chairs, tables or desks. Sit in comfortable chairs with good back support when rocking or holding children.
3. Ensure that diaper-changing tables are at an appropriate adult height. Offer toddlers a step-stool so they can climb up onto a change table (with your help) rather than being lifted.
4. Use a stroller for outings if there's a possibility that children might get too tired to walk.
5. Have proper footwear. Choose comfortable non-slip shoes that provide proper arch and foot support.
6. Store items for easy access, with the heaviest items at waist height. Use a stool when reaching for items on high shelves.
7. Don't move or lift heavy furniture by yourself.
8. Transport garbage in manageable loads, and use a cart for heavier loads.
9. Avoid prolonged bending. Reduce or eliminate bending by kneeling or squatting to face a child. Avoid being on the floor in uncomfortable positions for extended periods. When sitting on the floor, use a wall or furniture for back support.
10. Be aware. Educate staff about preventing back injuries and use an *Injury report form* (pages 97–99) to determine where and how an injury occurred.

Source: Canadian Child Care Federation. 2002. "Back Injury and Stress," *Interaction* 16(3). Adapted with permission.

Consult a doctor when back pain does occur, especially if it is severe. Resting the back for a few days, applying an ice pack and taking a non-steroidal anti-inflammatory drug such as acetylsalicylic acid (ASA or aspirin) or ibuprofen (e.g., Motrin or Advil), which reduce pain and improve mobility, are common treatments. An over-the-counter muscle relaxant can relieve stiffness and reduce muscle spasms. However, you will probably need to modify your work habits to avoid putting stress on the affected area. Back-strengthening exercises, yoga, massage, physiotherapy, chiropractic or acupuncture can also help. Surgery is not a recommended option for the vast majority of back problems.

Figure 15.1: Proper lifting techniques

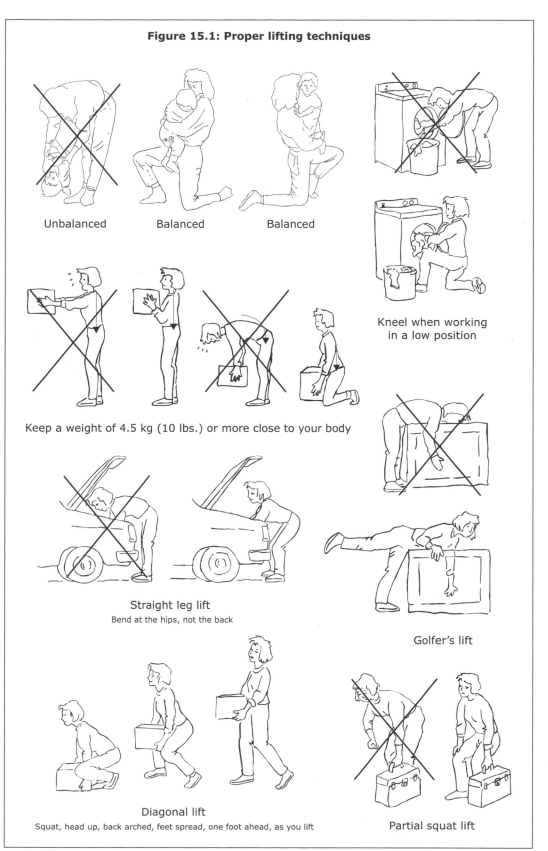

Unbalanced Balanced Balanced

Kneel when working in a low position

Keep a weight of 4.5 kg (10 lbs.) or more close to your body

Straight leg lift
Bend at the hips, not the back

Golfer's lift

Diagonal lift
Squat, head up, back arched, feet spread, one foot ahead, as you lift

Partial squat lift

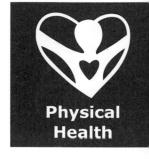

Physical Health

Source: Melnick, Michael S., H. Duane Saunders and R. Saunders, *Managing Back Pain: Self-help Manual*, 1998. Adapted with permission.

Neck and shoulder injury

Neck and shoulder injury is a generic description for conditions affecting muscles and connective tissue in the upper back, shoulders and neck. Poor posture and nervous tension tend to aggravate the two main causes of neck and shoulder pain: structural stress (stemming from chronic slouching or "forward head," which strains small neck muscles), and compression (pressure on the spinal discs in the neck caused by tight neck muscles). Both causes are also aggravated by the unconscious and sometimes chronic lifting of the shoulders to ease stress. Characteristic symptoms are pain when looking from side to side, and acute pain radiating from the upper back to the base of the skull. You should seek medical advice, especially if you are experiencing numbness or tingling in the arms or hands, along with neck and shoulder pain.

Slow, gentle and regular stretching of the muscles in the upper back, shoulders and neck can alleviate pain caused by structural stress and compression. A balanced series of professionally recommended exercises usually includes stretching on the front, sides and back of the neck, as well as the chest, upper back and shoulders (including under the arms): the whole "shoulder girdle." Other common treatments for neck and shoulder pain are consciously correcting posture when seated or in motion, using "back-friendly" furniture, and changing habits that contribute to stress.

For back pain, most doctors recommend that you resume daily routines gradually but as soon as possible. Bed rest for any longer than 2 or 3 days may do more harm than good. Doing regular, gentle back-strengthening exercises and sleeping on a firm mattress are effective preventive routines. Consult your doctor for advice on your particular situation.

Exercises to ease tension and tone muscle groups

1. Turn your head slowly and levelly from side to side.
2. Rotate your shoulders forward and back.
3. Slowly touch your left ear to your left shoulder, and repeat for the right side.
4. Shrug your shoulders toward your ears and down in a relaxed way.
5. Pull in your stomach muscles, hold for a count of 8, then slowly relax.
6. Lying on your back, bring both knees slowly up to your chest, tighten your stomach muscles, hold for a count of 20, then slowly relax.

Repetitive strain injuries

Bursitis: A bursa is a fluid-filled sac that separates hard bony surfaces from the tendons and muscles that glide over the top of a bone. The function of a bursa is to reduce friction.

Repetitive activity, especially while carrying heavy loads, may inflame the bursa, causing bursitis. The affected area becomes painful, tender and hot and may swell. In child care practitioners, common sites for bursitis include:

- shoulders, as a result of frequent lifting,
- hips, as a result of holding children on the hip,
- knees, as a result of kneeling down often to play.

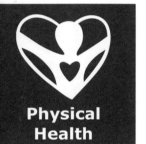

Physical Health

You can avoid bursitis by keeping muscles active through regular exercise and stretching. Seek medical advice if you experience pain or other symptoms of bursitis. Once diagnosed, bursitis is usually treated by rest, applying an ice pack and taking a non-steroidal anti-inflammatory drug such as acetylsalicylic acid (ASA or aspirin) or ibuprofen (e.g., Motrin or Advil). You will also need to modify your work habits to avoid putting stress on the affected area.

Carpal tunnel syndrome: Carpal tunnel syndrome (CTS) is a common and frequently diagnosed repetitive strain injury. It's brought on by extensive, repetitive hand and wrist movement involving the flexor muscles on the inside of the forearm and the median nerve. The median nerve controls sensation and muscle movement in the thumb and first three fingers. When the median nerve becomes compressed or inflamed through repetitive tasks such as drawing, sewing, playing an instrument or using a computer, CTS can develop. Early symptoms may include:

- a tingling or "burning" sensation,
- weakness, usually in the dominant hand,
- swollen or numb fingers on awakening in the morning, or
- an aching or painful wrist.

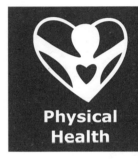

Physical Health

It is important to seek medical advice and treatment early on. Ignoring initial symptoms can result in loss of hand strength and dexterity, especially when forming a fist or grasping an object in a pinching motion (e.g., a pen or paintbrush). Loss of sensation (e.g., being less able to distinguish between hot and cold), as well as debilitating pain, can occur if CTS is left untreated.

Treating CTS often includes:

- resting the hand—avoiding activities that cause pain or using a wrist brace,
- applying ice packs to reduce swelling,
- stretching or other "tendon-gliding" exercises prescribed by a doctor or physiotherapist,
- taking frequent breaks to stretch and shift position when engaged in repetitive tasks,
- consciously correcting posture when seated or in motion, and
- taking anti-inflammatory medication or a corticosteroid injection.

If treatment does not relieve pain over time, surgery may be recommended.

Tendonitis: A tendon is a band of tissue connecting muscles to bone that can become strained through repetitive motion. Frequently lifting, holding or carrying children may inflame the tendons, resulting in tendonitis. Tendonitis commonly occurs in the upper arm, causing shoulder pain and tenderness. Keeping muscles strong, stretching regularly and avoiding repetitive actions in the workplace wherever possible help reduce the risk of developing tendonitis. Seek medical advice if you experience inflammation or other symptoms of tendonitis. Once diagnosed, tendonitis is usually treated by rest, applying an ice pack and taking a non-steroidal anti-inflammatory drug such as acetylsalicylic acid (ASA or aspirin) or ibuprofen (e.g., Motrin or Advil). You will also need to modify your work habits, at least temporarily, to avoid putting stress on the affected area.

Reporting workplace injuries

Staff have both the right and the responsibility to report all workplace injuries. The effects of even a minor injury are not always known until later. For example, a small cut can become infected and limit your ability to work. A more serious injury might mean being absent from work for anywhere from a few days to several weeks or months. Having a completed injury report on file is especially important if a claim needs to be filed with workers' compensation authorities or for insurance purposes.

An injury report should include the following:

- your name,
- the time and date of the injury and the time and date it was reported,
- the sequence of events leading up to the injury (e.g., where it occurred, what you were doing when it happened, and if equipment was involved),
- the type of incident (e.g., a fall, strain or overexertion, exposure to a substance via splashing or fumes, a child's bite, etc.),
- the nature and extent of the injury (e.g., scratching, bruising, bleeding),
- the names of adult witnesses,
- possible contributing conditions or factors (e.g., unsafe equipment, inadequate adult-to-child ratio, inadequate lighting, an unsafe surface or activity),
- the name of the person notified about the incident,
- first aid, if administered,
- the doctor's name and contact information, if a doctor was seen, and
- other treatment (if required).

The *Injury report form* used for children may also be used for staff. A line diagram can be used, if necessary, to indicate where on the body the injury occurred. Child care practitioners should report an injury to their employer within 72 hours. (For more about reporting injuries, see Chapter 5, *Keeping Children Safe*.)

Major injuries must be reported to the appropriate government agency, usually the provincial/territorial department of labour, within a specified time. This time limit varies across Canada, so you should find out what it is for your jurisdiction. Major injuries are those serious enough to require long-term recovery or to cause permanent physical disability or even death. If a child care facility is covered by workers' compensation, the injury should be reported

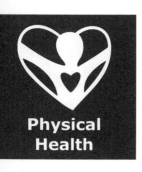

Physical Health

Employer self-assessment

To protect staff from workplace injury, do we:

1. Observe proper adult-to-child ratios at all times?
2. Provide orientation and in-service training in proper lifting techniques?
3. Provide orientation and in-service training in hazardous material handling and product safety?
4. Respond promptly to reported inadequacies in work space, equipment and furnishings?
5. Complete workplace injury reports in a timely and detailed manner?
6. Analyze each occurrence of injury and take measures to prevent recurrence?
7. Check equipment and spaces regularly to ensure they are safe and in good repair?

Employee self-assessment

To protect myself and others from workplace injury, do I:

1. Observe proper adult-to-child ratios at all times?
2. Practice proper lifting techniques?

immediately to that office as well. Check with your provincial/territorial child care office for specific directives on reporting.

Infections

Child care practitioners, especially those caring for children under 2 years of age, are exposed to many contagious germs. Routine practices, especially hand hygiene, are always the first and best protection against infections commonly found in child care settings. Immunization has also made it possible to protect child care practitioners, their co-workers and the children in their care from several illnesses.

Immunization and testing recommendations

Before starting work in a child care program, all staff, students and volunteers should be immunized according to the schedule recommended for the general adult population. For a current schedule, see the Public Health Agency of Canada website (www.phac-aspc.gc.ca). In many jurisdictions, tuberculosis (TB) screening is also required. A child care facility may require new employees to have a general medical examination. In some jurisdictions, the facility is also liable to pay for this examination and should be billed by the doctor accordingly.

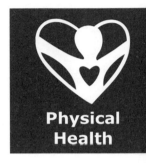

Physical Health

Standard immunization requirements for prospective child care practitioners are as follows:

1. Proof that immunizations against diphtheria, tetanus, polio and pertussis are up-to-date, with tetanus–diphtheria (as Td or dTap) received within the last 10 years and at least one dose of dTap received in adulthood.
2. Documentation of one MMR (measles, mumps and rubella) vaccination if a prospective child care employee was born after 1970. A laboratory-confirmed proof of immunity against these diseases is also acceptable.
3. Documentation of two doses of chickenpox (varicella) vaccine or a doctor's documentation of the person having had chickenpox or laboratory-confirmed proof of immunity against chickenpox.
4. Documentation of a negative TB skin test. Some child care facilities require a two-step skin test, to screen out false negative results. Two tests are completed 1 to 4 weeks apart, with the second test being the true result. Before beginning work in child care, a person testing positive must undergo further assessment and present a doctor's note confirming that active TB has been ruled out.
5. Annual influenza vaccine if the child care practitioner will be caring for children under 24 months of age or children with chronic diseases.

A prospective staff member may request an exemption from vaccination requirements for religious, philosophical or medical reasons. The employee needs to make this request in writing in cases of religious or philosophical objections, or must provide a doctor's note explaining the medical reasons for an exemption. These documents are kept in an employee's personal file and, if required, forwarded to the local public health unit. The facility must warn exempted employees that, if exposure to a vaccine-preventable illness occurs, they will be considered an infection risk (both to themselves and to children) and may be automatically excluded until the risk of infection has passed or public health authorities declare an outbreak to be over. Child care employers with questions or concerns about an applicant's immunization record or immune status may consult their local public health unit for guidance.

In addition to routine immunizations, there are a number of optional but recommended vaccinations. It is recommended that child care practitioners receive the following:

- **Hepatitis A vaccine**, especially in programs serving vulnerable communities (e.g., in rural or remote areas with inadequate water or sewage purification systems). A child care practitioner would receive two doses of hepatitis A vaccine, given 6 to 12 months apart.
- **Hepatitis B vaccine**, especially in programs where children whose families have come from countries where hepatitis B is common are present, or in communities where hepatitis B is common. The usual adult schedule is three doses: one at the first visit, a second one month later, and a final dose 6 months after that. Follow-up testing for antibody response may also be necessary to verify immunity.
- **Booster shots for mumps and measles.** While vaccines protecting against both these illnesses are universally administered in early childhood under the routine schedule, a booster shot may be required for those who received only one dose. Local public health recommendations should be followed. Child care practitioners can ask their doctor for advice.

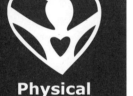

Physical Health

Employer self-assessment

To protect the health of our staff and prevent illness, do we:

1. Maintain complete and up-to-date immunization records for all staff?
2. Provide orientation and in-service training in:
   - infection control strategies (i.e., routine practices)?
   - safe food handling and preparation?
3. Provide appropriate space, equipment and time for staff to follow hand-hygiene, diapering and toileting protocols?
4. Post these protocols prominently in the relevant areas?

Employee self-assessment

To protect my co-workers and children from illness, do I:

1. Keep my immunizations completely up-to-date?
2. Get my annual influenza vaccine?
3. Follow hand-hygiene, diapering and toileting protocols at all times?

ALERT

Some vaccines contain a live, attenuated (weakened) form of the virus that they protect against and **are not** given to pregnant women or to children or adults whose immune system has been seriously weakened by another condition. These vaccines include:

- chickenpox,
- measles,
- mumps,
- rubella.

Women receiving these vaccines should avoid becoming pregnant for 4 weeks after vaccination. Preventive treatment of child care staff or community contacts with immune globulin (Ig) after a known exposure to chickenpox or measles is usually effective, providing it is given in time.

Keep copies of immunization records or proof of immune status on file for all employees, both past and present. These records need to be made available to public health authorities in the event of an outbreak or if concerns arise about an individual's exposure to a particular infection.

Guidelines for exclusion of employees with infections

As discussed in Chapter 8, *Preventing Infections*, every child care program should have a written illness policy that specifies when child care practitioners should be excluded. These guidelines are shared with new employees. The policy explains that a child care practitioner or other staff member will stay away from work if she:

- cannot fulfill her responsibilities because her illness compromises the care of the children.
- is sick with a respiratory infection. Facility supervisors should encourage an ailing staff member to stay home to prevent the spread of illness.
- has a gastrointestinal infection with diarrhea or vomiting.
- has any of the specific conditions requiring exclusion, listed in Appendix 9.2 (pages 225–34).

Occasionally, staff-to-child ratio requirements may determine that a child care practitioner who is feeling unwell with a mild respiratory or gastrointestinal infection needs to be at work. In that case, review and reinforce routine practices, especially hand hygiene, to help prevent the spread of germs. Those with respiratory infections must wash their hands after any contact with respiratory secretions or used tissues, and cover all coughs and sneezes. Those with gastrointestinal infections must practice meticulous hand hygiene after using the toilet and should not prepare or serve food on site.

The definition of an "outbreak" of infectious illness can depend on the type of illness, as well as normal seasonal variations and provincial/territorial guidelines. If you suspect an outbreak:

- Determine how many staff and children have similar symptoms. Include those who are absent in your count if they may be ill at home.
- Consult your local public health unit for guidance.

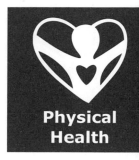

Physical Health

Infections of concern to child care practitioners who are of childbearing age or pregnant

While the following infections may cause severe disease in any adult, they are of special concern in pregnancy. Child care practitioners who are or may become pregnant should already be immunized against the vaccine-preventable infections that pose a risk to an unborn baby, such as rubella, chickenpox, mumps and measles. However, if they are unsure of their immune status for these specific infections, they should ask their doctor for antibody testing.

Chickenpox: The majority of Canadians have had chickenpox in childhood and are therefore immune to the disease. However, the dormant virus can cause shingles later on. Children or co-workers who are not immune can get chickenpox from contact with chickenpox or shingles. Adults who get chickenpox may become very ill. In addition, contracting chickenpox in the first half of pregnancy can pose serious risks to fetal health. A woman considering pregnancy can be tested for immunity and—if found to be susceptible—vaccinated against chickenpox. She should avoid becoming pregnant for 4 weeks after vaccination and should not receive the vaccine if she is already pregnant.

Her non-immune partner and other household contacts should be immunized at the same time. A non-immune pregnant woman should be encouraged to be vaccinated as soon as possible after her baby is born. She can still breastfeed her baby.

If you suspect that an exposure to chickenpox or shingles has occurred, be sure to:

- Follow all protocols set out in Chapter 9, *Managing Infections*.
- Advise non-immune non-pregnant staff or parents to be vaccinated against chickenpox immediately.
- Advise non-immune pregnant staff or parents to consult a doctor immediately.
- Advise non-immune employees with a weakened immune system, who are at risk of severe chickenpox, to consult a doctor as soon as possible. These individuals can be treated with immune globulin (Ig) containing a high concentration of antibody against chickenpox (varicella-zoster Ig) to prevent the disease or make it less severe. However, this must be given within 4 days (96 hours) of initial contact to be effective.
- Exclude a child care practitioner with chickenpox until the lesions have all dried and crusted, unless they can be covered with a secure dressing.

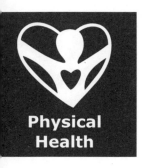

Physical Health

Rubella (German measles): Rubella is rarely seen in Canada thanks to immunization. However, if a non-immune mother is exposed to this disease in the first 3 months of pregnancy, it can pose serious risks to fetal health. A woman considering pregnancy can be tested for immunity and—if found to be susceptible—vaccinated against rubella. Because the rubella vaccine contains a live, attenuated (weakened) form of the virus, vaccination should be done at least 4 weeks before conception. If rubella is diagnosed in your child care community:

- Follow all protocols set out in Chapter 9, *Managing Infections*.
- Advise non-immune non-pregnant staff or parents to be vaccinated against rubella immediately.
- Advise non-immune pregnant staff or parents to consult a doctor immediately.
- Encourage a pregnant woman who has not been vaccinated against rubella to be immunized as soon as possible after her baby is born. She can still breastfeed her baby.
- If an infant is diagnosed with congenital rubella syndrome (acquired in the womb), refer the issue of exclusion (where non-immunized staff or parents are present) to the treating physician, who will decide on a case-by-case basis.

Mumps: Most people are immune to mumps, either from having had the illness in childhood or from receiving MMR vaccine. However, outbreaks do occur among adolescents and young adults, many of whom have received only one dose of the vaccine. Exposure to mumps in the first 3 months of pregnancy may increase the risk of miscarriage. A woman considering pregnancy can be tested for immunity and—if found to be susceptible—vaccinated against mumps, at least 4 weeks before conception. Her non-immune partner and other household contacts should be immunized at the same time. If mumps is diagnosed in your child care community:

- Follow all protocols set out in Chapter 9, *Managing Infections*.
- Advise non-immune non-pregnant staff or parents to be vaccinated against mumps immediately.

- Advise non-immune pregnant staff or parents to consult a doctor immediately.
- Encourage a pregnant woman who has not been vaccinated against mumps to be immunized as soon as possible after her baby is born. She can still breastfeed her baby.

Measles: Most people are immune to measles, either from having had the illness in childhood or from receiving MMR vaccine. However, outbreaks do occur among adolescents and young adults, many of whom have received only one dose of the vaccine. Measles causes severe disease in pregnant women and increases the risk of premature delivery. A woman considering pregnancy can be tested for immunity and—if found to be susceptible—vaccinated against measles, at least 4 weeks before conception. Her non-immune partner and other household contacts should be immunized at the same time. If measles is diagnosed in your child care community:

- Follow all protocols set out in Chapter 9, *Managing Infections*.
- Advise non-immune non-pregnant staff or parents to be vaccinated against measles immediately. Treatment with immune globulin (Ig) may be mandated by public health authorities.
- Advise non-immune pregnant staff or parents to consult a doctor immediately.
- Encourage a pregnant woman who has not been vaccinated against measles to be immunized as soon as possible after her baby is born. She can still breastfeed her baby.
- Exclude a non-immune child care practitioner for 2 weeks after the onset of a rash in the last case in the facility, unless she was vaccinated within 72 hours of the first exposure.

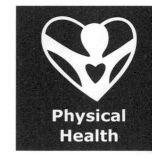

Physical Health

Hepatitis B virus (HBV): HBV is preventable by vaccination. All children in Canada are immunized either in infancy or at school. Child care practitioners may not be immune if they were born in Canada before the routine hepatitis B vaccination programs started or in a country where the vaccine is not given routinely.

The incidence of HBV transmission in child care settings is extremely low, and infection is preventable through routine practices. A child care practitioner who is bitten hard enough to break the skin, or whose non-intact skin or mucous membranes (e.g., nose, mouth) are exposed to blood or bloody body fluids without the protection of gloves or other barriers, should consult a doctor immediately. (See Chapter 9, *Managing Infections*.) Notify your local public health unit if any child care practitioner is bitten by a child and the skin is broken.

All expectant mothers are tested for HBV during an early prenatal visit, because HBV can pass from mother to child during pregnancy, regardless of whether the mother has an active form of the disease or no symptoms. Steps can then be taken to protect the baby.

REMEMBER

A blood-borne illness such as hepatitis B or C or HIV **cannot** be transmitted from person to person by child care activities such as changing diapers or clothing, toileting, nose blowing, feeding, washing hands and faces, holding hands or hugging. These infections can be spread only by direct contact (e.g., through a mucous membrane or open wound) with blood or body fluids containing the virus.

Source: Region of Peel (Ont.) Public Health, *Keep on Track: A Health and Resource Guide for Child Care Providers in Peel.* Adapted with permission.

Child care practitioners are **not** required to disclose their HBV status, but if an employee chooses to do so, a facility must do the following:

- Treat this information as absolutely confidential. That means it can be shared only with the caregiver's express permission.
- Make sure all staff are trained in routine practices to prevent the transmission of blood-borne diseases, and use them in any situation where blood or body fluids are involved.
- Ensure that all staff keep skin sores or lesions covered.
- Ask if the caregiver needs information or guidance on personal precautions that are necessary to prevent transmitting HBV to others. (See *Selected resources* for Chapter 9, *Managing Infections*.)
- Advise the caregiver to be vaccinated against hepatitis A.

There are antiviral treatments available for chronic HBV.

Hepatitis C virus (HCV): There have been no reports of HCV infection as a result of exposure in child care. Child care practitioners are **not** required to disclose their HCV status, but if an employee chooses to do so, a facility must take all of the steps set out for HBV (above), plus the following:

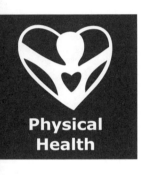

Physical Health

- Advise a staff member diagnosed with HCV to be vaccinated against hepatitis A and B.
- If a woman discloses her HCV status, ask if she needs information or guidance on personal precautions that are necessary to prevent transmitting HCV to others, including her baby, during pregnancy or while breastfeeding. The risk of transmission is low unless she is also infected with HIV, and there are no known measures to prevent transmission at present. (See *Selected resources* for Chapter 9, *Managing Infections*.)

Antiviral treatments are available for chronic HCV. There is no vaccine against HCV at this time.

Human immunodeficiency virus (HIV): There have been no reports of HIV infection as a result of exposure in child care. HIV is not very infectious and does not spread as a result of everyday contacts in the home, child care facility or school. It can be passed from an infected pregnant woman to her baby before or during birth, or by breastfeeding. Child care practitioners are **not** required to disclose their HIV status, but if an employee chooses to reveal that she is HIV-positive, a facility must take all of the steps set out for HBV (above), plus the following:

- Be aware that this employee may have a weakened immune system and may be more vulnerable to infection than others. She may also need longer to recover from illness.
- If a woman discloses her HIV status, ask if she needs information or guidance on personal precautions that are necessary to prevent transmitting HIV to others,

including her baby, during pregnancy or delivery or afterward. (See *Selected resources* for Chapter 9, *Managing Infections*.)

There are effective antiviral treatments for HIV. There is no vaccine against HIV at this time.

Pertussis (whooping cough): Outbreaks of pertussis still occur in child care settings where the immunization of children and staff is not adequate. Women in their third trimester of pregnancy are considered at risk, because forceful coughing may bring on labour prematurely. If pertussis is diagnosed in your child care community:

- Follow all protocols set out in Chapter 9, *Managing Infections*.
- Advise non-immune pregnant staff or parents to consult a doctor immediately. Vaccination and/or antibiotic treatment may be required.

Parvovirus B19: Parvovirus B19 (also known as fifth disease, erythema infectiosum or "slapped cheek" syndrome) is an infection that is very common in child care settings and the general community and that poses a measure of risk to fetal health. Routine practices, especially hand hygiene, effectively prevent child-to-caregiver transmission of this infection. It is not vaccine-preventable.

In adults, parvovirus B19 occasionally produces the lace-like rash that is so characteristic in children. In addition, adults may have arthritic symptoms that can persist for months. If a child care practitioner has a weakened immune system or a chronic form of anemia (e.g., sickle cell disease), this infection can be more severe. About half of women of childbearing age have had parvovirus B19 in early life and, having developed protective antibodies, will not be reinfected if they are exposed again. However, if a woman is infected with parvovirus B19 for the first time during pregnancy, there is a small risk that her infant will be affected *in utero*.

Parvovirus B19 is so pervasive in the community that, if it is diagnosed in your child care setting, the routine exclusion of non-immune pregnant staff is neither practical nor recommended. The following steps should be taken:

- Follow all protocols set out in Chapter 9, *Managing Infections*.
- Advise pregnant staff or parents to consult a doctor. If they do not know their immune status, antibody testing can be done.
- Review and reinforce routine practices with all staff.
- If you have children or adults in your program whose immune system may be weakened, consult your local public health unit for guidance.

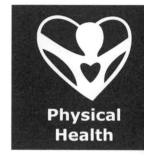

Physical Health

BEST PRACTICE

The best way to assess your risk and prevent exposure to any of these infections in a child care setting is to seek health counselling before becoming pregnant. Determine your immune status if you are unsure. If a blood test shows you are susceptible, consult your doctor about the best time to be immunized for a vaccine-preventable illness. For an infection for which there is no vaccine, find out what steps you can take to minimize exposure in the workplace. Usually, following routine practices is all it takes to protect both you and your baby.

While routine practices are considered effective protection against the spread of parvovirus B19, there is no treatment for this infection.

Cytomegalovirus (CMV): CMV is a common virus that can have serious effects on fetal health if a first infection occurs in the early stages of pregnancy. There is a risk that an infant will be infected *in utero*, and 5 to 15 per cent of affected infants will have serious disease at birth. There is also a small risk associated with re-exposure during pregnancy. Approximately 5 per cent of affected infants have mild but lasting effects, including moderate hearing loss and/or a developmental delay. Routine practices, especially hand hygiene, effectively prevent child-to-caregiver transmission of this infection. It is not vaccine-preventable.

CMV infection is already so pervasive in the community that, if it is diagnosed in your child care setting, the routine exclusion of pregnant staff is neither practical nor recommended. The following steps should be taken:

- Follow all protocols set out in Chapter 9, *Managing Infections*.
- Advise pregnant staff or parents to consult a doctor. If they do not know their immune status, antibody testing can be done.
- Review and reinforce routine practices with all staff, especially the need for proper hand hygiene after contact with saliva or urine.
- Review and reinforce toileting protocols with all staff, especially the need for careful handling and disposal of soiled diapers.
- Remind staff to avoid oral contact with children's saliva (e.g., kissing on the mouth).

Other infections of concern to child care practitioners

Hepatitis A virus (HAV): Child care programs can actually accelerate the spread of HAV in a community because infected children often have no symptoms. Their caregivers get much sicker, and the first sign of an outbreak is usually a child care practitioner with symptoms. If you suspect HAV, you need to confirm the diagnosis and notify your local public health unit immediately. All staff will need to be vaccinated or have a blood test to determine their immune status. Be sure to:

- Follow all protocols set out in Chapter 9, *Managing Infections*.
- Exclude the staff member diagnosed with HAV for at least one week after the onset of the illness, unless all children and staff have received preventive treatment.
- Ensure there is no sharing of towels and facecloths.
- Review and reinforce proper hand-hygiene, toileting and food-handling routines.

ALERT

The presence of pets in the workplace may cause difficulties for child care practitioners who are pregnant. For example, toxoplasmosis, an infection transmitted by contact with cat feces, is a risk for the fetus, especially in the first trimester. Long-time cat owners are usually immune, but it's best to take precautions. Avoid touching cat feces in the garden or sandbox, and delegate the cleaning of a litter box, as dust heightens the risk of exposure. If you must do these tasks, be sure to wear gloves.

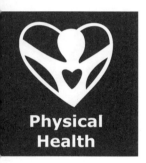

Physical Health

- Watch children and staff for symptoms and ask parents to report if they or any household members develop symptoms of HAV.

There is only a short period after exposure (one week) when vaccine can effectively prevent the spread of HAV. If more than one week but less than two has elapsed since exposure, or if a caregiver has a weakened immune system because of another condition, immune globulin (Ig) is given. Several provinces are considering a switch from hepatitis B vaccine to a combined vaccine for hepatitis A and B for school-based immunization programs.

Tuberculosis (TB): A caregiver with active pulmonary TB can infect children and co-workers in a child care setting, which is why testing is a condition of employment in many jurisdictions. In communities where local public health authorities have concerns about the presence or prevalence of pulmonary TB, periodic tuberculin skin testing may be routine. Pregnancy is not a reason to avoid a skin test. Any caregiver with a positive skin test, whether pregnant or not, must be referred to a doctor for evaluation. A child care practitioner found to have active TB should be excluded until treatment is completed and she has been declared non-infectious by a doctor.

For more about specific infections, see Chapter 9, *Managing Infections*.

Occupational health services

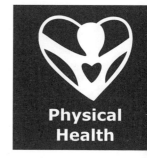

Physical Health

Promoting physical health in child care involves education for child care practitioners and easy access to occupational health services. Although far from being the norm in Canada, some child care centres or umbrella groups of facilities have an occupational health program that supports and protects staff and promotes health, such as offering fitness and nutrition counselling, heightening awareness of drug, alcohol or substance abuse, or helping staff to stop smoking. In these programs, health professionals (e.g., psychologists, occupational therapists, dietitians) may help child care practitioners to assess, prevent and treat work- and sometimes non-work-related health problems.

An occupational health program in child care can promote physical health by:

- providing training, counselling, health assessments, treatment and rehabilitation, as needed,
- communicating new public health information, or changes to safety regulations and standards, and helping to ensure full compliance,
- ensuring that individuals receive one-on-one counselling and/or medical care for work-related trauma or illness, as needed, and
- helping to protect staff against possible workplace health hazards, such as an infection or environmental exposure.

Some programs provide primary health care services for employees. A good occupational health program focuses on personal development, as well as the work environment.

To find out whether occupational health services are available for specific child care facilities, contact your provincial/territorial department of labour or the Canadian Centre for Occupational Health and Safety. (See *Selected resources* at the end of this chapter.)

Program directors' policies to protect and support staff health

Far more prevalent in Canada than occupational health services for child care practitioners are the basic administrative policies that program directors develop and share with their community. Policies that help to ensure the physical health of child care practitioners include:

- clear, fair and inclusive hiring practices, with specific provisions for applicants or staff who have a physical challenge,
- compensation for illness or injury,
- clear guidelines for work restriction (e.g., light duties) and possible exclusion for pregnant or injured workers,
- access to health education and counselling for all staff,
- regular assessment of the workplace for potential safety/health hazards,
- strategies for preventing and managing infections that are communicated and reinforced,
- routine reporting of workplace injuries and illnesses,
- regular maintenance of employee health records, and
- a strict policy of confidentiality where health records are concerned.

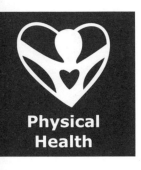

Physical Health

> ### Pregnant employee self-assessment
>
> To protect my own health and that of the child I am carrying:
>
> 1. Do I practice medically recommended precautions when performing physical duties at work (e.g., not carrying heavy loads, resting more often, avoiding exposure to household cleaning products)?
> 2. Am I aware of the terms and conditions of my maternity leave, if I take one?

Hiring practices and equal opportunity: Everyone has the right to work. This basic principle has driven Canadian legislation promoting equal opportunity for people with and without disabilities. It is discriminatory to disqualify a person from working in a child care setting on the basis of a physical impairment, unless it can be shown that the impairment puts co-workers or children at risk or prevents the individual from doing her job.

No clear standards of "fitness for work" have been established for the child care field. However, determining suitability would depend on answers to three questions:

1. Is the applicant capable of performing essential child care tasks?
2. Is this person put at physical risk by the nature of child care work?
3. Does this person pose a physical risk to children or co-workers?

While interviewing prospective employees, a facility director should discuss potential job hazards, such as the amount of lifting, carrying and holding required, and the demands of the daily cleaning routines.

A health review for new child care employees is often required by the employing facility or provincial/territorial regulations, but only once employment has been confirmed. To ensure objectivity, a doctor shouldn't be asked to complete a health review form until after a child care practitioner is hired.

The following steps are recommended:

- The employee has a health review form completed by a doctor, usually within two weeks of hiring. In regions where a health review or records of immunization are required by law, your local public health unit may have developed a specific health review form that needs to be completed.
- The employee returns a copy of the form to an occupational health professional, if this service is available, or to the local public health unit affiliated with the child care facility, who reviews the medical information and may recommend follow-up counselling, treatment or training. In the absence of such a person or service, the facility's director assumes this responsibility.

The health review form is kept in the employee's confidential personal file. File maintenance is the responsibility of the occupational health professional, the local public health unit or, in the absence of these authorities, the facility's director.

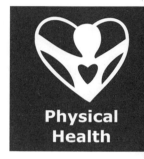

Physical Health

Self-assessment for an employee with an injury or disability

1. Does my disability require physical accommodation in the workplace?
2. Do I use workplace adaptations or accommodations to support my needs?
3. Have I made my employer aware of how best to support my needs?
4. If so, does my employer follow through on supporting my needs?

Compensation for illness or injury: Having to take time away from work due to injury, illness or surgery can have serious financial implications. Knowing which steps to take first—and promptly—in the event of an interruption of work can help minimize financial hardship. Child care facilities typically provide staff with sick leave as an employee benefit. But if the time away from work extends beyond the employee's allotted sick leave, a child care practitioner's options are limited.

After a specific term of work, Canadian workers are eligible for Employment Insurance (EI) Special Benefits, including sickness benefits, payable for up to 15 weeks to a maximum of 60 per cent of a worker's insurable earnings. These benefits are based on income from the last 20 weeks worked. There is a standard waiting period before payment begins, usually 2 weeks, and a child care practitioner may be back at work within this time. If the effects of injury or illness extend beyond the eligible number of weeks, EI Special Benefits payments will stop. In that case, the following options may be open to child care practitioners.

Workers' compensation is a provincial/territorial program. In some jurisdictions, participation in the program is voluntary, while in others it is compulsory. This relationship changes if the child care centre is affiliated with a corporate or institutional employer. Whether an employer contributes to the program or not, staff should be aware of their rights and responsibilities as employees.

Disability insurance is a benefit offered by insurance companies across Canada, although premiums for individuals are expensive. Group plans usually have lower premiums. Unfortunately, many child care centres don't employ enough people to qualify for a group disability insurance plan. However, it is sometimes possible to obtain coverage through a professional association. A regional association might serve as an umbrella group, where a child care practitioner's membership fee includes the premium for a disability insurance plan.

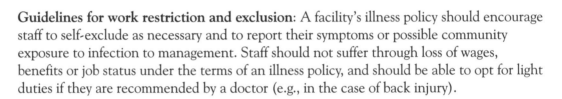

Employer self-assessment

To promote the health of staff, do we:

1. Provide a medical plan?
2. Provide a short- or long-term disability insurance plan?
3. Make staff fully aware of the benefits included under both plans?
4. Have a clear policy on when staff should stay home, and encourage them to do so when necessary?

Employee self-assessment

1. Am I familiar with the terms of my medical and/or disability plan?
2. Do I abide by the facility's illness policy?
3. Am I aware of what benefits I may be entitled to in the event of illness or injury?
4. Do I know whom to contact if I have questions about coverage?
5. Do I know what to do if I need to be off work for an extended period of time?

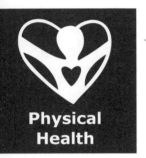

Physical Health

Guidelines for work restriction and exclusion: A facility's illness policy should encourage staff to self-exclude as necessary and to report their symptoms or possible community exposure to infection to management. Staff should not suffer through loss of wages, benefits or job status under the terms of an illness policy, and should be able to opt for light duties if they are recommended by a doctor (e.g., in the case of back injury).

Access to health education and counselling: Health counselling is especially important for women considering pregnancy and for workers with chronic medical conditions. Workplace support and assistance for child care practitioners with a physical disability should also be readily available. Workers suffering from job-related stress should be referred to an occupational health therapist or a doctor for assessment and counselling. Staff members who miss work frequently due to illness should also see a doctor. Where no occupational health professional is available, a local public health unit or personal physician can help with access to counselling services.

Maintenance of employee health records: Ideally, an occupational health professional would maintain current health records for all staff working at a child care facility or —better still—at a group of facilities. A more centralized health record system would make it easier for an occupational health professional to identify a pattern of outbreak for a particular infection, for example, and to coordinate a response with public health authorities. However, most often it is facility directors who maintain their former and current employees' immunization and health records and track time away from work due to illness or injury.

Under Canadian law, maintaining health information is largely the responsibility of those who collect it. Employers have a responsibility to keep records current and transferable. Child care practitioners have a right to the medical information in their records but not to the documents themselves. Many legal issues involving the preservation and disposal of health records have yet to be resolved, such as the number of years a facility is obligated to keep them secure.

Confidentiality: Under current privacy laws, an employer has the right to know whether an employee's state of health might affect her ability to do a particular job. However, an employer does not have the right to access private information about the nature of that person's disability or health problem. No information about the employee should be given to the employer without the employee's consent, unless the employee poses a risk to the public or to co-workers. Medical, including psychological, information can be given to a third party only with the written consent of the child care practitioner, to comply with a court order, or to comply with public health authorities in emergency situations. While the records themselves may belong to a child care facility, anyone having access to these records has an ethical obligation to ensure their absolute confidentiality.

The results of any medical examination should be communicated clearly to the person(s) examined, particularly if ongoing observation or treatment is required. Voluntary examinations are the norm, except where a risk to public health is at issue. Any occupational hazard identified as a result of an examination should be communicated clearly to both the employee and the employer, so that preventive measures can be taken.

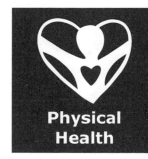

Physical Health

The need for an employer to collect information is balanced by an employee's right to privacy. For most personal employee information, including health, pay and benefit records, the following basic rules, listed on the federal government's privacy website (www.privcom. gc.ca), help to keep that balance:

- An employer must specify what personal information it collects from employees, why it is collected, and what is done with this information.
- The collection, use or disclosure of personal information should normally be done only with an employee's knowledge and consent.
- An employer may collect only the personal information that is necessary for its stated purpose, and must collect it by fair and lawful means.
- An employer may use or disclose personal information solely for the purpose for which it was collected, and must keep this information in a secure place for the term specified by provincial/territorial regulations, unless the employer obtains the employee's express consent to do something else with the information or is legally required to use or disclose it for another purpose.
- An employee's personal information must be accurate, complete and up-to-date.
- An employee must be able to access personal information, and be able to challenge its accuracy and completeness.

Healthy living

While facility directors and occupational health services have a vital role to play in promoting workplace health, healthy living is primarily a personal responsibility. Whether you work in a child care centre or home setting, periodic self-assessment can provide a simple reality check of your own physical well-being or of working conditions that may be affecting you physically. Self-awareness and a timely adjustment of your environment, lifestyle or work habits will often prevent potential health problems. Consider the following questions once each season.

Track your healthy living habits

1. Do I maintain a healthy diet according to *Canada's Food Guide*?
2. Do I get enough exercise? According to *Canada's Guide to Physical Activity*, that means a total of at least one hour of physical activity every day.
3. Do I get between 7 and 8 hours of sleep each night?
4. Do I live smoke-free?
5. Do I limit my alcohol intake to one drink per day (for women) or two drinks per day (for men)?
6. Do I have regular medical checkups?
7. Do I have any unexplained discomforts, aches or pains that I haven't had checked by a doctor?
8. Are my immunizations completely up-to-date?
9. Have I received my annual influenza vaccine?
10. Do I follow routine practices at all times?

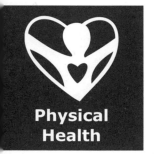

Physical Health

Workplace health and quality care

Promoting the health and well-being of child care practitioners in a setting designed or organized with their needs in mind has benefits far beyond comfort or convenience. Child–staff interaction, job satisfaction and staff retention levels all benefit from proactive and conscientious workplace health policies.

Selected resources

Baker, Carol J., Ed. 2007. *Red Book Atlas of Pediatric Infectious Diseases.* Elk Grove, IL: American Academy of Pediatrics. www.aap.org

Beach, Jane and Martha Friendly. 2005. Child care centre physical environments. Childcare Resource and Research Unit. An overview of research on physical environments in child care settings and regulations pertaining to physical environments in each jurisdiction in Canada. www.childcarequality.ca

Best Start and the Canadian Partnership for Children's Health and Environment. 2006. *Playing it safe: Service provider strategies to reduce environmental risks to preconception, prenatal and child health.* Toronto, Ont.: Best Start. www.beststart.org

Canadian Centre for Occupational Health and Safety. 2007. Back injury prevention. www.ccohs.ca. Site features courses and publications on workplace health and safety. Also information on federal/provincial/territorial legislation pertaining to occupational health and safety and contact information for each jurisdiction.

Canadian Child Care Federation. 2005. *Children's environmental health learning kit.* Ottawa, Ont.: CCCF. Includes research paper, articles, workshops. www.cccf.fcsge.ca

———. 2002. "Back injury and stress," by M. Mercer. *Interaction* 16(3): 29-31.

The Canadian Paediatric Society's website for parents and caregivers, Caring for Kids, has parent notes and information about the infections and immunizations discussed in this chapter. These can be downloaded at www.caringforkids.cps.ca and shared with families and child care staff.

Canadian Paediatric Society. 3rd ed., 2006. *Your Child's Best Shot: A Parent's Guide to Vaccination*. Ottawa, Ont.: Canadian Paediatric Society.

Canadian Partnership for Children's Health and Environment. 2005. *Child health and the environment: A primer*. Toronto, Ont.: CPCHE. www.healthyenvironmentforkids.ca

Centre for the Child Care Workforce (U.S.). www.ccw.org

Chandler, Karen. 3rd ed., 2008. *Administering for Quality: Canadian Early Childhood Development Programs*. Toronto, Ont.: Pearson Education.

Child Care Connection Nova Scotia. 2000. Universal classification standard work description for early childhood care teachers. www.ccns.org

Child Care Human Resources Sector Council. www.ccsc-cssge.ca

Harms, Thelma, Richard M. Clifford and Debby Cryer. 2nd ed., 2005. *Early Childhood Environment Rating Scale*. New York, NY: Teachers College Press.

Health Canada, Workplace Hazardous Materials Information System (WHMIS). www.hc-sc.gc.ca

Labour Canada, Workplace health and safety. www.labour.gc.ca
Federal laws, regulations, policies and standards and general information on prevention of workplace injuries.

Manitoba Child Care Association. 2007. *Human Resource Management Guide for Early Childhood Programs*. Winnipeg, Man.: MCCA. Includes a chapter on workplace health and safety. www.mccahouse.org

Melnik, Michael S., H. Duane Saunders and Robin Saunders. 1998. *Managing Back Pain: Self-help Manual*. Chaska, MN: Saunders Group.

National Advisory Committee on Immunization. 7th ed., 2006. *Canadian Immunization Guide*. Ottawa, Ont.: Public Health Agency of Canada. www.phac-aspc.gc.ca

Pimento, Barbara and Deborah Kernested. 4th ed., 2009. *Healthy Foundations in Early Childhood Settings*. Scarborough, Ont.: Nelson Education.

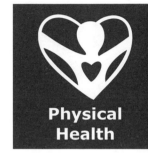

Physical Health

Provincial/territorial health and safety

Alberta
Workplace Health and Safety
Alberta Human Resources and Employment
General inquiries: (780) 415-8690; Workplace Health and Safety Call Centre: 1-866-415-8690
www.gov.ab.ca/hre/whs

British Columbia
Workers' Compensation Board of British Columbia
Health and Safety questions: (604) 276-3100; 1-888-621-SAFE (7233)
General inquiries: (604) 273-2266
www.worksafebc.com

Manitoba
Workplace Safety and Health Division
Manitoba Labour and Immigration
General inquiries: (204) 945-3446; 1-800-282-8069
www.gov.mb.ca/labour/safety

New Brunswick
Workplace Health, Safety and Compensation Commission of New Brunswick
General inquiries: (506) 453-2467; 1-800-442-9776 (from NB only)
www.whscc.nb.ca

Newfoundland and Labrador
Occupational Health and Safety Branch
Department of Government Services
General inquiries: (709) 729-7420; 1-800-563-5471 (in NL only)
www.gs.gov.nl.ca/ohs

Northwest Territories and Nunavut
Workers' Compensation Board of the Northwest Territories and Nunavut
General inquiries: (867) 920-3888; 1-800-661-0792
www.wcb.nt.ca

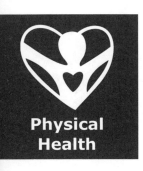

Physical Health

Nova Scotia
Occupational Health & Safety Division
NS Department of Labour and Workforce Development
General inquiries: (902) 424-5400; 1-800-9-LABOUR [1-800-952-2687] (in NS only)
www.gov.ns.ca/lwd/ohs

Ontario
Occupational Health and Safety Branch
Ministry of Labour
General inquiries: 1-800-268-8013 (in Ont. only)
www.labour.gov.on.ca/english/hs

Prince Edward Island
Occupational Health and Safety Division
Workers' Compensation Board
General inquiries: (902) 368-5680; 1-800-237-5049 (in PEI only)
www.wcb.pe.ca

Quebec
Commission de la santé et de la sécurité du travail du Québec
(Occupational Health and Safety Commission)
General inquiries: (514) 906-3060; 1-800-667-7585 (in QC only)
www.csst.qc.ca

Saskatchewan
Occupational Health and Safety Division
Saskatchewan Labour
General inquiries: (306) 787-4496; 1-800-567-7233
www.labour.gov.sk.ca

Yukon
Yukon Workers' Compensation, Health and Safety Board
Occupational Health and Safety Branch
General inquiries: (867) 667-5645; 1-800-661-0443
www.wcb.yk.ca

chapter

16

Caregivers' Emotional Health

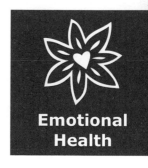

Emotional Health

Early childhood education and care is an important profession, and working with children and their families can be deeply rewarding. However, the very things that make the work so emotionally fulfilling—the close, personal relationships with children and parents, variety, stimulation and creativity—also pose unique challenges. Maintaining healthy daily routines for children is demanding, especially when combined with high activity, active supervision and the particular needs of each child and family.

Because you care so much about what you do, you may find yourself neglecting your own needs. However, emotional strength is the best asset you can bring to work every day. A healthy lifestyle, appropriate stress management, work–life balance, and a healthy and supportive working environment are all sources of emotional strength. Fortunately, they're also aspects of life over which you can exercise some control, at least most of the time. While Chapter 15, *Caregivers' Physical Health*, covers some physical aspects of working in child care, this chapter deals with emotional issues, recognizing that these two elements of professional life are closely intertwined.

Building professional self-confidence

Feeling that your profession is valued and respected is a crucial aspect of emotional well-being. Yet, working in child care often does not get the recognition or credit it deserves. Despite the tremendous societal value of what you do, accessing professional development, building community connections and fostering a sense of achievement in your field will probably depend as much on your own self-motivation as on external, societal or political support. This is true for both centre- and home-based child care practitioners.

Here are some steps you can take to build professional self-confidence:

1. Take time every day to think positively about yourself and your work. This means deliberately noticing the personal successes—even minor ones—that arise in almost any working day. If you keep a journal, jot them down. Taking note of your achievements helps to reinforce them, especially if you can determine why something you did worked well.
2. When you complete a task, give yourself a mental pat on the back. Focus on what gets done well in each day rather than on what is left undone. Accept that there will always be tasks left over, and keep your expectations realistic.
3. When a parent or a co-worker compliments your work, accept the praise and allow yourself to appreciate it. Let the person know how important positive feedback is and take the time to feel good about it.
4. Create an environment where everyone—children and staff—can receive and offer positive reinforcement. Strategies that help to build mutual support and appreciation among staff with different backgrounds, skills and abilities might include encouraging open discussion of these differences and finding ways to make them actively complementary—rather than competitive—in the workplace. Individual attempts to introduce new ideas into your program should be recognized and rewarded. This can even be done in a light and amusing way if things don't work out as well as anticipated. Create opportunities for staff to identify and express one another's strengths, and recognize special efforts and activities of staff members at meetings, when parents are present, or in other public ways. Celebrating the "small wins" and life passages of co-workers is important for staff morale, but save the biggest celebrations for achievements that were a team effort. People work best together when they feel valued as individuals, well informed and appreciated. An atmosphere of sharing, caring and cooperation among staff has the added benefit of modelling positive reinforcement for the children in your care.
5. Learn communication strategies (e.g., active listening, pausing for feedback) and styles (e.g., motivation interviewing, which is passive, eliciting and non-persuasive). Child care practitioners who develop and practice effective communication skills have lower stress levels.

A certain amount of conflict in any team is normal. By openly recognizing this, and presenting staff conflicts as opportunities to team-build by clarifying and solving a problem together, you can help defuse tension and keep expectations realistic.

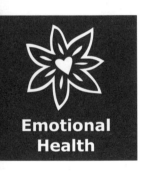

Emotional Health

6. Celebrate your strengths. Your patience, creativity, sense of fun and ability to multi-task, as well as your specialized training and communication skills, are all tremendous life assets. Whatever your strengths, sharing them outside of work and in the company of adults will affirm your professional self-esteem.

7. Promote respect for your profession. Share the value and rewards of child care not only with families connected with your program, but also with people less familiar with the field.

8. Look for professional development opportunities. Child care practitioners with an early childhood education diploma are eligible for further training through post-diploma programs in infant specialization, special needs, school-age programs and facility management/administration. The Canadian Child Care Federation (CCCF) has developed two guides to self-reflection for child care practitioners that can be used to evaluate a professional development plan. (See *Tools for Practitioners* in the *Selected resources* at the end of this chapter.) A practical plan sets achievable short-term objectives and long-term goals that are:

- regularly assessed for relevance,
- prioritized to have the most positive impact on your current practice, and
- adjusted to ensure continued progress.

9. Attend local workshops and conferences. They are forums for acquiring or updating skills, and for networking informally with other child care practitioners, sharing knowledge and learning how other child care programs operate.

10. Participate in professional organizations, locally, regionally and nationally. Child care associations provide support by advocating for higher standards, fair compensation and skills training. They also offer workshops, seminars and access to resources, and provide a sense of community in a profession that may feel isolating at times. You'll likely discover that many of the same issues you are facing are shared by others.

11. Maintain a healthy work–life balance.

Personal activities and leisure time are as important as the work you do. Balance work, play and rest. The quality of your care for children is enhanced by taking time for and caring for yourself.

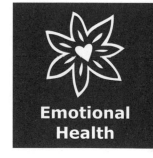

Emotional Health

Maintaining work–life balance

Relationship-building is at the core of child care. Child care practitioners care deeply about the well-being of children in their program and form close attachments with them and their families. The line between work and home life can easily blur, especially in home-based programs where work may spill over into personal life if parents are consistently late in picking up their children, or if your own family's needs conflict with program demands.

The CCCF's guides to self-reflection can help child care practitioners to evaluate their work–life balance. A proper balance allows you to nurture professional enthusiasm and share your expertise in the community, while:

- focusing on the positive and accepting the limitations inherent in your role,
- taking the time to "recharge" with people and activities outside of work,
- caring for your own physical and emotional needs,
- keeping expectations of yourself and others realistic, and
- learning to say "no" when demands on your time and energy are unreasonable.

For a child care practitioner in a home setting, interacting positively and effectively between your home and work roles involves the members of your own family, to the extent that:

- they understand and support your responsibilities,
- they are given opportunities to participate in your work (e.g., for special outings, family nights),
- their needs are considered when you plan programming, and
- they are kept "in the loop" as events, issues and routines arise or change.

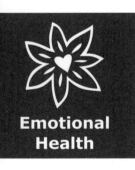

Emotional Health

Measure your work–life balance

Whether you agree or disagree, each answer is worth 1 point.

Does this statement apply to you?	Agree	Disagree
1. I feel like I have little or no control over my work life.	0	1
2. I regularly enjoy hobbies or interests outside of work.	1	0
3. I often feel guilty because I can't make time for everything I want to.	0	1
4. I often feel anxious or upset because of what's happening at work.	0	1
5. I usually have enough time to spend with my loved ones.	1	0
6. When I'm at home, I feel relaxed and comfortable.	1	0
7. I have time to do something just for me every week.	1	0
8. On most days, I feel overwhelmed and over-committed.	0	1
9. I rarely lose my temper at work.	1	0
10. I never use all my allotted vacation days.	0	1
Total		

What your score means:

0 to 3: Your life is out of balance. You need to make significant changes to find your equilibrium. But you can take control!

4 to 6: You're keeping things under control—but only barely. Now is the time to take action before you're knocked off balance.

7 to 10: You're on the right track! You've been able to achieve work–life balance—now, make sure you protect it.

Note: This quiz provides general information only. It is not a diagnostic test, and information provided is not a substitute for professional advice. If you feel that you may need advice, please consult a qualified health care professional.

Source: Canadian Mental Health Association, www.cmha.ca. With permission.

Balancing work with personal life takes practice. It means planning so that you can enjoy your free time. Be clear with children's families right from enrolment about drop-off and pick-up times. Help parents understand that your own family obligations are affected when they are late for pick-up. Staying silent may suggest that imposing on your time is all right and that you do not value your own time as much as your work life. Similarly, clarifying your role and responsibilities for your own family while other children or adults are present may sometimes be necessary. Inevitably, there will be times when forces beyond your control demand a longer day or an extra effort. Just make sure these don't become more frequent than necessary.

Managing emotional stress

Work-related stress is the second biggest occupational health problem after back pain. Stress among child care practitioners affects not only mental and physical heath, but also the quality of care you're able to give. Stress is a subjective experience, and people feel and cope with it differently. Physical responses such as headache, sweating or an accelerated heart rate, as well as emotional ones like irritability or the urge to escape, are extremely common. Major life occurrences, as well as stress arising from day-to-day routines, can cause entirely normal feelings of anxiety, vulnerability and self-doubt. Also, facing a particular or ongoing challenge—even an essentially positive one—can be stressful. A job promotion or a new relationship will cause stress if you feel unprepared to manage the changes it brings.

The causes of stress in child care settings can be short- or long-term. They can be job-specific (arising from the work itself), job-related (arising from the workplace context) or connected with work–life balance. **Job-specific** causes of stress might be a heavy workload, working hours (too long or too short), the pace of work (too fast or too slow), feelings of isolation (e.g., in home settings), a higher than adequate staff-to-child ratio or the immediacy of children's needs.

Job-related causes of stress might be a poor physical environment (e.g., poor ventilation or lighting, or high noise levels), a dysfunctional relationship with a co-worker, supervisor or parent, low wages, limited scope for professional advancement or confusion over expectations.

What's your stress level?

Early signs of emotional stress are easy to miss or to attribute to other things. Physical signs are harder to ignore. Hunching your shoulders is an almost automatic response to stress—and finding yourself in this protective posture a lot is a sure sign of tension.

However, some typical emotional or behavioural responses become so ingrained that you may not recognize them as being stress-related.

REMEMBER

The stress stretch

When you're under stress, tension builds up in your neck and jaw. Take a minute to gently and slowly roll your head from front to back, side to side, and then in a full circle. For your jaw, stretch your mouth open and slowly move your lower jaw from side to side and front to back.

Note: If you experience pain or if you have injured your back, neck or jaw, consult a doctor first.

Source: Canadian Mental Health Association, www.cmha.ca. With permission.

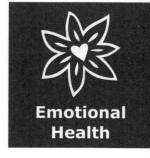

Emotional Health

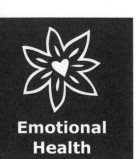

Emotional Health

Measure your stress levels

Do you often:		Yes	No
1.	Neglect your diet?	✓	
2.	Try to do everything yourself?	✓	
3.	Blow up easily?	✓	
4.	Set unrealistic goals?		✓
5.	Fail to see the humour in situations others find funny?		✓
6.	Sometimes act rude?	✓	
7.	Make a "big deal" of everything?	✓	
8.	Look to other people to make things happen?	✓	
9.	Have difficulty making decisions?		✓
10.	Feel disorganized?		✓
11.	Avoid people whose ideas are different from yours?		✓
12.	Keep everything inside?		✓
13.	Neglect exercise?		✓
14.	Have few supportive relationships?		✓
15.	Use sleeping pills or tranquilizers without a doctor's approval?		✓
16.	Get too little rest?	✓	
17.	Get angry when you're kept waiting?	✓	
18.	Ignore stress symptoms?		✓
19.	Put things off until later?		✓
20.	Think there's only one right way to do something?		✓
21.	Fail to build relaxation time into your day?		✓
22.	Gossip?	✓	
23.	Race through the day?		✓
24.	Spend a lot of time complaining about the past?		✓
25.	Fail to get a break from noise and crowds?		✓
Total			

If you've answered "yes" to 21 or more …

> … **you need to take time out and rethink how you're living**, and start paying more attention to diet, exercise and relaxation.

If you've answered "yes" to 14 to 20 …

> … **you may be suffering stress-related symptoms**, and relationships with others could be under strain. Review and think carefully about the choices you've made and take more breaks to relax.

Note: This quiz provides general information only. It is not a diagnostic test, and information provided is not a substitute for professional advice. If you feel that you may need advice, please consult a qualified health care professional.

Source: Canadian Mental Health Association, www.cmha.ca. With permission.

Understanding burnout

Burnout, defined as emotional exhaustion, is an occupational hazard for child care practitioners, as for many in people-oriented professions. Burnout is caused by experiencing work-related and/or personal stress for long periods, with little or no relief. It is characterized by a drop in productivity, and reduced interest and involvement in work. If you're suffering from burnout, you may become withdrawn, irritable or quick to anger. You may be less sensitive to the needs and feelings of others, express your lack of satisfaction with work, and fail to provide appropriate care, service and help to the children in the program or to other staff.

Signs of burnout

- low energy level
- absenteeism
- impaired job performance
- lack of self-esteem
- feeling incompetent
- conflicts in personal relationships
- feeling the need for social support but being unable to accept it

- substance abuse
- depression
- irritability
- a sense of helplessness
- being easily distracted
- preoccupation with meaningless tasks
- feeling disengaged
- inability to focus

Source: Canadian Mental Health Association, www.cmha.ca. With permission.

If you're suffering from burnout, professional counselling and work leave may be necessary. However, by actively managing stress, you can reduce the risk of burnout.

Coping mechanisms

While people experience and deal with stress differently, there are basic steps for handling personal stress.

1. Learn to recognize your own stress signals. Being irritable, losing your sense of humour and snapping may be signs. Physical symptoms such as butterflies in the stomach or sudden sweating are important indicators.
2. Be aware of your rights and obligations. In child care centres, you can advocate for changes to working conditions and expectations. Your job should be well defined and evaluated regularly through performance appraisals.
3. Recognize and accept realistic limitations in a stressful situation. You may not be able to change the world, but you can always try to appreciate small successes and celebrate improvements.
4. Manage time effectively. Overscheduling, under-delegating and omitting to set aside enough time for individual tasks are common tendencies that you can usually correct. Take charge of your day by prioritizing and organizing ahead of time. Have a wall calendar or daily agenda and use it to map out the next week or month in a visual way. When planning activities, make the delegation of tasks part of the plan. When estimating how long a task or activity should take, make a point of building in some extra time.
5. Take inventory. When you experience stress, record what you feel and the probable causes in writing. If possible, try not to react until you've taken some time and space.

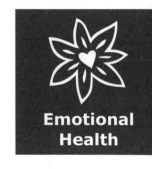

Emotional Health

6. Learn relaxation techniques, such as deep breathing, yoga and meditation. Practice these with children as part of the program routine.

7. Respect your own need for personal time and regular connection with friends and family. Avoid bringing work home, or home to work.

8. Exercise. Something as simple as a walk can put some needed distance between you and a stressful day. Exercise that is varied, fun or social can help you forget work completely, at least for a while. Caring for children offers many opportunities to be physically active. For more on physical activity, see Chapter 2, *Healthy Activities* and Chapter 15, *Caregivers' Physical Health.*

9. Take short, regular breaks. The need to maintain proper staffing ratios and to supervise continually can sometimes make scheduling breaks difficult. In child care centres, a "floating" staff member may be available to fill in during breaks and lunches. The space designated for breaks should be quiet, away from the children's activities and furnished comfortably. Taking breaks is more difficult in home settings. Try to take time for yourself while children are napping. Make a point of seeking out community resources, such as drop-in playgroups. You might also arrange for occasional or regular respite care. This means finding a qualified caregiver in the community to take on some or all duties for short periods. Parents should be informed of this arrangement well in advance and have the opportunity to meet the alternate caregiver.

10. Follow healthy routines. It's easy to skip meals or lose sleep at extremely busy or stressful times, but keeping to a regular schedule as much as possible helps to reduce stress. For more on healthy routines, see Chapter 15, *Caregivers' Physical Health.*

11. Create opportunities to laugh—for yourself and for the children in your care. Laughter releases stress-relieving chemicals in the brain. Appreciate the natural humour of children and share it. Sharing a joke or a fun activity with co-workers can dispel workplace tension. Relax at home with movies, TV or pastimes you enjoy.

12. Remember your social network. Make the time to stay in touch with friends.

13. Plan fun in your day by scheduling activities that you enjoy (e.g., perhaps singing with the children, but then taking a half-hour to read your book or magazine or listen to music on a lunch break).

14. Change your approach. If you're someone who answers every request for help, try saying "no" occasionally. If you're easily drawn into arguments, ask yourself why. If there's a pattern to your interactions with children or co-workers that's repetitive or troubling to you, try adjusting it.

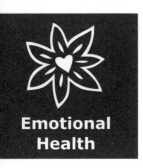

Emotional Health

REMEMBER

Set a SMART goal and achieve it

Unrealistic goals add to stress. Try setting yourself one goal a week that is:

Small and specific. Write it down.

Measurable. Is it tangible enough to be counted or checked off a list?

Achievable. Is it realistic? If you have your doubts, make it smaller.

Rewardable. Think of a way to reward yourself for achieving it.

Time-limited. Set a specific, realistic time-frame for finishing the task or achieving your goal.

Discovering your favourite age

Some child care practitioners prefer working with children of a certain age, while others enjoy the interaction among multi-aged preschoolers. Your own preference might emerge through experience and training with one age group, or a sense that your personality is better suited to working with children of a certain age. Whatever the age or grouping of ages you work with, it's essential for staff to do the following:

Walk away from stress instead of sitting down with another cup of coffee. On your lunch break or at home, try to walk every day. If you don't like walking by yourself, try forming a regular walking group with a few co-workers or friends.

- Maintain appropriate staff-to-child ratios. What is mandatory for your jurisdiction isn't necessarily best practice. Where there's the option, aim for the lowest workable staff-to-child ratio. It means more personal time with every child and greater flexibility when planning activities.
- Work as a team. Having co-workers with complementary strengths in one room may work better than having (for example) two talented animators. Make sure that each person has scheduled breaks. In a home setting, connecting with other local caregivers for daily walks or regular outings is an opportunity for information-sharing and mutual support. Take advantage of community drop-in programs for child care practitioners.
- Speak with families often and share details of their child's day. This exchange is as affirming as it is practical. Sharing information about child development and behaviour, as well as policies and upcoming events—through newsletters, brochures, family nights and bulletin board postings—builds a supportive community environment.
- Keep up-to-date with current knowledge on child development. The more you know about ages and stages, child psychology and normal behaviour patterns, the better you can plan activities and respond to children, or their parents' questions or expectations.

Each age group has its own basic dynamics and requirements:

- Caring for **infants and babies** is both physically demanding (e.g., lots of lifting and bending) and emotionally intense (e.g., one-on-one contact, natural bonding and nurturing). The parents of babies may be more involved with, and possibly anxious about, the day-to-day details of their child's routine care, especially if they're new to parenting. You'll want to set aside time to read, speak and sing with children this age.
- **Toddlers** are energetic, activity-oriented and impulsive. Constant supervision and the principles of child guidance help to shape your program day. You'll bring patience, sensitivity and respect for age-appropriate behaviours (including defiance and the occasional tantrum) to this group. You'll share observations and updates with families each day, and recognize that their methods (e.g., for guidance and toilet learning) may be different at home. Program planning includes lots of age-appropriate activities and discussion with children about what they would like to do. Listen to their ideas and let their interests guide program plans. Ensure that your facility has a variety of quality, age-appropriate craft materials, toys and play equipment.

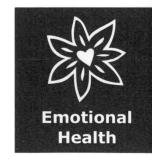

Emotional Health

- **Preschoolers** are energetic, curious and talkative. This is the age when children begin to develop peer friendships and other social behaviours. They become increasingly independent, but active play, social games and learning about the world around them are highlights of the program day. You'll bring energy, creativity and flexibility to this group, and be prepared to answer lots of questions. Consistency is still key, but this age group looks forward to and appreciates a special occasion. Build these events into your program and involve families whenever possible.

Building partnerships with families

Establishing and maintaining collaborative relationships with families is essential to quality child care and to a sense of professional self-esteem. A trusting and supportive relationship between program staff and families provides stability, consistency and support for all concerned. Although parents are the leading experts on their child's needs, what they do may occasionally be quite different from what you would do in the same situation. Your interpersonal and problem-solving skills—and emotional maturity—will be called upon at times to keep these relationships strong.

The CCCF's guides to self-reflection can help child care practitioners and facility directors to evaluate how well they're supporting parenting strategies. (See *Selected resources* at the end of this chapter.) Working in partnership with each child's family means:

- openly respecting differences in child-rearing values, practices and expectations, and learning more about the cultures or traditions that support different approaches.
- listening attentively and non-judgmentally to parents' views and concerns.
- recognizing the parents' role as primary caregivers, encouraging them to use their caregiving strengths, and inviting them to share their unique knowledge of their child with you.
- helping parents to define their wishes, needs and goals for their child.
- communicating information in a variety of ways about your program's philosophy and policies.
- freely exchanging information about the child at drop-off and pick-up times.
- welcoming parents' visits any time their child is attending your program, and encouraging involvement with program activities or planning.
- encouraging families connected with the program to socialize and share.
- making sure that program activities are appropriate to every child's cultural or religious background or lifestyle.
- responding promptly and appropriately when requests for assistance or information are received, and when differences of opinion occur.

Respecting, understanding and empathizing with parents on issues they may experience— such as cultural adjustment, financial stress and overwork—are ongoing tasks for child care practitioners. These all-too-common pressures can strain family and working relationships. Parents may:

- feel guilty about not caring for their child themselves, particularly if a child is unwell. These guilty feelings may be manifested as questions about and/or criticisms of your work.

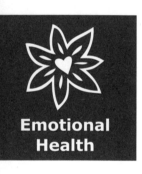

Emotional Health

- feel vulnerable or insecure about their parenting skills, especially first-time parents. This may make them defensive about suggestions you may have.
- worry about a program's value system, or wonder how different your beliefs are from theirs. They may ask more personal questions than you're accustomed to.
- fail to always properly understand or respect your role. You'll need to be a strong advocate of your profession.
- be overwhelmed by their own responsibilities, and unable to parent adequately. You could be one of the first people to suspect that a child is at risk of neglect. (See also Chapter 14, *Protecting Children from Maltreatment*.)

Building open, positive, two-way relationships with parents can relieve pressures on the family. The following offer proven opportunities for shared input, participation and education:

- Have an orientation package or website setting out the program's philosophy, basic policies and procedures that parents can read and consider in advance.
- Schedule at least one interview before enrolment and regular meetings during the year where parents are encouraged to share opinions, ideas and concerns.
- Send home newsletters or a monthly calendar of upcoming events, some of which families can participate in socially (e.g., family nights).
- Record children's activities in a book for parents to review periodically, with photos or an occasional video to document their child's participation in daily routines or special events.
- Make sure that parents feel welcome to visit the facility at any time, and encourage or invite them to drop in at particular times.
- Encourage parents to participate in the program by joining a facility's board of directors or parent advisory committee.
- Share information and knowledge about child health, development, guidance and everyday child care topics (e.g., separation anxiety). Invite parents to share their knowledge individually or during group sessions.
- Link up with family services and resources in the community.
- Learn from families. Encourage them to share information about their cultural background or parenting strategies. Understanding a child's home life can be vital to understanding what she needs most from your program.
- Have a clear reporting process. When there is a conflict with a parent, knowing who to report to, when and how, can reduce stress for both sides.

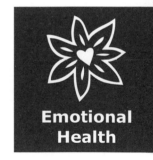

Emotional Health

Relating to co-workers

As with any profession, work relationships in child care are a major determinant of job satisfaction and emotional well-being. The nature of child care (hands-on, highly interactive and emotional at times) and its workplace (shared spaces, clutter and high noise levels at times) is intimate. The personalities, temperaments and daily rhythms of staff become quickly obvious. By sharing a common purpose, child care philosophy and cooperative spirit, and by communicating openly, child care practitioners can thrive on these differences as much as the children in their care.

The CCCF's guides to self-reflection can help child care practitioners evaluate the quality of their workplace relationships. (See *Selected resources* at the end of this chapter.) Collaborative working relationships with colleagues, supervisors, assistants and alternate caregivers involve:

- perceiving your group as a team,
- providing practical and verbal support to one another, and welcoming feedback from others,
- being open to new ideas and approaches, and incorporating them in practice,
- openly communicating concerns, and responding to the concerns of others in a calm and respectful way, and
- keeping personal information private, by preserving confidentiality and discouraging gossip.

A positive workplace possesses the following organizational strengths:

1. **Clear and open lines of communication**, including:
   - regular staff meetings to discuss work issues that affect everyone,
   - regular job performance evaluations and frequent feedback, so that individuals feel both appreciated and included in group decision-making.
2. **Clear expectations and tasks**, including policies, procedures and responsibilities that are well defined and understood. However, these should also be responsive to the needs of staff and change as collective priorities evolve.
3. **A common vision.** Both overall program objectives and goals for individual children should be shared, celebrated and, as needs arise, reassessed for relevance and effectiveness.
4. **Professional growth.** In-service training opportunities and professional development should be supported, and meaningful, empowering tasks delegated to reinforce organizational strength and direction.
5. **Staff participation in decisions** that affect the program.
6. **Flexibility and openness** to staff input in matters of scheduling, goal-setting and problem-solving. Staff should be invited to choose activities and program themes.
7. **Recognition of individual endeavours or successes and celebration of collective achievements**.
8. **Teamwork**, including staying focused, actively supporting each other's strengths and abilities, and sharing feelings and resources.
9. **A fair and equitable system for compensation**, benefits and opportunities to advance.
10. **One-on-one conflict resolution.** Staff members should feel comfortable with trying to resolve a problem themselves, but also with involving management if needed.

Strategies for conflict resolution are beyond the scope of this chapter, but if you're having trouble communicating with a co-worker or parent, the following questionnaire may help pinpoint what isn't working between you. Both parties should answer the following questions, and then meet to share and discuss the responses. An objective mediator, to ease discussion or ensure fairness, may be requested by either party.

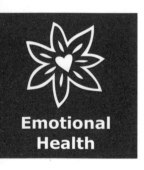

Emotional Health

Are you listening?

When you and I are talking together ...	Always	Often	Sometimes	Never
1. You make me feel as if this is the most important thing you could be doing right now and that your time is truly mine.	❏	❏	❏	❏
2. Your attention is divided. You interrupt our conversation by answering the phone or addressing the needs of others.	❏	❏	❏	❏
3. You begin shaking your head or saying "no" before I finish.	❏	❏	❏	❏
4. You make references to other conversations. There is a history to our communication.	❏	❏	❏	❏
5. You fidget and squirm and look at the clock as though you cannot wait to get on to other, more important projects and conversations.	❏	❏	❏	❏
6. You begin asking questions before I finish my message.	❏	❏	❏	❏
7. You look me in the eye and really focus your attention on me.*	❏	❏	❏	❏
8. You ask questions that let me know you weren't really listening.	❏	❏	❏	❏
9. You finish my sentences for me as though nothing I have to say could be new to you.	❏	❏	❏	❏
10. You express interest by asking thoughtful questions and by contributing your insights.	❏	❏	❏	❏
11. You change the agenda by taking over and changing the content of the conversation.	❏	❏	❏	❏
12. You follow up on what we discussed and keep me posted on what is happening.	❏	❏	❏	❏
13. You are sensitive to the tone of what I have to say and respond respectfully.	❏	❏	❏	❏
14. You give me credit for ideas and projects that grow out of our communications.	❏	❏	❏	❏
15. You try to speed things up and leap ahead with ideas or conclusions as though we're in a rush.	❏	❏	❏	❏
16. You smile at me and make me feel comfortable and valued.	❏	❏	❏	❏
17. You make jokes about things that are serious to me and thereby belittle my concerns.	❏	❏	❏	❏
18. You get defensive and argue before I can fully explain my point.	❏	❏	❏	❏
19. You ask questions that demonstrate an effort to understand what I have to say.	❏	❏	❏	❏
20. Whether or not you agree with me, you make me feel that my opinions and feelings are respected.	❏	❏	❏	❏

* Making eye contact during conversation is considered disrespectful in some cultures. Lack of eye contact doesn't necessarily indicate poor communication.

Source: Child Care Exchange, www.childcareexchange.com. Adapted with permission.

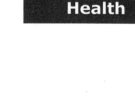

Emotional Health

Evaluating working conditions

As in any field, a child care practitioner's emotional well-being is influenced by work environment and conditions. The work itself poses unique challenges, both physical (e.g., the demands of staffing ratios and group size, and the time and energy expended in lifting children and play equipment, feeding, cleaning spills and tidying play areas) and psychological (e.g., limited provision for breaks and respite, constant supervision, high staff turnover and parental expectations).

This checklist may help you to evaluate some very basic workplace conditions that are known to affect job satisfaction.

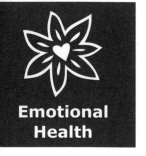

Emotional Health

Does your employer...	Yes	No	Sometimes
... support healthy eating habits by:			
ensuring adequate break times?	☐	☐	☐
providing a comfortable place to eat and relax?	☐	☐	☐
... recognize the importance of balancing work, rest and exercise by:			
maintaining adequate staff-to-child ratios?	☐	☐	☐
ensuring that all staff take regular breaks each day?	☐	☐	☐
incorporating sufficient time into the daily schedule for program planning and record-keeping?	☐	☐	☐
curtailing overtime and discouraging staff from taking work home?	☐	☐	☐
... promote collegiality and emotional well-being by:			
providing written job descriptions for each position and ensuring that all understand one another's role?	☐	☐	☐
establishing clear lines of communication and reporting?	☐	☐	☐
providing adequate supervision?	☐	☐	☐
conducting regular performance evaluations?	☐	☐	☐
organizing staff meetings and in-service training in communication, conflict resolution, etc.?	☐	☐	☐
providing a comprehensive employee benefit package that includes family responsibility leave?	☐	☐	☐
providing time and, possibly, financial support for professional development?	☐	☐	☐
actively participating as a member in a regional or national child care association?	☐	☐	☐
encouraging opportunities for staff to socialize?	☐	☐	☐

Source: Barbara Pimento and Deborah Kernested, *Healthy Foundations in Early Childhood Settings*. 3rd ed., 2004. Adapted with permission.

Positive basic workplace conditions in child care include:

- Appropriate staffing ratios for smaller groups, permitting meaningful and individualized adult-to-child interaction.
- A fair and equitable division of tasks related to cleaning and maintenance.

- Thorough on-site orientation and training for new staff.
- A physical environment that protects the health and safety of both children and adults, and supports developmentally appropriate programming.
- Program supplies and equipment that are regularly replenished, kept clean and in good repair.
- Storage space for staff's personal belongings, and some adult-sized furniture in the children's play and eating areas.
- Record-keeping and information storage that is reliable, organized and accessible as needed.
- Routine procedures for child care that are written down, regularly reinforced and, when there is a change, promptly communicated to all staff members.
- Clear organizational lines of authority/reporting that are known to everyone associated with the program.
- An annual review of the facility's physical environment, policies and procedures, and programming, where requirements or desirable changes are identified, and a plan of action promptly implemented.

Practicing self-care

Child care is among the most demanding of the caring professions. Being physically and emotionally healthy helps immeasurably to make working with children the truly rewarding experience it can be.

Selected resources

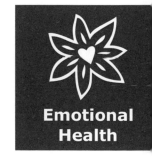

Emotional Health

Child care-specific

Canadian Child Care Federation. 2000. *Tools for Practitioners in Child Care Settings* and *Tools for Administrators in Child Care Settings.* These guides to self-reflection were developed under the Partners in Quality project, and examine standards of policy, practice and ethics. www.cccf-fcsge.ca

———. 2008. *Supporting our children's social well-being: It's a team effort.* Ottawa, Ont.: CCCF. Online resource kit includes articles, resource sheets and workshops on building practitioner–family partnerships in support of children's social well-being. Covers specific topics such as behaviour guidance, communication, self-esteem, resiliency and cultural identity. www.cccf-fcsge.ca

———. 2003. Caring for the caregiver: Setting your personal goals.

———. 2002. Self-reflection quiz: Personal and work role balance.

———. 1995. Team-building in the child care work place.

Canadian Mental Health Association and the Hincks-Dellcrest Treatment Centre. 2004. *Handle with Care: Strategies for Promoting the Mental Health of Young Children in Community-based Child Care*, Chapter 6. Booklet. Ottawa, Ont.: CMHA. www.cmha.ca

Child Care Human Resources Sector Council. Includes reports, statistics on wages and working conditions of child care workforce. www.ccsc-cssge.ca

Doherty, Gillian, Donna Lero, et al. 2000. *You Bet I Care: Reports 1-4*. Guelph, Ont.: Centre for Family, Work and Well-being, University of Guelph. www.worklifecanada.ca

Elliot, Enid. 2006. *We're Not Robots: The Voices of Daycare Providers*. Albany, NY: State University of New York Press.

Jorde-Bloom, Paula. 2007. *From the Inside Out: The Power of Reflection and Self-Awareness*. Washington, DC: National Association for the Education of Young Children.

———. 1997. *A Great Place to Work: Improving Conditions for Staff in Young Children's Programs*. Lakeforest, IL: New Horizons.

———. 1989. *Avoiding Burnout: Strategies for Managing Time, Space, and People in Early Childhood Education*. Lakeforest, IL: New Horizons.

Manitoba Federation of Labour Occupational Health Centre and Day Nursery Centre. *A Guide to Workplace Health, Safety and Wellness for Child Care Workers*. DVD. Winnipeg, Man.: Authors.

Partners in Practice. 1999. *The Partners in Practice Mentoring Model: Reflection, Caring and Sharing*. Halifax, N.S.: PIP.

Pimento, Barbara and Deborah Kernested. 3rd ed., 2004. *Healthy Foundations in Early Childhood Settings*. "Promoting your emotional and social well-being," pp. 70-82. Toronto, Ont.: Nelson Education.

Rodrigues, M. 2002. Walking the tightrope: Taking care of oneself. www.cccf-fcsge.ca

Talan, Teri N. and Paula Jorde-Bloom. 2004. *Program Administration Scale: Measuring Early Childhood Leadership and Management*. New York, NY: Teachers College Press.

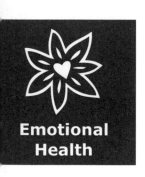

Emotional Health

General

Canadian Centre for Occupational Health and Safety. www.ccohs.ca

———. 2006. Violence in the workplace: Negative interactions.

———. 2002. Workplace stress—general.

———. 2000. Work/life balance.

Canadian Mental Health Association. Includes resources on emotional well-being, stress, work–life balance. www.cmha.ca

Canadian Women's Health Network. Includes a database of health topics, links, a monthly bulletin, and women's health initiatives. www.cwhn.ca

Human Resources and Social Development Canada, Work–life balance in Canadian workplaces. Includes tools to help employers create workplaces that support work–life balance. www.labour.gc.ca

Index

A page number in *italics* indicates an illustration, table or sidebar.

Health Canada
    food recommendations, 35
    hazardous materials information, 366-67
    physical activity recommendations, 13
    product safety regulations, *63*, 65, 91
healthy activities *see* activity
hearing, *see also* otitis media
    developmental milestones, *335-36*
    disorders, 334-38, 346
heart conditions, 249-50, 252-53
heart health, 10
hedgehogs, 161
helmets, 73-75, 80-81, 101, 105
hemophilia, 250-51, 253
hepatitis A, 189-90, *229*, 374, 378, 380-81
hepatitis B, 143, 212-14, *229*, 374, 377-78
hepatitis C, 143, 216, *230*, 377-78
herpes, genital, 217
Hib (*Haemophilus influenzae* type b) disease, 206-07, *229*
hiccups, 135
high chairs
    cleaning, 46, *165*
    safety, 87-88, 100, 102
hiring practices, 361, 382-83
HIV (human immunodeficiency virus), *see also* AIDS, 143, 215-16, *230*, 378-79
housekeeping tips, 158-59
HPV (human papillomavirus), 217
human immunodeficiency virus (HIV), *see also* AIDS, 143, 215-16, *230*, 378-79
human papillomavirus, 217
humidifiers, *177*
hunger cues
    and emotional attachment, 297-98
    and healthy eating, 27
    babies
        breast or bottle feeding, 29, 297
        solid foods, 33-34
    overweight children, 43
hyperactivity, 326
hypoglycemia, *246*, 247, *262*, *267*, 285
hypothermia, 282

I

ibuprofen
    do not use with acetaminophen, *173*
    for back pain (staff), 368
    for bursitis (staff), 371
    for fever, 173
    for tendonitis (staff), 371
    no prescription required, 220
ICF (International Classification of Functioning, Disability and Health), 316
IEP (Individual Education Plan), 317
IFSP (Individual Family Service Plan), 317
immune globulin
    for chickenpox, 198-99, *227*, *374*, 376
    for hepatitis A infection, 189, *229*, 381
    for measles, 201, *231*, *374*, 377

immunization
    for chickenpox, 198, 373, 376
    for diphtheria, 185, 373
    for hepatitis A, 189, 374, 378, 380
    for hepatitis B, 213, 374, 377-78
    for influenza, 175, 373
    for measles, 200-01, 373-74, 377
    for meningitis, 205
    for meningococcal disease, 208, *231*
    for mumps, 184, 373-74, 376
    for pertussis, *182*, 374, 379
    for pneumococcal disease, 209
    for polio, 217-18
    for rubella (German measles), 203, 373, 376
    for tetanus, 217, 373
    no connection with ASDs, 324
    of care providers, 373-74
    of children, 151
    resources, 163
    role in outbreak prevention, 175
impetigo, 194-95, 211-12, *228*, *230*
inclusion
    special needs children, 8, 316, 320-21
        plans, 317-18
        resources, 343
        rights and benefits, 321-22, 342
        strategies for specific concerns, 322-42
Individual Education Plan (IEP), 317
Individual Family Service Plan (IFSP), 317
Individual Program Plan (IPP), 317
indoors
    activities, 18-19
    garbage disposal, 87, 100, *102-03*, 158
    safety, 65-69, 93
    supervision, 66
infant formula, 31-33
infants (birth to 6 months)/babies
    and infection spread, 142
    caring for, 397
    car seats, 115-16
    choking first aid, 276
    colic, 127-29
    constipation, 129-30
    cradle cap, 130
    DEET, do not use, 78
    dehydration, 132, 170, *174*, 186-87
    dental cleaning routine, 55-56
    developmental milestones, *26*, *348-49*
    developmental patterns, 11-12
    diapering routines, 151-53
    diaper rash, 130-31, 196-97, *234*
    diarrhea, 131-32, 170, 186-88
    drooling, 132, 138, 194
    drowning, *76*
    eczema, 132-33
    encouraging attachment, 297
    febrile seizures, 173, 175, 203, 287
    feeding
        and attachment, 29, 297
        breastfeeding support, 29-30
        breast milk, storage and handling, 30-31
        principles, 28-29
        solid foods, 33-37
        water and juice, 33

weight
excessive, 42-43
healthy, 10
West Nile virus, 145
wheelchairs, 77, 328-29
wheezing, 169
whooping cough, 144, 182-83, *232*, 379
wind chill, 81
window blinds, 85-86
windows
in car, 114
in house, 85-86, 100-01, *166*
window screens, *86*, 104
wood stoves, 84
work–life balance, 391-93
workplace
infections, 383-85
injuries, 372-73
World Health Organization, ICF model, 316

Y

Yersinia infection, 186-87, *226*
yogurt *see* milk products

Z

zinc
foods with, *35*, 36
in creams, 131